Coagulation/ Endothelial Dysfunction

Editors

HERNANDO GOMEZ DANIES
JOSEPH A. CARCILLO

CRITICAL CARE CLINICS

www.criticalcare.theclinics.com

Consulting Editor
JOHN A. KELLUM

April 2020 • Volume 36 • Number 2

ELSEVIER

1600 John F. Kennedy Boulevard • Suite 1800 • Philadelphia, Pennsylvania, 19103-2899

http://www.theclinics.com

CRITICAL CARE CLINICS Volume 36, Number 2
April 2020 ISSN 0749-0704, ISBN-13: 978-0-323-71253-8

Editor: Colleen Dietzler
Developmental Editor: Casey Potter

Critical Care Clinics (ISSN: 0749-0704) is published quarterly by Elsevier Inc., 360 Park Avenue South, New York, NY 10010-1710. Months of issue are January, April, July, and October. Business and Editorial Offices: 1600 John F. Kennedy Blvd., Suite 1800, Philadelphia, PA 19103-2899. Customer Service Office: 6277 Sea Harbor Drive, Orlando, FL 32887-4800. Periodicals postage paid at New York, NY and additional mailing offices. Subscription prices are $250.00 per year for US individuals, $683.00 per year for US institutions, $100.00 per year for US students and residents, $285.00 per year for Canadian individuals, $856.00 per year for Canadian institutions, $318.00 per year for international individuals, $856.00 per year for international institutions, $100.00 per year for Canadian students/residents, and $150.00 per year for foreign students/residents. To receive student/resident rate, orders must be accompanied by name of affiliated institution, date of term, and the signature of program/residency coordinator on institution letterhead. Orders will be billed at individual rate until proof of status is received. Foreign air speed delivery is included in all *Clinics* subscription prices. All prices are subject to change without notice. POSTMASTER: Send address changes to *Critical Care Clinics*, Elsevier Periodicals Customer Service, 11830 Westline Industrial Drive, St. Louis, MO 63146. **Customer Service: 1-800-654-2452 (US). From outside of the US, call 1-314-447-8871. Fax: 1-314-447-8029. E-mail: journalscustomerservice-usa@elsevier.com (for print support) or journalsonlinesupport-usa@elsevier.com (for online support).**

Reprints. For copies of 100 or more of articles in this publication, please contact the Commercial Reprints Department, Elsevier Inc., 360 Park Avenue South, New York, NY 10010-1710. Tel.: 212-633-3874; Fax: 212-633-3820; E-mail: reprints@elsevier.com.

Critical Care Clinics is also published in Spanish by Editorial Inter-Medica, Junin 917, 1er A, 1113, Buenos Aires, Argentina.

Critical Care Clinics is covered in *MEDLINE/PubMed (Index Medicus), EMBASE/Excerpta Medica, Current Concepts/ Clinical Medicine, ISI/BIOMED, and Chemical Abstracts.*

Contributors

CONSULTING EDITOR

JOHN A. KELLUM, MD, MCCM
Professor, Critical Care Medicine, Medicine, Bioengineering and Clinical and Translational Science, Director, Center for Critical Care Nephrology, The Clinical Research Investigation and Systems Modeling of Acute Illness (CRISMA) Center, Vice Chair for Research, Department of Critical Care Medicine, University of Pittsburgh School of Medicine, Pittsburgh, Pennsylvania, USA

EDITORS

HERNANDO GOMEZ DANIES, MD, MPH
Assistant Professor, Critical Care Medicine, Emergency Medicine and Clinical and Translational Science, Department of Critical Care Medicine Center for Critical Care Nephrology, Cardiopulmonary Physiology Laboratory, Clinical Research, Investigation and Systems Modeling of Acute Illness (CRISMA) Center and the Vascular Medicine Institute, University of Pittsburgh, Pittsburgh, Pennsylvania, USA

JOSEPH A. CARCILLO, MD
Professor of Critical Care Medicine, Division of Pediatric Critical Care Medicine, Department of Critical Care Medicine, Children's Hospital of Pittsburgh, Center for Critical Care Nephrology and Clinical Research Investigation and Systems Modeling of Acute Illness (CRISMA) Center, University of Pittsburgh, Pittsburgh, Pennsylvania, USA

AUTHORS

MARINE ARNAUD, MSc
INSERM U976, Saint-Louis Teaching Hospital, Paris, France

EDEN ARRII
INSERM U976, Saint-Louis Teaching Hospital, Paris, France

ELIE AZOULAY, MD, PhD
Medical Intensive Care Unit, Saint Louis University Hospital, Assistance Publique des Hôpitaux de Paris, Paris, France

ROBERT A. BALK, MD
J. Bailey Carter, MD Professor of Medicine, Division of Pulmonary, Critical Care, and Sleep Medicine, Rush University Medical Center, Rush Medical College, Chicago, Illinois, USA

BERNHARD F. BECKER, MD, PhD
Walter-Brendel-Centre of Experimental Medicine, Ludwig-Maximilians-University, Munich, Germany

NAVIN P. BOEDDHA, MD, PhD
Department of Pediatrics, Erasmus MC-Sophia Children's Hospital, University Medical Center Rotterdam, Rotterdam, The Netherlands

THOMAS BYCROFT, MD
St Mary's Hospital, Imperial College Healthcare NHS Trust, London, United Kingdom

PEDRO CABRALES, PhD
Department of Bioengineering, University of California, San Diego, La Jolla, California, USA

DANIEL CHAPPELL, MD, PhD
Department of Anaesthesiology, University Hospital of Munich (LMU), Munich, Germany

ANTHONY R. CYR, MD, PhD
Resident Physician, Department of Surgery, University of Pittsburgh Medical Center, F679 Presbyterian University Hospital, Pittsburgh, Pennsylvania, USA

DANIEL DE BACKER, MD, PhD
Professor, Department of Intensive Care, CHIREC Hospitals and Université Libre de Bruxelles, Brussels, Belgium

GASPAR DEL RIO-PERTUZ, MD
Center for Critical Care Nephrology, The Clinical Research Investigation and Systems Modeling of Acute Illness (CRISMA) Center, Department of Critical Care Medicine, University of Pittsburgh School of Medicine, Pittsburgh, Pennsylvania, USA

ALLAN DOCTOR, MD
Professor, Department of Pediatrics, Director, Center for Blood Oxygen Transport and Hemostasis, University of Maryland School of Medicine, HSF III, Baltimore, Maryland, USA

CASSANDRA FORMECK, MD
Center for Critical Care Nephrology, The Clinical Research Investigation and Systems Modeling of Acute Illness (CRISMA) Center, Department of Critical Care Medicine, University of Pittsburgh School of Medicine, Department of Nephrology, Children's Hospital of Pittsburgh of UPMC, Pittsburgh, Pennsylvania, USA

HERNANDO GOMEZ DANIES, MD, MPH
Assistant Professor, Critical Care Medicine, Emergency Medicine and Clinical and Translational Science, Department of Critical Care Medicine Center for Critical Care Nephrology, Cardiopulmonary Physiology Laboratory, Clinical Research, Investigation and Systems Modeling of Acute Illness (CRISMA) Center and the Vascular Medicine Institute, University of Pittsburgh, Pittsburgh, Pennsylvania, USA

JAN A. HAZELZET, MD, PhD
Department of Public Health, Erasmus MC, University Medical Center Rotterdam, Rotterdam, The Netherlands

LAUREN V. HUCKABY, MD
Resident Physician, Department of Surgery, University of Pittsburgh Medical Center, F679 Presbyterian University Hospital, Pittsburgh, Pennsylvania, USA

CAN INCE, PhD
Professor, Department of Intensive Care, Laboratory of Translational Intensive Care, Erasmus MC, University Medical Center, Rotterdam, The Netherlands

JAN JEDLICKA, MD
Department of Anaesthesiology, University Hospital of Munich (LMU), Munich, Germany

RAM KALPATTHI, MD
Division of Pediatric Hematology Oncology, Associate Professor, Department of Pediatrics, UPMC Children's Hospital of Pittsburgh, Pittsburgh, Pennsylvania, USA

JOHN A. KELLUM, MD, MCCM
Professor, Critical Care Medicine, Medicine, Bioengineering and Clinical and Translational Science, Director, Center for Critical Care Nephrology, The Clinical Research Investigation and Systems Modeling of Acute Illness (CRISMA) Center, Vice Chair for Research, Department of Critical Care Medicine, University of Pittsburgh School of Medicine, Pittsburgh, Pennsylvania, USA

JOSEPH E. KISS, MD
Division of Hematology Oncology, Professor, Department of Medicine, Medical Director, Clinical Apheresis and Blood Services, Vitalant Northeast Division, University of Pittsburgh School of Medicine, Pittsburgh, Pennsylvania, USA

JESSICA KUPPY, MD
Instructor of Medicine, Division of Pulmonary, Critical Care, and Sleep Medicine, Rush University Medical Center, Rush Medical College, Chicago, Illinois, USA

DANIEL D. LEE, PhD
Indiana University School of Medicine, South Bend, Indiana, USA

MAUD LOISELLE, MD
INSERM U976, Saint-Louis Teaching Hospital, Paris, France

ALFREDO LUCAS, MS
Department of Bioengineering, University of California, San Diego, La Jolla, California, USA

CARLOS L. MANRIQUE-CABALLERO, MD
Center for Critical Care Nephrology, The Clinical Research Investigation and Systems Modeling of Acute Illness (CRISMA) Center, Department of Critical Care Medicine, University of Pittsburgh School of Medicine, Pittsburgh, Pennsylvania, USA

ERIC MARIOTTE, MD
Medical ICU, Saint Louis University Hospital, Assistance Publique des Hôpitaux de Paris, Paris, France

PHILIP R. MAYEUX, PhD
Professor, Department of Pharmacology and Toxicology, University of Arkansas for Medical Sciences, Little Rock, Arkansas, USA

CARLOS J. MUNOZ, MS
Department of Bioengineering, University of California, San Diego, La Jolla, California, USA

SIMON NADEL, MD
St Mary's Hospital, Imperial College Healthcare NHS Trust, Department of Paediatrics, Faculty of Medicine, Imperial College London, South Kensington Campus, London, United Kingdom

TRUNG C. NGUYEN, MD
Associate Professor, Department of Pediatrics, Critical Care Medicine Section, Texas Children's Hospital/Baylor College of Medicine, The Center for Translational Research on Inflammatory Diseases (CTRID), Houston, Texas, USA

SAMIR M. PARIKH, MD
Department of Medicine, Center for Vascular Biology Research, Beth Israel Deaconess Medical Center, Harvard Medical School, Boston, Massachusetts, USA

ROBERT I. PARKER, MD
Professor Emeritus, Renaissance School of Medicine, Department of Pediatrics, Pediatric Hematology/Oncology, Stony Brook University, Stony Brook, New York, USA

SADUDEE PEERAPORNRATANA, MD
Center for Critical Care Nephrology, The Clinical Research Investigation and Systems Modeling of Acute Illness (CRISMA) Center, Department of Critical Care Medicine, University of Pittsburgh School of Medicine, Pittsburgh, Pennsylvania, USA; Excellence Center for Critical Care Nephrology, Division of Nephrology, Department of Medicine, Faculty of Medicine, Department of Laboratory Medicine, Chulalongkorn University, Bangkok, Thailand

STÉPHANIE PONS, MD
INSERM U976, Saint-Louis Teaching Hospital, Paris, France

STEPHEN ROGERS, PhD
Assistant Professor, Department of Pediatrics, Center for Blood Oxygen Transport and Hemostasis, University of Maryland School of Medicine, Baltimore, Maryland, USA

KELSEY D. SACK, MD, PhD
Department of Medicine, Center for Vascular Biology Research, Beth Israel Deaconess Medical Center, Harvard Medical School, Boston, Massachusetts, USA

MARGARET A. SCHWARZ, MD
Professor of Pediatrics, Indiana University School of Medicine, South Bend, Indiana, USA

SRUTI S. SHIVA, PhD
Associate Professor of Pharmacology and Chemical Biology, Vascular Medicine Institute, University of Pittsburgh, Pittsburgh, Pennsylvania, USA

SARAH SUNGURLU, DO
Assistant Professor of Medicine, Division of Pulmonary, Critical Care, and Sleep Medicine, Rush University Medical Center, Rush Medical College, Chicago, Illinois, USA

SANDRINE VALADE, MD
Medical ICU, Saint Louis University Hospital, Assistance Publique des Hôpitaux de Paris, Paris, France

TOM VAN DER POLL, MD, PhD
Amsterdam University Medical Centers, Location Academic Medical Center, University of Amsterdam, Center of Experimental and Molecular Medicine and Division of Infectious Diseases, Amsterdam, The Netherlands

ALEXANDER T. WILLIAMS, BS
Department of Bioengineering, University of California, San Diego, La Jolla, California, USA

LARA ZAFRANI, MD, PhD
INSERM U976, Medical Intensive Care Unit, Saint-Louis Teaching Hospital, Paris, France

BRIAN S. ZUCKERBRAUN, MD
Professor, Department of Surgery, University of Pittsburgh Medical Center, F1281 Presbyterian University Hospital, Pittsburgh, Pennsylvania, USA

Contents

Guided by organ-specific signals in both development and disease response, the heterogeneous endothelial cell population is a dynamic member of the vasculature. Functioning as the gatekeeper to fluid, inflammatory cells, oxygen, and nutrients, endothelial cell communication with its local environment is critical. Impairment of endothelial cell-cell communication not only disrupts this signaling process, but also contributes to pathologic disease progression. Expanding our understanding of those processes that mediate endothelial cell-cell communication is an important step in the approach to treatment of disease processes.

Lethal features of sepsis and acute respiratory distress syndrome (ARDS) relate to the health of small blood vessels. For example, alveolar infiltration with proteinaceous fluid is often driven by breach of the microvascular barrier. Spontaneous thrombus formation within inflamed microvessels exacerbates organ ischemia, and in its final stages, erupts into overt disseminated intravascular coagulation. Disruption of an endothelial signaling axis, the Angiopoietin-Tie2 pathway, may mediate the abrupt transition from microvascular integrity to pathologic disruption. This review summarizes preclinical and clinical results that implicate the Tie2 pathway as a promising target to restore microvascular health in sepsis and ARDS.

The endothelial glycocalyx (EG) is the most luminal layer of the blood vessel, growing on and within the vascular wall. Shedding of the EG plays a central role in many critical illnesses. Degradation of the EG is associated with increased morbidity and mortality. Certain illnesses and iatrogenic interventions can cause degradation of the EG. It is not known whether restitution of the EG promotes the survival of the patient. First trials that focus on the reorganization and/or restitution of the EG seem promising. Nevertheless, the step "from bench to bedside" is still a big one.

In sepsis, coagulation is activated and there is an increased risk of developing a consumptive coagulopathy with attendant increase in mortality. The processes that regulate hemostasis evolved as a component of the inflammatory response to infection. Many points of interaction occur on the endothelial cell surface linking the 2 cell types in the initiation and regulation of hemostasis and inflammation. Consequently, inflammation stimulates both platelets and endothelial cells in ways that affect both hemostasis and the immune response. Platelets are also prime drivers of the inflammatory response. This article discusses the pathways wherein inflammation regulates platelet and endothelial cell function.

The pathobiology of the septic process includes a complex interrelationship between inflammation and the coagulations system. Antithrombin (AT) and tissue factor are important components of the coagulation system and have potential roles in the production and amplification of sepsis. Sepsis is associated with a decrease in AT levels, and low levels are also associated with the development of multiple organ failure and death. Treatment strategies incorporating AT replacement therapy in sepsis and septic shock have not resulted in an improvement in survival or reversal of disseminated intravascular coagulation.

Oxygen (O2) delivery, which is fundamental to supporting patients with critical illness, is a function of blood O2 content and flow. This article reviews red blood cell (RBC) physiology and dysfunction relevant to disordered O2 delivery in the critically ill. Flow is the focus of O2 delivery regulation: O2 content is relatively fixed, whereas flow fluctuates greatly. Thus, blood flow volume and distribution vary to maintain coupling between O2 delivery and demand. This article reviews conventional RBC physiology influencing O2 delivery and introduces a paradigm for O2 delivery homeostasis based on coordinated gas transport and vascular signaling by RBCs.

The microcirculation is a complex network of vessels ranging from as large as 100 µm to as small as 5 µm. This complex network is responsible for the regulation of oxygen to the surrounding tissues and ensures metabolite washout. With a more complete understanding of the microcirculation's physiologic and pathologic tendencies, engineers can create new solutions to combat blood pathologies and shock-related diseases. Over the last number of decades a grown interest in the microcirculation has resulted in the development of fundamental techniques to quantify the microvasculature flow and the release of oxygen to tissues.

complex disease states, such as thrombotic microangiopathic syndromes, and can be associated with a wide range of conditions, including trauma, surgery, acute disease processes, cardiopulmonary bypass, and exposure to drugs and blood products. Prompt identification of underlying causes is important because treatment strategies vary. Moreover, prompt initiation of both supportive and specific treatments is vital to decrease the morbidity and mortality in the intensive care unit.

Thrombocytopenia-associated multiple organ failure is a clinical phenotype encompassing a spectrum of syndromes associated with disseminated microvascular thromboses. Autopsies performed in patients that died with thrombotic thrombocytopenic purpura, hemolytic uremic syndrome, or disseminated intravascular coagulation reveal specific findings that can differentiate these 3 entities. Significant advancements have been made in our understanding of the pathologic mechanisms of these syndromes. Von Willebrand factor and ADAMTS-13 play a central role in thrombotic thrombocytopenic purpura. Shiga toxins and the complement pathway drive the hemolytic uremic syndrome pathology. Tissue factor activity is vital in the development of disseminated intravascular coagulation.

Meningococcemia is notorious for evasion of the host immune system and its rapid progression to fulminant disease, and serves as a unique model for pediatric sepsis. Illness severity is determined by complex interplays among host, pathogen, and environment. The inflammatory host response, including proinflammatory and anti-inflammatory responses in innate and adaptive immunity, skews toward a proinflammatory state. This leads to endothelial dysfunction and activation of the hemostatic response, which may lead to disseminated intravascular coagulation. This article reviews the pathogenesis of sepsis, in particular the inflammatory and hemostatic response in meningococcal sepsis.

The vascular endothelium provides a direct interface between circulating blood cells and parenchymal cells. Thus, it has a key role in vasomotor tone regulation, primary hemostasis, vascular barrier, and immunity. In the case of systemic inflammation, endothelial cell (EC) activation initiates a powerful innate immune response to eliminate the pathogen. In some specific conditions, ECs may also contribute to the activation of adaptive immunity and the recruitment of antigen-specific lymphocytes. However, the loss of EC functions or an exaggerated activation of ECs during sepsis can lead to multiorgan failure.

Sandrine Valade, Eric Mariotte, and Elie Azoulay

Hemophagocytic lymphohistiocytosis (HLH) is a rare and severe condition
that can lead patients to the intensive care unit. HLH diagnosis may be
challenging, as it relies on sets of aspecific criteria. Several organ dysfunctions have been described during HLH, including hemostasis impairment
found in more than half of the patients. The most frequently reported
anomaly is a decrease in the fibrinogen level, which has been associated
with higher mortality rates. Coagulation impairment study in patients with
HLH represents an interesting field of research, as little is known about the
mechanism leading to hypofibrinogenemia.

CRITICAL CARE CLINICS

SERIES OF RELATED INTEREST

Hematology/Oncology Clinics
https://www.hemonc.theclinics.com/

THE CLINICS ARE AVAILABLE ONLINE!
Access your subscription at:
www.theclinics.com

Preface

Toward a Better Mechanistic Understanding of Critical Illness: Endothelial, Microvascular and Coagulation Dysfunction

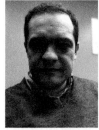

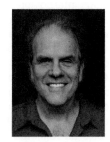

Hernando Gomez Danies, MD, MPH   Joseph A. Carcillo, MD
Editors

Few physiologic processes are closer to the "heart and soul" of critical care practice as tissue perfusion. Matching oxygen delivery to metabolic demand is arguably the quintessential physiologic essence of the practice of critical care medicine and one of the central daily struggles of every intensivist. It is no surprise that a deep understanding of how the cardiovascular system functions and how its components articulate to achieve efficient perfusion and oxygen delivery is central to the craft of the practicing clinician caring for the critically ill.

Major advancements have been made in our understanding of cardiovascular physiology, the dynamics of blood flow distribution, and the how, when, and where of oxygen delivery from the microvascular network to the tissues. However, only a fraction of this knowledge has been effectively translated into clinical tools that help clinicians guide therapeutic decisions at the bedside, in part because development of bedside tools that assess microvascular and endothelial function has lagged behind development of tools that assess macrocirculatory function.

Despite healthy controversy about whether available clinical tools measuring the macrocirculation improve outcomes,[1-4] assessment of systemic parameters of cardiac pump function, macrovascular tone, arterioventricular coupling, fluid responsiveness, gas exchange, oxygen consumption, and oxygen delivery are readily available to the

Crit Care Clin 36 (2020) xv–xvii
https://doi.org/10.1016/j.ccc.2020.01.001
0749-0704/20/© 2020 Published by Elsevier Inc.

practicing intensivist today and remain key guiding principles in the management of the critically ill patient. The increasing sophistication of these tools for assessment of these "macro" components of cardiovascular function at the bedside contrasts with the stark absence of monitoring techniques and therapeutic interventions for the "micro" components of the cardiovascular system, namely, the microvasculature and its regulatory organ, the endothelium. The "micro" level is critical because this is where the microvasculature meets cells in need of oxygen and nutrients. It is the location where everything that matters happens. It is where oxygen is delivered to match cellular metabolic demand.

While new bedside technologies are under development, attempts at filling the void of usable information about bedside microvascular and endothelial function have come from rather ingenious interpolation of systemic physiologic parameters and biomarkers, including plasma lactate, the arteriovenous content of carbon dioxide or P_{CO_2} gap, gastric tonometry, and more recently, hand-held microscopy to assess microvascular flow directly. In addition, there is increasing appreciation that microvascular and endothelial function is influenced by circulating red blood cell, white blood cell, and platelet interactions, particularly during states of inflammation and complement production. Clinicians can monitor these cellular components directly. Bedside clinicians can also assess endothelial activation as reflected by increasing von Willebrand factor (vWF) antigen levels, by proclivity to platelet-endothelial microvascular thrombosis as reflected by decreasing ADAMTS-13 activity (also known as vWF cleaving protease activity), and by assessing complement activation as reflected by decreasing complement levels and increasing activated components.

Clinical presentation of any given critical condition related to microvascular and endothelial dysfunction may be determined by diverse underlying pathologic mechanisms, and thus, tailored approaches targeted to these mechanistic underpinnings may be needed to improve outcome. This is how, for instance, in children with sepsis, much progress has been made at identifying subpopulations of patients with altered microvascular or microangiopathic disorders, that make them susceptible to specific, nonconventional treatments, like plasmapheresis or C5A monoclonal antibody. The focus is on the microvasculature, the critical intersection of endothelial function, coagulation, complement activation, and inflammation where tissue perfusion occurs. Never in history has medicine and scientific research been so close to the fundamental mechanistic underpinnings governing the processes by which tissues communicate with microvascular networks and their feeding arterioles to regulate the delicate balance between oxygen delivery, demand, and consumption, as we are now.

This issue of the *Critical Care Clinics* underscores the critical role of endothelial and coagulation dysfunction in critical illness by providing a comprehensive review of the current knowledge on mechanisms driving endothelial and microvascular dysfunction, elucidating how these mechanisms link to distinct clinical presentations during critical illness, and how these mechanisms are actively driving the search for novel supportive and mechanism-targeted therapies that hold the promise of more efficient treatment and better outcomes for our patients.

Finally, we want to thank the fantastic panel of authors that contributed their work to make this issue possible. We hope that this compilation will be a consultation aid to the practicing clinician at the bedside and a catalyst for renewed enthusiasm in the research community to advance our understanding of critical care physiology.

Hernando Gomez Danies, MD, MPH
Department of Critical Care Medicine
Center for Critical Care Nephrology
Cardiopulmonary Physiology Laboratory
Clinical Research, Investigation and Systems Modeling of Acute Illness (CRISMA)
Center and the Vascular Medicine Institute
University of Pittsburgh
3347 Forbes Avenue, Suite 220, Room 207
Pittsburgh, PA 15213, USA

Joseph A. Carcillo, MD
Critical Care Medicine
Division of Pediatric Critical Care Medicine
Department of Critical Care Medicine
Children's Hospital of Pittsburgh
Center for Critical Care Nephrology and
Clinical Research Investigation and
Systems Modeling of Acute Illness Center
University of Pittsburgh
Faculty Pavilion
UPMC Childrens' Hospital of Pittsburgh
4400 Penn Avenue, Suite 2000
Pittsburgh, PA 15421, USA

E-mail addresses:
gomezh@upmc.edu (H. Gomez Danies)
carcilloja@ccm.upmc.edu (J.A. Carcillo)

REFERENCES

1. De Backer D, Vincent JL. Early goal-directed therapy: do we have a definitive answer? Intensive Care Med 2016;42:1048–50.
2. Vincent JL, De Backer D. From early goal-directed therapy to late(r) Scvo2 checks. Chest 2018;154:1267–9.
3. Angus DC, Barnato AE, Bell D, et al. A systematic review and meta-analysis of early goal-directed therapy for septic shock: the ARISE, ProCESS and ProMISe Investigators. Intensive Care Med 2015;41:1549–60.
4. Protti A, Masson S, Latini R, et al. Persistence of central venous oxygen desaturation during early sepsis is associated with higher mortality: a retrospective analysis of the ALBIOS Trial. Chest 2018;154:1291–300.

Cell-Cell Communication Breakdown and Endothelial Dysfunction

Daniel D. Lee, PhD, Margaret A. Schwarz, MD*

KEYWORDS

- Endothelium • Dysfunction • Signaling • Disease • Heterogeneity • Development

KEY POINTS

- Metabolism and organ-specific signaling steer endothelial cell heterogeneity.
- Disruption of the vascular endothelial cell lining contributes to disease progression.
- The endothelium has an active role in local inflammatory and thrombotic response.

INTRODUCTION

Winding and twisting over 100,000 miles, a vascular network composed of more than 1 trillion stitched together endothelial cells (ECs) represents the functionally largest organ system within the human body. Operating as a dynamic semiselective barrier, endothelial-lined vessels are geared for different roles with smooth muscle–bound arteries delivering pulsatile oxygen-rich blood, capillaries serving as distribution sites for nutrients and oxygen before up taking waste, and the venous system, managed by a series of valves, facilitating vascular return of oxygen-poor blood. Within this maze, ECs are geared for organ-specific functions and *cell-cell communication* with continuous endothelial boundaries found in skeletal muscle, heart, lung, and brain tissue, fenestrations between ECs in endocrine glands, the gastrointestinal mucosal and renal glomeruli, and discontinuous endothelium in the liver and spleen.[1] As such, this diverse and heterogeneous organ system serves as a delivery system and first line of defense in disease processes.

Orchestrated from migrating primitive embryonic splanchnic mesoderm,[2] angioblast-derived blood islands guided by growth factor gradients, such as vascular endothelial growth factor (VEGF) and placental growth factor, merge together forming vasculogenic lumens while sprouting angioblasts activated by VEGF, guides sensitive tip cells to extend from endothelial stalk cells to form angiogenic extensions.[3] Coalescence of these branching networks, pruned by remodeling, are directed by distinctive

Funding: (M.A. Schwarz) NIH R21 HD090227.
Indiana University School of Medicine, 1234 Notre Dame Avenue, South Bend, IN 46617, USA
* Corresponding author.
E-mail address: schwarma@iu.edu

environmental cues creating a tissue-specific vascular bed designed to meet the diverse needs of each organ. A fundamental requirement for endothelium in normal organ development and maturation[4–6] suggests that distinct environmental cues within the developing tissues guide EC function. Indeed, recent studies using unbiased transcriptional profiling through single-cell analysis of ECs from different organs identified distinct organ-specific endothelial genetic profiles that not only define EC heterogeneity, but also suggests that epigenetic footprints control basal expression of EC-specific genes.[7–11] Guided by metabolic needs of the tissue,[12] ECs are the vascular building blocks essential for embryogenesis, organ development, and tissue regeneration. Disruption in the foundation of the endothelial network contributes to the evolution of pathologic disease processes, such as hypoperfusion, sepsis, vasculopathies associated with diabetes, and atherosclerosis and myocardial infarction.

CHARACTERISTICS OF THE NORMAL ENDOTHELIUM

Tissue homeostasis of the human body requires an adequate flow of blood for not only immune cell surveillance and nutrients but also oxygen delivery. To meet the demands, an elaborate vasculature lined by endothelium develops through the following nuanced processes: (1) *vasculogenesis*; (2) *angiogenesis*; (3) *arteriogenesis*; (4) and the lesser-known *lymphoangiogenesis*. Beginning from vasculogenesis, the angioblast-derived blood islands are specified through precisely timed and spatially coordinated networks of signaling pathways not only between themselves but also among other types of cells, which is collectively referred to as *cell-cell communication*.

The first 2 of the 4 processes are typically described in normal physiology, whereas altered mechanisms can occur in pathology due to *endothelial dysfunction*. *Vasculogenesis* is a 2-step sequential process of blood vasculature that grows anew from the primitive embryonic splanchnic mesoderm: first, fate determination of the endothelium and differentiation of endothelial progenitor cells that range from hemangioblast to the differentiated EC; second, the organization that occurs into primitive angioblast-derived blood islands.[13,14] Fate determination is largely genetically determined by transcription factors (eg, ETS transcription factor variant 2, ETV2; ER71) that it responds to factors secreted from neighboring endoderm, such as fibroblast growth factors (eg, FGF2) and bone morphogenic proteins (eg, BMP4). As fate is assigned, VEGF signaling regulates endothelial organization into blood islands and tubular formation, a process that has been documented to be both genetically prepatterned and self-organizing.[15] *Angiogenesis* is the remodeling and emerging of vessels from the existing vasculature, which can be further subdivided into 2 types: sprouting and nonsprouting.[16,17] Sprouting refers to the migration, proliferation, and 3-dimensional organization of ECs into tubes, whereas nonsprouting is the division and remodeling of existing vessels by transluminal invagination. Following tubular formation and cardiovascular development, the resulting blood flow creates vectors of physical force that can activate other forms of vascular growth.[18,19]

The latter 2 of the 4 processes, arteriogenesis and lymphoangiogenesis, are frequently described as compensatory in context of pathology that limit oxygen delivery, including, but not limited to, tissue damage and ischemia. As an adaptive response to ischemia, *arteriogenesis*, also known as collateral artery growth, is the proliferation and formation of collateral arteries from preexisting arterial connections.[16] *Lymphoangiogenesis* is the growth of lymphatic vessels from existing ones.[20]

With such a vast network of vessels that cover the human body, the endothelium is influenced by location-specific physiologic mechanisms, referred to as EC heterogeneity. The location thereby dictates their genetic and phenotypic characteristics along with cell-cell communication. Originally discovered by electron microscopy, EC heterogeneity was defined by structural characteristics like the presence of plasmalemmal vesicles, which are now called caveolae.[21] Since then, experimental techniques (eg, confocal microscopy), have defined the classical markers of the endothelial lineage as follows: hemangioblast (CD133$^+$/VEGFR2$^+$); neonatal angioblast (CD34$^+$/VEGFR2$^+$/VE-Cadherin$^-$); adult endothelial progenitor cell (CD34/VEGFR2$^+$VE-Cadherin$^+$); matured endothelium (CD34$^+$/CD31$^+$/VEGFR2$^+$/VE-Cadherin$^+$). Technological advances in RNA sequencing at the single-cell level have made it possible to further describe endothelial populations based on antigen composition along with the respective gene expression. Studies using single-cell RNA sequencing further support EC heterogeneity as being organ-specific.[8,11,22] For example, the endothelium in the heart and lung express higher levels of von Willebrand Factor (vWF) than do the kidney and liver.[11] More specifically, within the heart, vWF expression is higher in arterioles than capillaries or venules while it is a mosaic pattern within the aorta of the adult heart.[22] These studies support EC heterogeneity and an organ-specific identity.

The endothelium is not an inert tubelike delivery system functioning in isolation, but rather a metabolically active regulator of adequate blood flow. In constant communication with circulating factors, the endothelium can respond dynamically to its (micro) environment, further highlighting the importance of EC location and heterogeneity. Exposed to such a wide range of signals, the collective heterogeneous endothelium selectively processes and responds (signal) while minimizing spontaneous activity (noise), thus modulating cell-cell communication with other cells, such as pericytes or leukocyte.[23] Emerging evidence supports a dynamic metabolic shift within the endothelium during vessel formation, an important distinction from the dogma that genetic signaling cascades determined these processes. With relatively low mitochondrial counts,[24] tip cells of sprouting endothelium in vitro rely on changes to glycolytic flux, whereas stalk cells rely on changes to fatty acid oxidation. Therefore, emerging evidence supports the importance of ensuring the availability of essential metabolic components to maintain EC well-being and vessel stability.

FUNCTIONS OF THE ENDOTHELIUM

Governed by mechanical and humoral forces, ECs function as the gatekeeper of fluid, circulating cells, and solutes. Functionally, physiologic solutes and fluid transporting are reliant on 2 mechanisms: the paracellular process based on cell-cell junctions and transcellular vesicle-based pathways.[25,26] Acting as the dominant avenue, paracellular transport is mediated by the cooperation between 2 junction types: tight junctions and adherens junctions. Tight junctions (TJ), also known as zonulae occludens, are composed of a series of proteins, including claudins, occludins, junctional adhesion molecules (JAMs), and EC-selective adhesion molecules and are responsible for the structural actin cytoskeletal foundation of the EC. Varying in amount and organization based on vascular region, a higher concentration of TJs is required for the blood brain barrier, large arteries, and vessels with continuous networks, whereas fewer TJs present are found where ECs facilitate transport, such as capillaries and venules. Although the TJs are known to be preferential sites for basal transport, they are also susceptible to plasma protein and leukocyte extravasation.

Working in conjunction with TJs, adherens junctions (AJs) are protein complexes linked together by a cytoplasmic actin cytoskeleton that connects the cytoskeleton of one EC to the adjacent EC through an endothelial-specific adhesion protein called vascular endothelial (VE) cadherin. Stabilization of the Ca^{2+} dependent extracellular domain of VE-cadherin through its binding to the catenin family proteins, results in its maintenance at the juxtamembrane domain, providing membrane competence and preventing its destabilizing internalization. Together, TJs and AJs provide EC stability by regulating junctional tension through carefully organized crosstalk between these 2 interdependent mechanisms. However, when disruption of this organized cell-cell interface through either disconnection of the junction complexes or through clustering of the junctional complexes forming focal junctional connections occurs, it can create voids between the cells that contribute to vessel permeability.

Transcellular transport is dependent on vesicle-based mechanisms where macromolecules and fluid navigate across the EC through endocytosis, fusion, and vesiculo-vacuolar transport. For example, endocytosis of proteins such as albumin via its receptor clusters requires direct interaction with caveolin-1, resulting in caveolae-mediated albumin transport, whereas fusion of albumin-containing vesicles to the basal membrane uses SNARE proteins. Vesiculo-vacuolar organelles, predominately found in the capillary venules of tumors, form a transendothelial highway from plasma extravasation through interconnecting vesicles and vacuoles that span the luminal to abluminal surface. An alternative mechanism of transport is the paracellular transportation at the cell-cell junctions called transcellular diapedesis. This method allows for the extravasation of leukocytes and tumor cells at sites of EC adhesion molecules, including intracellular adhesion molecule-1 and platelet-EC adhesion molecule-1, CD99, or JAM-A. These finely regulated mechanisms are vital in the maintenance of vascular integrity and when inflammation or injury occurs, yield to movement of vessel contents into surrounding tissue.

Vascular injury to the EC barrier triggers a cascading chain reaction through a combination of inflammatory and wound healing processes in an attempt to regain hemostasis that in part is regulated by the disrupted endothelium.[27] Within intact vessels, quiescent EC hold transmembrane tissue factor (TF), a major initiator of hemostatic clot formation, inactive. Following EC disturbance, the extrinsic coagulation cascade is initiated through TF activation of factor (F) VII significantly augmenting the proteolytic activity of FVIIa that contributes to conversion of FX to FXa. FXa promotes transformation of prothrombin to thrombin whose function as a protease activates fibrinogen to the protein polymer fibrin. Once initiated, an amplification of the process ensues with circulating platelet aggregation, whereas the propagation phase results in the production of large amounts of insoluble fibrin that when crosslinked forms an organized clot or thrombus, sealing the site of injury.[27–30] Although vital in the repair process, TF also contributes to pathogenic processes such as atherosclerotic plaques and thromboembolisms. Once a wound is repaired, ECs regulate vessel recanalization through release of pro-fibrinolytic molecules, such as tissue plasminogen activator (PA) and urokinase-type PA and platelet cleaving metalloproteases, resulting in clot degradation.

Beyond barrier and integrity, the endothelium is positioned as a pivotal regulator of vascular contractile forces. Through the release of vasodilator substances, ECs modulate the state of adjacent smooth muscle by way of endothelium-derived relaxing factor, also known as nitric oxide (NO). Regulated by circulating neurohumoral mediators such as histamine, acetylcholine, bradykinin, thrombin, and growth factors, endothelial L-arginine is enzymatically converted by NO synthase to produce NO. Counteracting the relaxing effects of NO, "physiologic stimuli such as physical forces, circulating hormones (catecholamines, melanocortin, vasopressin) platelet derived substances (serotonin, adenosine diphosphate), and autacoids (histamine, bradykinin, prostacyclin, prostaglandin E_4) share with acetylcholine"[31] the ability to mediate endothelial release of vasoconstrictor substances called endothelium-derived contracting factors resulting in perivascular smooth muscle cell contraction. Although NO release can be chronically upregulated through exercise, dietary factors, and estrogen, similarly it can be downregulated in response to oxidative stress, vascular diseases such as diabetes and hypertension, and aging. As a result of endothelial-dependent dysregulation of vascular contractile forces, it contributes to progression of disease processes associated with aged individuals and patients with hypertension and diabetes.[31]

ENDOTHELIAL DEVELOPMENT AND CELL-CELL COMMUNICATION

The clinical importance of signaling networks that coordinate the heterogeneous endothelium regulation of cardiovascular activity, and its dependence on EC-cell communication is enormous. With such a key role as an effector, the endothelium must detect and process the numerous local and circulating cues presented from an average of 6 neighboring cells.[32] Exposed to such a wide range of signals, the collective of EC heterogeneity selectively processes and responds (signal) while minimizing spontaneous activity (noise). Thereby, modulating input with a coordinated signaling output with other neighboring cells is fundamental to maintain vessel homeostasis.

The endothelium heterogeneity of a vascular bed acquires specialization by adapting to environment-specific variance in shear stress and cues. Early experimental approaches, particularly in isolation such as organ baths or vessel isolation studies, had supported the notion that the endothelium was relatively homogeneous in its function. For specialization to occur, it dictates that there is an expression of specific receptors that sense transdifferential cues. For example, postcapillary venules highly express surface protein markers for classical leukocyte adhesion, such as E-cadherin, P-selectin, and VCAM1, whereas it does not express the endothelial protein C receptor that is found on large vessels.

Extracellular cues are sensed through their respective receptors, which are then transmitted as broadly defined to be either functional or proliferative-migratory signals. The breadth of signals for cell-cell communication is extensive yet growing. In addition to classical growth factors such as VEGF and platelet-derived growth factor (PDGF) isoforms, lipids such as sphingosine-1-phosphate (S1P) or ceramide-1-phosphate (C1P) metabolites secreted such as succinate and exosomes have been found to dictate signaling in the endothelium.[32–39]

The cell-cell communication that exists between endothelium and neighboring cells is transmitted through the following ways: endocrine, neurotransmitter, paracrine, and autocrine. Historically, Bayliss and Starling,[40] who showed a substance secreted into the bloodstream from the jejunum evoked a response in the pancreas, first illustrated endocrine signaling in 1902. Neurotransmitter signaling was then described, where an extracellular cue was directly exerted by the nervous system onto effector tissue. Methods to initiate transmission of local signaling occur through paracrine signaling to neighboring cells or self-activating autocrine signaling. Many cues, such as the ligands VEGF, PDGF, S1P, and C1P, are distributed in a concentration gradient that are recognized by their respective receptors and signal through multiple transmission methods in a context-dependent manner. For example, gradients of autocrine VEGF isoforms are essential for vascular homeostasis, whereas paracrine VEGF isoforms guide tip formation.[41–43]

Ligands bind to receptors that are generally classified into the following 3 types: G protein–coupled, ion channel–linked, or enzyme-linked. G protein–coupled receptors (GPCRs) are named for the heterotrimeric guanosine triphosphate–binding proteins that mediate their cellular actions; they contain 7 membrane-spanning alpha helices and a cytosolic C-terminal tail that is involved in receptor desensitization. Ligands binding to ion channel–linked receptors cause an open conformation to a channel that allows specific ions to pass through. Finally, enzyme-linked receptors bound to their respective ligand activate an intracellular enzyme, typically a kinase including, but not limited to, receptor tyrosine kinase and receptor guanylyl cyclases. The time-dependent consequences of the ligand-receptor binding can be grouped as follows: (1) short-term, functional; (2) long-term, proliferative signaling.

The same ligand-receptor binding can result in more than one output and is thereby context-dependent. Take S1P binding to 1 of its 5 GPCRs, S1PR1-5, as an example. S1P levels in plasma range from 0.1 to 1 μM.[44,45] Mid-range levels of S1P secreted by the endothelium can bind to S1PR1 on leukocytes to mediate their short-term homing.[34] However, increased amounts over time are needed for vascular maintenance by inducing proliferation.[33] In the following section, examples of various important cell-cell communications are described.

Mural Cell (ie, Pericyte, Vascular Smooth Muscle Cells)/Endothelium

Critical to vascular foundation, mural cells are essential for development and homeostasis of blood vessels. Alterations or disruption in mural cells contribute to endothelial dysfunction. Composed of pericytes and vascular smooth muscle cells (vSMC), similar to EC heterogeneity, the heterogeneity of mural cells is found through various vascular beds and tissue, differing by morphology and antigen expression. Whereas pericytes associate with blood vessels of smaller diameter, vSMCs associate with those of larger diameter vessels to directly control vasodilation and vasoconstriction. The ratio of pericyte to endothelium can range between 1:1, found in neural tissue, to 1:10, found in skeletal muscle.[46]

During angiogenesis, sprouting endothelium secretes PDGF-B to chemoattract pericytes that express the respective receptor PDGFR-β, stimulate proliferation of vSMCs, and initiate maturation of undifferentiated mesenchymal cells. Conversely, pericytes secrete angiopoietin-1 that binds to Tie2 and VEGF that binds to VEGFR2,[41] found on endothelium in a paracrine manner to promote its survival and attachment to mural cells. Recent studies describe exosomes secreted from vSMCs to endothelium increased its permeability and worsened atherosclerosis progression.[38]

Monocyte/Macrophage-Endothelium

Monocytes/macrophages are an important cellular source of hallmark-secreted factors, such as VEGF-A, that are essential for blood vessel growth. During vascular growth, cell-cell communications from tissue-resident macrophages regulate interlock sprouting of angiogenic vessels through direct cell-to-cell contact.[47,48] The classic view of monocyte egression in an injury context is described in (Tom van der Poll and Robert I. Parker's article, "Platelet Activation and Endothelial Cell Dysfunction"; and Sarah Sungurlu and colleagues' article, "Role of Antithrombin III and Tissue Factor Pathway in the Pathogenesis of Sepsis"; and Sandrine Valade and colleagues' article, "Coagulation disorders in Hemophagocytic LymphoHistiocytosis/Macrophage activation syndrome," in this issue). The regulation of the sources of cytokine secretion is important to be understood. For example, in tissue repair, macrophages that are matured from recruited CCR2$^+$Ly6-c$^+$ monocytes are essential for secreting VEGF-A, contributing to vessel growth.[49]

Still controversial is the notion that macrophages are a source of circulating endothelial progenitors through transdifferentiation. On one hand, evidence supporting the transdifferentiation of macrophage-endothelium is through overlapping gene expression profiles of leukocyte subpopulations and endothelium; as certain monocyte populations express the classic endothelial marker CD31.[50,51] On the other hand, studies suggest that the monocyte subpopulations defined to express classic endothelial markers are rather simply a subpopulation of macrophages, which are also highly plastic and known to acquire markers in their environment. Further studies are necessary to define the contribution of macrophages to vascular endothelium.

Endothelial-to-Mesenchymal Transition

Endothelial-to-Mesenchymal Transition (EndMT) is a process in which matured endothelium undergoes signaling cascades to acquire characteristics of mesenchymal cells (eg, myofibroblasts); it is analogous to its corollary counterpart, epithelial-to-mesenchymal transition (EMT) that has been described to a much greater and deeper extent. This phenomenon has become highlighted recently for its involvement in endothelial dysfunction and subsequent adult cardiovascular disease pathogenesis.[52] Whether it is causative in disease pathology remains unclear due to discrepancies and lack of standardization in experimental approaches to study EMT. Secreted transforming growth factor (TGF)-β is a potent factor for EndMT. An alteration in the signaling leads to endothelial dysfunction and contributes several pathogeneses as seen in the retina, where pericyte-derived TGF-β maintains endothelial integrity and stabilizes the structure.[53,54]

The functions of the endothelium through signaling processes of cell-cell communication are clearly complex yet interconnected. With the development of highly sensitive and specific techniques and assays, such as single-cell RNA sequencing, the identity of endothelial heterogeneity has become apparent; it also has allowed for experimental approaches to consider the cell-to-cell variability and the signaling networks there within. The heterogeneity contributes to the impaired cell-cell communication that results in endothelial dysfunction. Ultimately, the clinician's perspective to alter blood flow to meet the metabolic demands remains a daunting task that may be improved through a deeper appreciation of the endothelial heterogeneity and targeting to improve outcomes of the disrupted signaling machineries that lead to diseases.

MECHANISMS OF ENDOTHELIAL DYSFUNCTION CONTRIBUTING TO DISEASE PROGRESSION

Guardian of vascular homeostasis and tone, ECs are the first-line regulators of the proinflammatory and immune responses, whereas in tissue repair, they govern the reparative vessel rebuilding process of neovascularization. As the body ages, cellular components, including the endothelium, are also declining with EC morphology and functionality tightly coupled with self-imposed risk factors, such as smoking, obesity, and diabetes, driving this process. Recent studies highlight the pathophysiologic changes associated with the aging endothelium. For example, EC aging or senescence plays a key role in arterial stiffing and hypertension.[55] As cells age, they lose their ability to replicate, are prone to apoptosis, and demonstrate reduced regenerative ability. This in part is due to irreversible cell cycle arrest, where in the G1 phase, they no longer respond to cyclin-dependent kinase regulated cell growth stimuli.[55] Mediated in part by activity of p53, telomere dysfunction and DNA damage contribute to cell senescence, whereas p16/retinoblastoma gene product pathways are associated more with chromatin disruptions and mitogenic stress and are associated with atherosclerotic plaques.[56–58]

Cellular production of reactive oxygen species (ROS), such as hydrogen peroxide and hydroxyl radicals, contribute to EC oxidative stressors that are deleterious to

DNA transcription and redox sensitive signaling pathways. Not limited to classic ROS alone, ECs also are vulnerable to uncoupled forms of NO that give rise to damage-inducing peroxynitrites. When free radical scavengers, such as glutathione synthase and superoxide synthases, balance cellular ROS, premature EC senescence is avoided. Unchecked ROS expression contributes to inflammation, organ dysfunction, and inhibition of NO-dependent relaxation. In conjunction with ROS, circulating inflammatory biomarkers promote EC dysfunction. From prolonged low-grade inflammation arising from sustained venous hypertension and valvular incompetence of chronic venous disease[59] to life-threatening sepsis, recruitment of leukocytes perpetuates the inflammatory cascade.[60–62] As the interface between circulating proinflammatory mediators, such as interleukin-6, tumor necrosis factor-α, and monocyte chemoattractant protein-1 and body tissues, ECs function as innocent bystanders, as activated inflammatory pathways triggered by release of inflammatory cytokines promote vascular injury. Not limited to bacterial and viral etiologies, chronic inflammatory and oxidative states also have been identified in dysregulated endocrine and paracrine states, such as obesity, in which adipocyte-derived factors and adipo-cytokines contribute to adipose tissue inflammation, reduction of NO bioavailability, insulin resistance, and oxidized low-density lipoproteins.[63]

In conjunction with the release of cytokines, microthrombosis is induced. Stemming from exocytosis of large amounts of von Willebrand factor multimers (ULVWF) and platelet activation, they form platelet-ULVWF complexes resulting in disseminated intravascular microthrombosis, a reduction in microcirculation, and tissue hypoxia. This circular amplification process of inflammation, microthrombosis, hypoxia, and oxidative stress gives rise to the "2-activation theory of the endothelium," in which the endotheliopathy of sepsis promotes the activation of the 2 independent endothelial pathways: inflammatory and microthrombotic.[64,65]

Although disruption of the microcirculation due to collaboration between inflammatory and microthrombotic processes is a hallmark of immune-regulated sepsis, ECs also secrete a gellike substance called endothelial glycocalyx that supports healthy microvascular flow. Found on the luminal surface of vascular endothelium, glycocalyx is composed of glycosaminoglycans, glycoproteins, and glycolipids, where they modulate "vascular resistance to maintain homogeneity in microcirculation, mechanotransducing fluid shear stress to endothelium, modulating vascular permeability, and buffering ECs from plasma oxidants, cytokines, and circulating immune cells."[66] However, during the aging process, glycocalyx deteriorates, contributing to microvascular dysfunction and cardiovascular disease. When combined with dysregulation of endothelial NO and altered redox states, recruitment of proper endothelial progenitor cells and modulation of the inflammatory process begins to become unbalanced, leading to endothelial dysfunction and pathologic progression of disease processes.[67]

In contrast to vessel maintenance, tumor growth and progression are dependent on vessel formation. Influenced by tumor metabolic needs, vascular growth, extension, and remodeling actively guide tumor neovascularization. Previously quiescent ECs are recruited into hypoxic and necrotic regions where there is a disregard for immune surveillance, and vessel growth occurs in a sea of hypoxia, inflammation, and ROS. As a result of this volatile environment, tumor vasculature has increased amounts of leakage and anergy. Stabilization of the endothelium through use of antiangiogenic therapy allows for improvement in vessel stability, perfusion, oxygen delivery, and, importantly, distribution of tumor-targeting drugs. Therefore, normalization of the EC barrier within tumors is a critical in cancer therapy.[68]

SUMMARY AND PERSPECTIVES

Complex partners in the maintenance of vascular integrity, ECs in conjunction with supporting mural cells are an essential foreman guiding the egress of circulating cells, oxygen, and nutrients to meet tissue metabolic needs. Interference in endothelial-EC-cell communication and signaling contributes to progression of pathologic disease processes. Expanding our understanding of those factors that modulate this diverse and heterogeneous EC population is critical to improving our understanding of disease progression and the identification of novel therapeutic approaches.

DISCLOSURE

There are no commercial or financial conflicts of interest for the authors.

REFERENCES

1. Aird WC. Phenotypic heterogeneity of the endothelium: I. structure, function, and mechanisms. Circ Res 2007;100(2):158–73.
2. Coffin JD, Harrison J, Schwartz S, et al. Angioblast differentiation and morphogenesis of the vascular endothelium in the mouse embryo. Dev. Biol 1991; 148(1):51–62.
3. Betz C, Lenard A, Belting HG, et al. Cell behaviors and dynamics during angiogenesis. Development 2016;143(13):2249–60.
4. Abrahamson DR. Development of kidney glomerular endothelial cells and their role in basement membrane assembly. Organogenesis 2009;5(1):275–87.
5. Schwarz MA, Zhang F, Gebb S, et al. Endothelial monocyte activating polypeptide II inhibits lung neovascularization and airway epithelial morphogenesis. Mech Dev 2000;95(1–2):123–32.
6. Villasenor A, Cleaver O. Crosstalk between the developing pancreas and its blood vessels: an evolving dialog. Semin Cell Dev Biol 2012;23(6):685–92.
7. Daniel E, Cleaver O. Vascularizing organogenesis: lessons from developmental biology and implications for regenerative medicine. Curr Top Dev Biol 2019; 132:177–220.
8. Guo M, Du Y, Gokey JJ, et al. Single cell RNA analysis identifies cellular heterogeneity and adaptive responses of the lung at birth. Nat Commun 2019;10(1):37.
9. Khan S, Taverna F, Rohlenova K, et al. EndoDB: a database of endothelial cell transcriptomics data. Nucleic Acids Res 2019;47(D1):D736–44.
10. Lukowski SW, Patel J, Andersen SB, et al. Single-cell transcriptional profiling of aortic endothelium identifies a hierarchy from endovascular progenitors to differentiated cells. Cell Rep 2019;27(9):2748–58.e3.
11. Marcu R, Choi YJ, Xue J, et al. Human organ-specific endothelial cell heterogeneity. iScience 2018;4:20–35.
12. Draoui N, de Zeeuw P, Carmeliet P. Angiogenesis revisited from a metabolic perspective: role and therapeutic implications of endothelial cell metabolism. Open Biol 2017;7(12) [pii:170219].
13. Risau W, Lemmon V. Changes in the vascular extracellular matrix during embryonic vasculogenesis and angiogenesis. Dev. Biol 1988;125(2):441–50.
14. Risau W, Sariola H, Zerwes HG, et al. Vasculogenesis and angiogenesis in embryonic-stem-cell-derived embryoid bodies. Development 1988;102(3):471–8.
15. Czirok A, Little CD. Pattern formation during vasculogenesis. Birth Defects Res C Embryo Today 2012;96(2):153–62.

16. Carmeliet P. Mechanisms of angiogenesis and arteriogenesis. Nat Med 2000; 6(4):389–95.
17. Chung AS, Ferrara N. Developmental and pathological angiogenesis. Annu Rev Cell Dev Biol 2011;27:563–84.
18. Eilken HM, Adams RH. Dynamics of endothelial cell behavior in sprouting angiogenesis. Curr Opin Cell Biol 2010;22(5):617–25.
19. Song JW, Munn LL. Fluid forces control endothelial sprouting. Proc Natl Acad Sci U S A 2011;108(37):15342–7.
20. Escobedo N, Oliver G. Lymphangiogenesis: origin, specification, and cell fate determination. Annu Rev Cell Dev Biol 2016;32:677–91.
21. Weibel ER, Palade GE. New cytoplasmic components in arterial endothelia. J Cell Biol 1964;23:101–12.
22. Yuan L, Chan GC, Beeler D, et al. A role of stochastic phenotype switching in generating mosaic endothelial cell heterogeneity. Nat Commun 2016;7:10160.
23. Eelen G, de Zeeuw P, Simons M, et al. Endothelial cell metabolism in normal and diseased vasculature. Circ Res 2015;116(7):1231–44.
24. Groschner LN, Waldeck-Weiermair M, Malli R, et al. Endothelial mitochondria–less respiration, more integration. Pflugers Arch 2012;464(1):63–76.
25. Radeva MY, Waschke J. Mind the gap: mechanisms regulating the endothelial barrier. Acta Physiol 2018;222(1).
26. Wettschureck N, Strilic B, Offermanns S. Passing the vascular barrier: endothelial signaling processes controlling extravasation. Physiol Rev 2019;99(3):1467–525..
27. Yau JW, Teoh H, Verma S. Endothelial cell control of thrombosis. BMC Cardiovasc Disord 2015;15:130.
28. Budnik I, Brill A. Immune factors in deep vein thrombosis initiation. Trends Immunol 2018;39(8):610–23.
29. Hoffman M. The tissue factor pathway and wound healing. Semin Thromb Hemost 2018;44(2):142–50.
30. Witkowski M, Landmesser U, Rauch U. Tissue factor as a link between inflammation and coagulation. Trends Cardiovasc Med 2016;26(4):297–303.
31. Vanhoutte PM, Shimokawa H, Feletou M, et al. Endothelial dysfunction and vascular disease - a 30th anniversary update. Acta Physiol 2017;219(1):22–96.
32. McCarron JG, Wilson C, Heathcote HR, et al. Heterogeneity and emergent behaviour in the vascular endothelium. Curr Opin Pharmacol 2019;45:23–32.
33. Jung B, Obinata H, Galvani S, et al. Flow-regulated endothelial S1P receptor-1 signaling sustains vascular development. Dev. Cel 2012;23(3):600–10.
34. Rosen H, Stevens RC, Hanson M, et al. Sphingosine-1-phosphate and its receptors: structure, signaling, and influence. Annu Rev Biochem 2013;82:637–62.
35. Diebold LP, Gil HJ, Gao P, et al. Mitochondrial complex III is necessary for endothelial cell proliferation during angiogenesis. Nat Metab 2019;1(1):158–71.
36. Sapieha P, Sirinyan M, Hamel D, et al. The succinate receptor GPR91 in neurons has a major role in retinal angiogenesis. Nat Med 2008;14(10):1067–76.
37. Toma I, Kang JJ, Sipos A, et al. Succinate receptor GPR91 provides a direct link between high glucose levels and renin release in murine and rabbit kidney. J Clin Invest 2008;118(7):2526–34.
38. Zheng B, Yin WN, Suzuki T, et al. Exosome-mediated miR-155 transfer from smooth muscle cells to endothelial cells induces endothelial injury and promotes atherosclerosis. Mol Ther 2017;25(6):1279–94.
39. Arana L, Gangoiti P, Ouro A, et al. Ceramide and ceramide 1-phosphate in health and disease. Lipids Health Dis 2010;9:15.

40. Bayliss WM, Starling EH. The Mechanism of pancreatic secretion. J Physiol 1902; 28(5):325–53.
41. Franco M, Roswall P, Cortez E, et al. Pericytes promote endothelial cell survival through induction of autocrine VEGF-A signaling and Bcl-w expression. Blood 2011;118(10):2906–17.
42. Gerhardt H, Golding M, Fruttiger M, et al. VEGF guides angiogenic sprouting utilizing endothelial tip cell filopodia. J Cell Biol 2003;161(6):1163–77.
43. Lee S, Chen TT, Barber CL, et al. Autocrine VEGF signaling is required for vascular homeostasis. Cell 2007;130(4):691–703.
44. Ksiazek M, Chacinska M, Chabowski A, et al. Sources, metabolism, and regulation of circulating sphingosine-1-phosphate. J Lipid Res 2015;56(7):1271–81.
45. Winkler MS, Martz KB, Nierhaus A, et al. Loss of sphingosine 1-phosphate (S1P) in septic shock is predominantly caused by decreased levels of high-density lipoproteins (HDL). J Intensive Care 2019;7:23.
46. Armulik A, Genove G, Betsholtz C. Pericytes: developmental, physiological, and pathological perspectives, problems, and promises. Dev. Cel 2011;21(2): 193–215.
47. Cattin AL, Burden JJ, Van Emmenis L, et al. Macrophage-induced blood vessels guide Schwann cell-mediated regeneration of peripheral nerves. Cell 2015; 162(5):1127–39.
48. Fantin A, Vieira JM, Gestri G, et al. Tissue macrophages act as cellular chaperones for vascular anastomosis downstream of VEGF-mediated endothelial tip cell induction. Blood 2010;116(5):829–40.
49. Willenborg S, Lucas T, van Loo G, et al. CCR2 recruits an inflammatory macrophage subpopulation critical for angiogenesis in tissue repair. Blood 2012; 120(3):613–25.
50. Barnett FH, Rosenfeld M, Wood M, et al. Macrophages form functional vascular mimicry channels in vivo. Sci Rep 2016;6:36659.
51. Kim SJ, Kim JS, Papadopoulos J, et al. Circulating monocytes expressing CD31: implications for acute and chronic angiogenesis. Am J Pathol 2009;174(5): 1972–80.
52. Kovacic JC, Dimmeler S, Harvey RP, et al. Endothelial to mesenchymal transition in cardiovascular disease: JACC state-of-the-art review. J Am Coll Cardiol 2019; 73(2):190–209.
53. Kumarswamy R, Volkmann I, Jazbutyte V, et al. Transforming growth factor-beta-induced endothelial-to-mesenchymal transition is partly mediated by microRNA-21. Arterioscler Thromb Vasc Biol 2012;32(2):361–9.
54. Walshe TE, Saint-Geniez M, Maharaj AS, et al. TGF-beta is required for vascular barrier function, endothelial survival and homeostasis of the adult microvasculature. PLoS One 2009;4(4):e5149.
55. Jia G, Aroor AR, Jia C, et al. Endothelial cell senescence in aging-related vascular dysfunction. Biochim Biophys Acta Mol Basis Dis 2019;1865(7):1802–9.
56. Bhayadia R, Schmidt BM, Melk A, et al. Senescence-induced oxidative stress causes endothelial dysfunction. J Gerontol A Biol Sci Med Sci 2016;71(2):161–9.
57. Holdt LM, Sass K, Gabel G, et al. Expression of Chr9p21 genes CDKN2B (p15(INK4b)), CDKN2A (p16(INK4a), p14(ARF)) and MTAP in human atherosclerotic plaque. Atherosclerosis 2011;214(2):264–70.
58. Sung JY, Lee KY, Kim JR, et al. Interaction between mTOR pathway inhibition and autophagy induction attenuates adriamycin-induced vascular smooth muscle cell senescence through decreased expressions of p53/p21/p16. Exp Gerontol 2018; 109:51–8.

59. Castro-Ferreira R, Cardoso R, Leite-Moreira A, et al. The role of endothelial dysfunction and inflammation in chronic venous disease. Ann Vasc Surg 2018; 46:380–93.

60. Chang JC. Sepsis and septic shock: endothelial molecular pathogenesis associated with vascular microthrombotic disease. Thromb J 2019;17:10.

61. Opal SM, van der Poll T. Endothelial barrier dysfunction in septic shock. J Intern Med 2015;277(3):277–93.

62. Khaddaj Mallat R, Mathew John C, Kendrick DJ, et al. The vascular endothelium: a regulator of arterial tone and interface for the immune system. Crit Rev Clin Lab Sci 2017;54(7–8):458–70.

63. Engin A. Endothelial dysfunction in obesity. Adv Exp Med Biol 2017;960:345–79.

64. Chang JC. TTP-like syndrome: novel concept and molecular pathogenesis of endotheliopathy-associated vascular microthrombotic disease. Thromb J 2018; 16:20.

65. Chang JC. Thrombogenesis and thrombotic disorders based on 'two-path unifying theory of hemostasis': philosophical, physiological, and phenotypical interpretation. Blood Coagul Fibrinolysis 2018;29(7):585–95.

66. Machin DR, Phuong TT, Donato AJ. The role of the endothelial glycocalyx in advanced age and cardiovascular disease. Curr Opin Pharmacol 2019;45:66–71.

67. Premer C, Kanelidis AJ, Hare JM, et al. Rethinking endothelial dysfunction as a crucial target in fighting heart failure. Mayo Clin Proc Innov Qual Outcomes 2019;3(1):1–13.

68. Klein D. The tumor vascular endothelium as decision maker in cancer therapy. Front Oncol 2018;8:367.

The Angiopoietin-Tie2 Pathway in Critical Illness

Kelsey D. Sack, MD, PhD[a], John A. Kellum, MD, MCCM[b,1], Samir M. Parikh, MD[a,*,1]

KEYWORDS

- Angiopoietin • Tie2 • Sepsis • ARDS • Vascular leakage • Coagulation • VE-PTP

KEY POINTS

- Cardinal clinical features of sepsis, such as vascular leakage and coagulation, relate to microvascular health. A vascular signaling pathway anchored by Tie2 actively promotes quiescence.
- During sepsis, the endogenous Tie2 antagonist protein called Angiopoietin-2 is induced, leading to rapid reduction in Tie2 signaling. This renders microvessels leaky, proinflammatory, and prothrombotic.
- Experimental models of sepsis, acute lung injury, and other acute stressors collectively demonstrate that restoration of Tie2 signaling exerts a protective effect and enhances survival.
- Intensive care unit studies consistently demonstrate early and progressive elevation of circulating Angiopoietin-2 that is associated with worsening oxygenation, increased risk of disseminated intravascular coagulation, and other adverse outcomes.
- Human genetic studies suggest that common variants in ANGPT2 and TIE2 genes may be linked to the risk of acute lung injury.

INTRODUCTION

Homeostasis of small blood vessels exerts a powerful influence on the disease course in critically ill patients. In systemic inflammation, dysregulated microvessels throughout the body leak their contents into the surrounding tissue, potentiate the penetration of inflammatory cells into major organs, promote the formation of in situ thrombi, and disrupt the vascular tone necessary to deliver oxygen and nutrients where they are needed. Vascular dysfunction arising from systemic inflammation may impact clinically meaningful adverse outcomes in the intensive care unit (ICU).

Funded by: National Institutes of Health. Grant numbers: R01 HL125275; R35 HL139424.
[a] Department of Medicine, Center for Vascular Biology Research, Beth Israel Deaconess Medical Center, Harvard Medical School, 330 Brookline Avenue, RN330C, Boston, MA 02215, USA;
[b] Department of Critical Care Medicine, CRISMA Center, University of Pittsburgh, University of Pittsburgh, School of Medicine, 3347 Forbes Avenue, Suite 220, Room 202, Pittsburgh, PA 15213, USA
[1] These authors contributed equally to the work.
* Corresponding author.
E-mail address: sparikh1@bidmc.harvard.edu

Crit Care Clin 36 (2020) 201–216
https://doi.org/10.1016/j.ccc.2019.12.003
0749-0704/20/© 2019 Elsevier Inc. All rights reserved.

Table 1 Factors modulating TIE2 signaling	
Quiescence [activated Tie2]	Systemic inflammation [suppressed Tie2]
Angpt-1 (tetramers)	Angpt-2 (dimers)
TIE1	TIE1 cleavage
Integrins [alpha5beta1, alphavbeta3]	Cytokines TIE2 [cleavage, reduced expression]

The morbidity, mortality, and cost from these pathophysiologic processes is vast, while clinical care in the ICU remains largely supportive rather than targeted at the underlying pathophysiologic mechanisms.[1–3] Mechanisms that regulate the transition between microvascular homeostasis and dysregulation are therefore of substantial fundamental and translational interest.

The vascular endothelium receives signals from the circulating inflammatory milieu and responds to these signals to control tone, barrier function, adhesiveness to leukocytes, and coagulation. When inflammation arises locally, the transition from homeostasis to the activated state is likely adaptive: in response to local tissue injury, the breakdown of the microvascular barrier enables humoral and cellular effectors of immunity to access the parenchyma; local vasorelaxation increases the flux of such effectors into the target region; and thrombus formation limits the dissemination of pathogens from the portal of entry. However, when the very same sequence proceeds unchecked or unfolds simultaneously across multiple vascular beds, the results look like the septic patient: edematous soft tissues, inflamed and swollen major organs, vasoplegia, and disseminated intravascular coagulation (DIC).

Molecular pathways within the vascular endothelium collaborate to facilitate homeostasis of blood vessels. Involved pathways include, but are not limited to, the Tie2-Angiopoietin axis[4–6]; vascular endothelial growth factor (VEGF) interactions with its receptors, VEGFR-2 and VEGFR-1[7–9]; sphingosine-1 kinase and its receptors[10]; and mechanical regulators, such as shear stress generated by the flow of blood.[11,12] Among vascular signaling pathways, the Tie2 receptor is unique in that its phosphorylation provides an active signal to promote quiescence and counteract the "activated" state of endothelium.[13–15] Furthermore, Tie2 signaling is exquisitely fine-turned by an array of factors (**Table 1**). Perhaps not surprisingly, diverse critical illness syndromes, including sepsis, DIC, shock, acute respiratory distress syndrome (ARDS), myocardial infarction, and acute kidney injury (AKI), have all been linked to suppression of Tie2 signaling.[4,6,16–21]

BIOLOGY OF THE ANGIOPOIETIN-TIE2 AXIS
Overview

As a transmembrane tyrosine kinase, Tie2 is the central molecule in this axis. An orthologous protein called Tie1 is also expressed in endothelium, but does not directly bind Angiopoietins (Angpts) and remains an orphan receptor.[22,23] A third transmembrane protein, vascular endothelial–protein tyrosine phosphatase (VE-PTP), is also expressed in the endothelium, where it closely associates with Tie2 to regulate its signaling.

In the quiescent state, Angiopoetin-1 (Angpt-1) binds to Tie2, an event that clusters individual Tie2 molecules into a cross-phosphorylating complex. Downstream of phosphorylated Tie2, the second messenger AKT is activated, preventing endothelial apoptosis and enhancing cellular quiescence.[24] During times of stress (eg, inflammation signaled by cytokines such as tumor necrosis factor [TNF-α]) Angiopoietin-2 (Angpt-2) levels increase and competitively bind to the Tie2 receptor blocking Angpt-1-mediated phosphorylation.[25,26] Because Angpt-2 is less efficient than Angpt-1 at clustering Tie2 monomers, the net effect of Angpt-2 induction in the context of inflammation is to suppress tonic Tie2 signaling. Loss of Tie2 signaling releases an important "brake" in the endothelium, enabling it to rapidly shift its phenotype toward the activated state: weakened junctions,[27,28] expression of adhesion molecules for leukocytes, including ICAM1 and VCAM1,[26] and enhancement of procoagulant proteins at the luminal surface.[4,29] Each of these molecular-cellular events maps to major clinical manifestations in sepsis and ARDS. Weakened junctions lead to edema. Adhesion molecule induction promotes secondary inflammatory injury, and disruption of normal hemostatic mechanisms culminates in DIC. The subsequent sections summarize the molecular and cell biology of each major component in the Tie2 pathway.

Angiopoietin-1

Angpt-1 is the canonical agonist ligand for the Tie2. Angpt-1 has a modular structure, starting at the amino-terminus with a superclustering domain, then a coiled-coil domain, and finally, a fibrinogen-like domain. The N-terminal regions of Angpt-1 organize individual molecules into homotetramers and higher-order oligomers. The fibrinogen-like domain on the C-terminus is responsible for binding Tie2. Angpt-1 binds Tie2 very tightly at nanomolar affinity.[25,30] The oligomeric status of Angpt-1 promotes the clustering of Tie2 monomers at the endothelial surface. The resulting molecular complex becomes an efficient signaling unit.[31–33]

Angpt-1 knockout mice die in utero at ~E12.5 with a dilated, rudimentary vasculature that lacks branching and the support cells, such as pericytes that are characteristic of a matured vasculature.[30,34] The embryos exhibit edema and hemorrhage. Consistent with its role as an agonist, these features phenocopy global knockout of Tie2.[35] Conversely, upregulation of Angpt-1 results in an increased quantity of branched vasculature that is no longer leaky.[36–38]

Angpt-1 is expressed by platelets, mesenchymal cells, vascular smooth muscle cells, and pericytes.[25,34,39,40] The last 2 cell types bathe the extracellular matrix surrounding endothelial cells in Angpt-1. Moreover, Angpt-1 is naturally adhesive to the matrix.[41,42] The matrix-bound Angpt-1 provides a constant stimulus for Tie2 activation in the quiescent state. As discussed later, Tie2 activation plummets during inflammation with the induction of Angpt-2. However, in this latter context of endothelial "dyshomeostasis," Angpt-1-derived platelet granules may play an adaptive role. Platelets store large quantities of Angpt-1 protein, releasing it from granules under the influence of inflammatory modulators, such as thrombin. Degranulation of platelets could thereby help restore vascular homeostasis.[4,29,39,43,44]

Angiopoietin-2

In contrast to the stabilizing actions of Angpt-1, Angpt-2 is a context-dependent antagonist of the Tie2 receptor despite significant primary sequence homology to Angpt-1.[25] Indeed, overexpression of Angpt-2 results in an analogous phenotype to the Angpt-1 knockout model. Specifically, the vasculature is discontinuous and the endothelial cells themselves appear to have poor connection to the underlying extracellular matrix as noted by their spherical appearance.[25] Angpt-2 knockout mice remain relatively normal during the embryonic period, but exhibit poor vasculature remodeling in the postembryonic period and do not survive past 2 weeks of age secondary to lymphatic defects.[25,45]

Although Angpt-1 has a slightly higher binding affinity than Angpt-2 for the Tie2 receptor, when mixed together, Angpt-2 antagonizes the Tie2 receptor.[15,46,47] The basis for this signaling difference may be that Angpt-2 exists as a dimer rather than the higher-order oligomers of Angpt-1.[31–33] Therefore, at molar excess, the fibrinogen-like domain of Angpt-2 may compete with Angpt-1 for Tie2 binding, leaving Tie2 molecules in a more dispersed (ie, less phosphorylated) state on the endothelial surface.

Endothelial cells of the small vasculature express Angpt-2.[45,48] Preformed Angpt-2 protein is stored in the Weibel-Palade bodies of these cells, making Angpt-2 readily available for secretion after endothelial cells are stressed by triggers, including hypoxia, TNF-α, turbulent flow, and thrombin.[48–54] Therefore, noxious stimuli trigger the endothelium to release preformed Angpt-2 protein. This Angpt-2 acts in a local, or paracrine, fashion to unseat Angpt-1, thereby deactivating Tie2 signaling. The switch from quiescence to disruption is fortified because activated Tie2 tonically inhibits the transcription of the ANGPT2 gene by keeping the transcription factor FoxO1 sequestered in the endothelial cytoplasm.[46,48,55] Therefore, when Tie2 phosphorylation is switched off by the rapid release of preformed Angpt-2 protein, that endothelial cell then commences to synthesize more Angpt-2 protein through FoxO1-mediated gene transcription.

Tie2

Tie2 knockout is embryonically lethal at E10.5 because of a poorly developed heart and dilated leaky vessels that lack an investment of support cells[13,35] (**Figs. 1** and **2**). These features are similar to the Angpt-1 knockout model.[30,34] Tie2 is expressed in both active and quiescent endothelium and is necessary for adult vasculature. The quantity of receptor is downregulated in sprouting and inflamed vasculature.[14,56,57] Loss of Tie2 in vivo and in vitro results in a dysfunctional endothelium with impaired barrier function.[4,48,58]

In confluent or quiescent cells, Angpt-1 activates Tie2 at cell-cell borders in a *trans* configuration.[42] Tie2 activation at cell-cell junctions signals PI3 kinase and Akt. Akt phosphorylates FoxO1 on key residues that inhibit its translocation to the nucleus and its binding of the ANGPT2 gene.[46,48,52,55,59] Activated Akt also signals the molecular apparatus regulating the contractility of the endothelial cell and the essential junctional barrier protein VE-cadherin.[6,28,60–62] Expression of inflammatory adhesion molecules, including ICAM1, VCAM1, and E-selectin, is attenuated.[63] Finally, activated Akt suppresses key triggers of coagulation, including phosphatidylserine and tissue factor.[4] The net output of these molecular events downstream of Tie2 activation is an endothelial layer that forms an effective barrier, suppresses the production of Angpt-2, inhibits leukocyte adhesion, and prevents the activation of coagulation.

Because of its critical function, Tie2 is regulated at multiple levels. Angpt-1 binding results in receptor ubiquitylation, which triggers receptor internalization and degradation.[64] Minimal receptor internalization occurs in the presence of Angpt-2. Tie2 releases both Angpt-1 and Anpt-2 after engagement, allowing for further activation of additional receptors.[65] Together, this indicates the system remains poised for recovery during critical insult as a quantity of Tie2 receptor remains available for phosphorylation during dysfunctional, Angpt-2 predominant states. Additional regulation of Tie2 is mediated by shedding of its extracellular domain. Matrix metalloproteinase cleavage facilitates both Angpt-1- and Angpt-2-induced shedding. Shed receptor binds additional ligand, preventing further receptor activation, ultimately resulting in a smaller more directed pool of ligand and receptor.[66,67]

Tie1 and Vascular Endothelial–Protein Tyrosine Phosphatase

Further regulation of Tie2 receptor signaling occurs via transmembrane proteins that closely associate with Tie2. Although Tie1 does not directly bind Angpts, it is

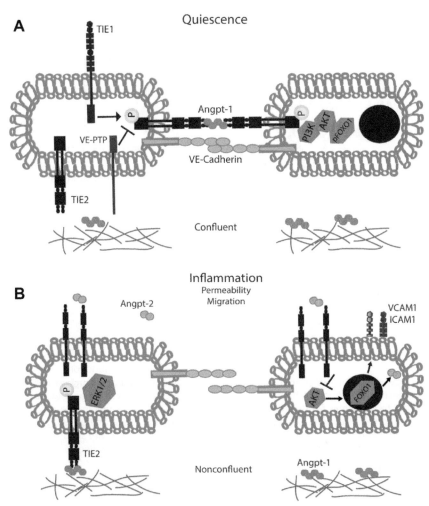

Fig. 1. Angiopoietin balance in quiescence and inflammation. (*A*) Endothelial cell Tie2 signaling during quiescence. Tie2 receptors cluster together and engage tetramers of Angpt-1, which results in activation of the receptor in a *trans* configuration. Furthermore, Tie1 binding further potentiates Tie2 activation. Downstream of activated Tie2, VE-cadherin is stabilized to strengthen barrier function. (*B*) Endothelial cell Tie2 signaling during inflammation. Tie2 receptor binds Angpt-2 dimers resulting in dephosphorylation and FOXO1 migration to the nucleus resulting in translation of inflammatory mediations and additional Angpt-2.

nonetheless critical for embryonic survival.[68] In in vitro and in vivo, Tie1 binding to Tie2 enhances the agonistic signaling of Angpt. Rapid cleavage of Tie1 occurs in response to inflammatory mediators, such as TNF-α and phorbol esters.[22,69]

VE-PTP enzymatically removes phosphates from proteins with which it associates. These proteins include VEGFR-2, VE-cadherin, and Tie2.[70–72] VE-PTP knockout mice die in utero of angiogenesis defects.[73] Inhibition of VE-PTP enhances Tie2 phosphorylation and strengthens the microvascular barrier against inflammatory triggers of permeability.[27] This barrier-enhancing effect of VE-PTP inhibition appears to require

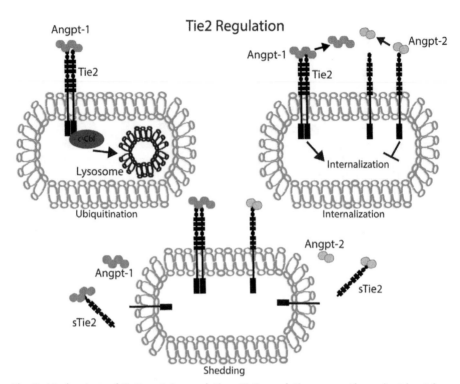

Fig. 2. Mechanisms of Tie2 protein regulation. Tie2 regulation occurs through at least four known mechanisms. Angpt-1 binding to Tie2 results in c-Cbl ubiquitination and resulting trafficking to lysosomes for destruction. Angpt-1 binding to Tie2 results in internalization, whereas Angpt-2 binding is only able to minimally internalize receptor. Both Angpt-1 and Angpt-2 are released from receptor after engagement. Tie2 receptors are shed from endothelial cells (sTie2) following cleavage by metalloproteinase, resulting in decreased receptor pool available for engagement. Finally, TIE2 gene transcription is attenuated during inflammation, also resulting in decreased receptor pool available for engagement (not depicted).

Tie2. Tie2 activation via VE-PTP inhibition is currently being explored in ocular conditions.[74,75]

PRECLINICAL EVIDENCE OF TIE2 REGULATING VESSELS DURING INFLAMMATION

Tie2 signaling appears to be a major determinant of the vascular response to a broad array of noxious stimuli. The earliest studies of the barrier-promoting effect of Tie2 stimulation demonstrated that Angpt-1 counteracts vascular leakage induced by unrelated triggers, including VEGF, serotonin, and mustard oil.[36,38] Since then, evidence from many laboratories testing diverse models of organ damage has coalesced around the central concept that Tie2 activation prevents vascular leakage, attenuates cellular inflammation, reduces spontaneous thrombus formation, and improves survival. As described next, this concept has been tested in preclinical models of sepsis, acute lung injury, and AKI. It has also been tested in experimental malaria, anthrax, and hemorrhagic fevers, including Ebolavirus disease. The volume and diversity of the experimental settings convincingly propose that Tie2 signaling is a major determinant of outcomes across settings that acutely destabilize the vasculature.

Sepsis

In the earliest report focusing on sepsis, Angpt-1 overexpression was shown to defend blood pressure, prevent leakage, attenuate inflammation, and improve survival in a model of endotoxic shock.[76] Angpt-1-mediated defense of vascular barrier function in the context of systemic endotoxin was thereafter shown to require p190RhoGap, a regulator of endothelial cell contraction,[60] and p47phox, an upstream signal transducer.[77] Intravenous Angpt-1 administration improved multiorgan dysfunction and survival in a model of polymicrobial abdominal sepsis induced by cecal ligation and perforation (CLP).[78] Acquired acute deficiency of Tie2 was found to be sufficient to weaken the vascular barrier in vivo.[77] Compared with wild-type littermates, loss of 1 Tie2 allele worsened vascular leakage and survival following either systemic endotoxin or CLP.[77] Tie1 expression must also be intact to counteract sepsis,[22] and VE-PTP inhibition or genetic deletion has been shown to strengthen the vascular barrier against systemic inflammation.[27]

Finally, Angpt-2 has been inhibited in several ways, all of which implicate this molecule as a mediator of adverse outcomes in experimental sepsis. First, partial genetic deletion of ANGPT2 was shown to protect CLP-induced mice from vascular leakage and to improve survival.[18] This result was verified by a second group, which also demonstrated protection against experimental sepsis with an Angpt-2 binding antibody.[79] The importance of the feed-forward loop that sustains Angpt-2 biosynthesis after the onset of inflammation was demonstrated in 2 studies that applied RNA interference to limit de novo production of Angpt-2.[59,80] Both reports demonstrated a positive impact on survival, suggesting that even a relatively late intervention (ie, after preformed Angpt-2 protein has already been released) could still improve outcomes. The most recent work in this area has focused directly on the question of oligomerization by showing that a novel antibody that can "cluster" Angpt-2 also improves survival in 2 different models of sepsis.[81] Together, these studies propose that targeted manipulations to favor Tie2 signaling enhance organ function and survival, whereas manipulations that weaken Tie2 signaling impair the organismic response to sepsis.

Lung Injury/Acute Respiratory Distress Syndrome

The Tie2 axis has been shown repeatedly to defend animals against disparate triggers of acute or chronic lung injury: this list includes intratracheal instillation of lipopolysaccharides[82]; parenteral lipopolysaccharides[27,60,76]; abdominal sepsis CLP[58,78,80,81,83]; hyperoxia in young animals[84]; the chemical warfare agent phosgene[85,86]; and pulmonary hypertension following monocrotaline, serotonin, or interleukin-6.[87,88] The salutary effect of Tie2 stimulation against unrelated noxious insults suggests a conserved role for Tie2 in the pathogenesis of lung injury.

Acute Kidney Injury

The Tie2 axis has been tested in animal models of AKI arising from sepsis. Angpt-2 deficiency was shown to protect against CLP-induced AKI.[18] Furthermore, intravenous Angpt-1 administration after the onset of CLP was shown to attenuate renal inflammation and expression of vascular adhesion molecules.[78] In models of acute injury that progress to fibrosis, administration of a recombinant Angpt-1 modified for better pharmacokinetic characteristics has been shown to ameliorate long-term outcomes.[89,90]

Disseminated Intravascular Coagulation

Only 2 published studies have examined targeted manipulations of the Tie2 axis in the context of DIC. One study reported coagulation parameters in the CLP mouse model with and without treatment with the clustering antibody that converts Angpt-2 into a Tie2 agonist. That study demonstrated beneficial effects on sepsis-induced DIC with the use of the clustering antibody.[81] A second study examined the effects of partial Tie2 deletion and Angpt-1 addition in the early stages of endotoxemia or CLP.[4] Loss of 1 Tie2 allele was found to potentiate injury-induced fibrin deposition in vivo in the absence of inflammation. In the context of endotoxemia, the tendency of Tie2 heterozygotes to develop fibrin-rich clots was more severe than their wild-type littermates. Conversely, when Angpt-1 was administered in either the endotoxemia model or CLP, the tendency to clot formation was markedly attenuated.

Nonsepsis States of Acute Vascular Destabilization

Studies in models of acute vascular destabilization that do not involve sepsis collectively suggest that stimulation of Tie2 can defend or restore vascular quiescence in diverse contexts. These diseases include experimental models of hemorrhagic fevers (Puumala, hantavirus, Ebola, dengue), anthrax, malaria, influenza,[58] chronic mycobacterial infection,[48,91] and systemic capillary leak syndrome.

Hantavirus-infected endothelial cells are sensitized to triggers of permeability, such as VEGF, an effect counteracted by Angpt-1.[92] A study seeking to address causes of variation in the outcomes to Ebolavirus infection applied an experimental version of the virus to numerous outcrossed strains of mouse, then conduced genetics in the outliers. This study found that mice bearing hypomorphic alleles of TIE2 were more vulnerable to prolonged coagulation times, visceral hemorrhages, and early death.[93] Certain TIE1 alleles were associated with increased weight loss, earlier death, and increased overall mortality.[93] In a mouse model of dengue infection, treatment with Angpt-1 improved survival.[94] In a mouse model of malaria that develops cerebral edema, Angpt-1 was shown to restore vascular integrity, reduce edema, and improve survival.[95]

Systemic administration of anthrax lethal toxin downregulated Tie2 signaling and increased vascular leakage in mice.[96] Partial deletion of Angpt-2 improved survival in this model. Partial loss of Angpt-2 attenuated survival, and administration of Angpt-1 by gene transfer improved survival in this model. Finally, in primates infected with an attenuated strain of Bacillus anthracis that nonetheless provokes vascular collapse, circulating Angpt-2 levels increased rapidly, whereas Angpt-1 levels decreased. The changes in circulating Angpts were proportional to the inoculum of bacteria.[96]

CLINICAL EVIDENCE IMPLICATING THE TIE2 AXIS
Overview

Clinical studies of the Tie2 axis have primarily involved measurement of circulating levels of Angpt-1 and Angpt-2, although there are some reports on soluble levels of Tie2 and Tie1. Genetic polymorphisms influencing Angpt-2 and Tie2 expression have also been linked to risk of ARDS in the setting of both sepsis and nonsepsis.

Sepsis and Acute Respiratory Distress Syndrome

Early work in sepsis focused on the lung and showed that high circulating Angpt-2 was associated with impaired gas exchange, perhaps the result of vascular leak.[6] Subsequent studies in severe sepsis showed that Angpt-2 can increase dramatically in the circulation early in the course of disease and associated well with loss of vascular integrity in various organs.[97,98] Angpt-2 levels even spike with infusion of low-dose endotoxin in healthy volunteers,[99] leading many to propose that it could be a useful biomarker of infection. Furthermore, as Angpt-2 increases with systemic inflammation, Angpt-1 decreases. Thus, the ratio of Angpt-2/Angpt-1 in the circulation may be a better indicator of Tie2 signaling impairment than either protein alone.[98,100] However, "sterile inflammation" syndromes, such as trauma or major surgery, can also disrupt Tie2 signaling, making it less specific for sepsis.[101–103] Finally, genetic polymorphisms linked to Angpt-2 oversecretion have shown an increased risk for ARDS.[104] Common variants reducing TIE2 gene expression itself have also been linked to the development of ARDS.[58]

SEPSIS AND DISSEMINATED INTRAVASCULAR COAGULATION

Disruption of the endothelial Tie2 axis also appears to be a sentinel event in septic DIC. The authors recently described proteomic analysis in septic DIC patients that revealed a network involving inflammation and coagulation with Angpt-2, occupying a central node.[4] Angpt-2 was strongly associated with traditional DIC markers, including platelet counts, yet more accurately predicted mortality in 2 large independent cohorts (combined $N = 1077$). Similarly, in endotoxemic mice, reduced Tie2 signaling preceded signs of overt DIC. Intravital imaging of the microvascular revealed excessive fibrin accumulation in a pattern reminiscent of Tie2 deficiency. Conversely, Tie2 activation normalized prothrombotic responses by inhibiting endothelial tissue factor and phosphatidylserine exposure. Importantly, Tie2 activation in this model had no adverse effects on bleeding. Given that interventions targeting Tie2 can normalize coagulation without increasing bleeding risk, this approach could prove superior to current DIC therapies.

Cardiopulmonary Bypass and Acute Kidney Injury

One study measured serum Angpt-2 from 25 adult patients before and after cardiopulmonary bypass (CPB) and compared it with indices of organ dysfunction, duration of mechanical ventilation, length of stay in the ICU, and hospital mortality. Angpt-2 levels steadily increased from 2.6 ± 2.4 ng/mL at 0 hours up to 7.3 ± 4.6 ng/mL at 24 hours following CPB ($P<.001$). The release of Angpt-2 correlated with the duration of CPB, aortic cross-clamp time, and post-CPB lactate levels. Changes in Angpt-2 during follow-up correlated with Pao_2/Fio_2 ratios, hemodynamics, fluid balance, and disease severity measures. Angpt-2 levels at 12 hours predicted the durations of mechanical ventilation and ICU stay, and hospital mortality.[105] Another study of 21 patients who experienced a 50% or greater increase in serum creatinine after cardiac surgery compared circulating levels of Angpt-1, Angpt-2, and Tie2 with propensity-matched controls. The investigators also measured kidney injury molecule-1 (KIM-1) and N-acetyl-β-D-glucosaminidase (NAG) in the urine. Angpt-2 plasma levels increased over time in patients with AKI (from 4.2 to 11.6 ng/mL) but did so as well in control patients (from 3.0 to 6.7 ng/mL). Plasma levels of Tie2 and Angpt-1 also decreased in both AKI patients and controls. However, there was a positive correlation between plasma levels of Angpt-2 and urinary levels of NAG but not KIM-1.[21] Although circulating Angpt-2 levels were predictive of AKI and renal failure in patients with acute pancreatitis, the relationship may be nonspecific.[106] Angpt-2 significantly correlated with acute phase proteins as well.

Other States of Vascular Destabilization

In patients with certain hemorrhagic fevers, including hanta virus, dengue, and Crimean-Congo hemorrhagic fever, the serum quantity of Angpt-2 increases in a similar fashion to that in septic patients.[107–109] In Clarkson disease (systemic capillary leak syndrome), patients have transient episodes of vascular leakage resulting in hemoconcentration and hypotension. Angpt-2 increases during disease flares and returns to baseline during remission.[110] Angpt-1 and Tie2 are both dysregulated in blood-outgrowth endothelial cells from affected humans, suggesting a further role of this pathway in the systemic process.[111] Finally, *P. falciparum* cerebral malaria has also been associated with Angpt/Tie derangements. Once again, as levels of Angpt-2 serum levels increased, the severity of falciparum malaria worsened.[112]

SUMMARY AND FUTURE DIRECTIONS

Vascular disruption underlies cardinal features of critical illness that culminates in death. A body of work spanning biochemistry, cell biology, rodent and primate models, human observational studies, and human genetics collectively proposes that the Tie2 axis may be an important determinant of the vascular response to acute destabilizing stressors. Although successful translation of preclinical observations to the bedside has been a major challenge in critical care medicine, the evidence emerging from laboratories around the world proposes several routes to clinical realization.

Genetic markers of the Tie2 axis and/or circulating Angpt measurements could 1 day inform clinicians regarding the susceptibility of a given patient to adverse vascular-related outcomes. In turn, such knowledge could be used to guide routine clinical care (eg, fluid-conservative vs liberal resuscitation strategies or adjustment of ventilator settings to avoid secondary damage) or inform the selection of patients for trials of investigational agents that target the vasculature. Because circulating Angpt-2 levels indirectly report Tie2 signaling, sequential Angpt-2 measurements could be used to monitor the response to investigational therapies targeting Tie2. Such a surrogate marker of target engagement amenable to evaluation in a phase 1b setting can significantly impact clinical development. As a circulating protein, Angpt-2 is amenable to neutralization with an antibody. A clinical-stage Angpt-2 neutralizing antibody has already been developed for cancer testing.[113] Conversely, Angpt-1 could be delivered as a modified recombinant protein or by gene transfer or even cell-based therapy that is already being tested in ARDS.[114] VE-PTP inhibition is also being tested in patients with retinal edema.[75,115] Therefore, multiple "shovel-ready" approaches exist to test this promising hypothesis in patients.

Translational pursuit of the Tie2 axis could result in new ways to diagnose, stratify, and treat ICU patients. Any such advance would constitute a breakthrough for the many patients affected by sepsis, ARDS, and related conditions.

DISCLOSURE

S.M. Parikh is a member of the Scientific Advisory Board for Aerpio.

REFERENCES

1. Cohen J, Vincent JL, Adhikari NKJ, et al. Sepsis: a roadmap for future research. Lancet Infect Dis 2015;15(5):581–614.

2. Iwashyna TJ, Ely EW, Smith DM, et al. Long-term cognitive impairment and functional disability among survivors of severe sepsis. JAMA 2010;304(16):1787–94.

3. Liu V, Escobar GJ, Greene JD, et al. Hospital deaths in patients with sepsis from 2 independent cohorts. JAMA 2014;312(1):90–2.

4. Higgins SJ, De Ceunynck K, Kellum JA, et al. Tie2 protects the vasculature against thrombus formation in systemic inflammation. J Clin Invest 2018; 128(4):1471–84.

5. Thamm K, Schrimpf C, Retzlaff J, et al. Molecular regulation of acute Tie2 suppression in sepsis. Crit Care Med 2018;46(9):e928–36.

6. Parikh SM, Mammoto T, Schultz A, et al. Excess circulating angiopoietin-2 may contribute to pulmonary vascular leak in sepsis in humans. PLoS Med 2006; 3(3):e46.

7. van der Flier M, van Leeuwen HJ, van Kessel KP, et al. Plasma vascular endothelial growth factor in severe sepsis. Shock 2005;23(1):35–8.

8. Opal SM, van der Poll T. Endothelial barrier dysfunction in septic shock. J Intern Med 2015;277(3):277–93.

9. Olsson AK, Dimberg A, Kreuger J, et al. VEGF receptor signalling–in control of vascular function. Nat Rev Mol Cell Biol 2006;7(5):359–71.

10. Li X, Stankovic M, Bonder CS, et al. Basal and angiopoietin-1–mediated endothelial permeability is regulated by sphingosine kinase-1. Blood 2008;111(7): 3489–97.

11. De Backer D, Creteur J, Preiser JC, et al. Microvascular blood flow is altered in patients with sepsis. Am J Respir Crit Care Med 2002;166(1):98–104.

12. Heo K-S, Fujiwara K, Abe J-I. Disturbed-flow-mediated vascular reactive oxygen species induce endothelial dysfunction. Circ J 2011;75(12):2722–30.

13. Sato TN, Tozawa Y, Deutsch U, et al. Distinct roles of the receptor tyrosine kinases Tie-1 and Tie-2 in blood vessel formation. Nature 1995;376(6535):70–4.

14. Wong AL, Haroon ZA, Werner S, et al. Tie2 expression and phosphorylation in angiogenic and quiescent adult tissues. Circ Res 1997;81(4):567–74.

15. Yuan HT, Khankin EV, Karumanchi SA, et al. Angiopoietin 2 is a partial agonist/ antagonist of Tie2 signaling in the endothelium. Mol Cell Biol 2009;29(8): 2011–22.

16. Lee KW, Lip GYH, Blann AD. Plasma angiopoietin-1, angiopoietin-2, angiopoietin receptor Tie-2, and vascular endothelial growth factor levels in acute coronary syndromes. Circulation 2004;110(16):2355–60.

17. Davis JS, Yeo TW, Piera KA, et al. Angiopoietin-2 is increased in sepsis and inversely associated with nitric oxide-dependent microvascular reactivity. Crit Care 2010;14(3):R89.

18. David S, Mukherjee A, Ghosh CC, et al. Angiopoietin-2 may contribute to multiple organ dysfunction and death in sepsis*. Crit Care Med 2012;40(11): 3034–41.

19. Liu K-L, Lee KT, Chang C-H, et al. Elevated plasma thrombomodulin and angiopoietin-2 predict the development of acute kidney injury in patients with acute myocardial infarction. Crit Care 2014;18(3):R100.

20. Kümpers P, Hafer C, David S, et al. Angiopoietin-2 in patients requiring renal replacement therapy in the ICU: relation to acute kidney injury, multiple organ dysfunction syndrome and outcome. Intensive Care Med 2010;36(3):462–70.

21. Jongman RM, van Klarenbosch J, Molema G, et al. Angiopoietin/Tie2 dysbalance is associated with acute kidney injury after cardiac surgery assisted by cardiopulmonary bypass. PLoS One 2015;10(8):e0136205.

22. Korhonen EA, Lampinen A, Giri H, et al. Tie1 controls angiopoietin function in vascular remodeling and inflammation. J Clin Invest 2016;126(9):3495–510.

23. Savant S, La Porta S, Budnik A, et al. The orphan receptor Tie1 controls angiogenesis and vascular remodeling by differentially regulating Tie2 in tip and stalk cells. Cell Rep 2015;12(11):1761–73.

24. Papapetropoulos A, Fulton D, Mahboubi K, et al. Angiopoietin-1 inhibits endothelial cell apoptosis via the akt/survivin pathway. J Biol Chem 2000;275(13): 9102–5.
25. Maisonpierre PC, Suri C, Jones PF, et al. Angiopoietin-2, a natural antagonist for Tie2 that disrupts in vivo angiogenesis. Science 1997;277(5322):55–60.
26. Fiedler U, Reiss Y, Scharpfenecker M, et al. Angiopoietin-2 sensitizes endothelial cells to TNF-α and has a crucial role in the induction of inflammation. Nat Med 2006;12(2):235–9.
27. Frye M, Dierkes M, Küppers V, et al. Interfering with VE-PTP stabilizes endothelial junctions in vivo via Tie-2 in the absence of VE-cadherin. J Exp Med 2015; 212(13):2267–87.
28. Gamble JR, Drew J, Trezise L, et al. Angiopoietin-1 is an antipermeability and anti-inflammatory agent in vitro and targets cell junctions. Circ Res 2000; 87(7):603–7.
29. Daly C, Qian X, Castanaro C, et al. Angiopoietins bind thrombomodulin and inhibit its function as a thrombin cofactor. Sci Rep 2018;8:505.
30. Suri C, Jones PF, Patan S, et al. Requisite role of angiopoietin-1, a ligand for the TIE2 receptor, during embryonic angiogenesis. Cell 1996;87(7):1171–80.
31. Davis S, Papadopoulos N, Aldrich TH, et al. Angiopoietins have distinct modular domains essential for receptor binding, dimerization and superclustering. Nat Struct Biol 2003;10(1):38–44.
32. Kim K-T, Choi HH, Steinmetz MO, et al. Oligomerization and multimerization are critical for angiopoietin-1 to bind and phosphorylate Tie2. J Biol Chem 2005; 280(20):20126–31.
33. Procopio WN, Pelavin PI, Lee WMF, et al. Angiopoietin-1 and -2 coiled coil domains mediate distinct homo-oligomerization patterns, but fibrinogen-like domains mediate ligand activity. J Biol Chem 1999;274(42):30196–201.
34. Davis S, Aldrich TH, Jones PF, et al. Isolation of angiopoietin-1, a ligand for the TIE2 receptor, by secretion-trap expression cloning. Cell 1996;87(7):1161–9.
35. Dumont DJ, Gradwohl G, Fong GH, et al. Dominant-negative and targeted null mutations in the endothelial receptor tyrosine kinase, tek, reveal a critical role in vasculogenesis of the embryo. Genes Dev 1994;8(16):1897–909.
36. Thurston G, Rudge JS, Ioffe E, et al. Angiopoietin-1 protects the adult vasculature against plasma leakage. Nat Med 2000;6(4):460–3.
37. Suri C, McClain J, Thurston G, et al. Increased vascularization in mice overexpressing angiopoietin-1. Science 1998;282(5388):468–71.
38. Thurston G, Suri C, Smith K, et al. Leakage-resistant blood vessels in mice transgenically overexpressing angiopoietin-1. Science 1999;286(5449):2511–4.
39. Huang Y-Q, Li J-J, Karpatkin S. Identification of a family of alternatively spliced mRNA species of angiopoietin-1. Blood 2000;95(6):1993–9.
40. Mammoto T, Jiang A, Jiang E, et al. Platelet rich plasma extract promotes angiogenesis through the angiopoietin1-Tie2 pathway. Microvasc Res 2013;89:15–24.
41. Xu Y, Yu Q. Angiopoietin-1, unlike angiopoietin-2, is incorporated into the extracellular matrix via its linker peptide region. J Biol Chem 2001;276(37):34990–8.
42. Saharinen P, Eklund L, Miettinen J, et al. Angiopoietins assemble distinct Tie2 signalling complexes in endothelial cell-cell and cell-matrix contacts. Nat Cell Biol 2008;10(5):527–37.
43. Li JJ, Huang YQ, Basch R, et al. Thrombin induces the release of angiopoietin-1 from platelets. Thromb Haemost 2001;85(02):204–6.
44. Ho-Tin-Noé B, Goerge T, Cifuni SM, et al. Platelet granule secretion continuously prevents intratumor hemorrhage. Cancer Res 2008;68(16):6851–8.

45. Gale NW, Thurston G, Hackett SF, et al. Angiopoietin-2 is required for postnatal angiogenesis and lymphatic patterning, and only the latter role is rescued by angiopoietin-1. Dev Cell 2002;3(3):411–23.

46. Daly C, Pasnikowski E, Burova E, et al. Angiopoietin-2 functions as an autocrine protective factor in stressed endothelial cells. Proc Natl Acad Sci U S A 2006; 103(42):15491–6.

47. Kim I, Kim J-H, Moon S-O, et al. Angiopoietin-2 at high concentration can enhance endothelial cell survival through the phosphatidylinositol 3′-kinase/ Akt signal transduction pathway. Oncogene 2000;19(39):4549–52.

48. Kim M, Allen B, Korhonen EA, et al. Opposing actions of angiopoietin-2 on Tie2 signaling and FOXO1 activation. J Clin Invest 2016;126(9):3511–25.

49. Fiedler U, Scharpfenecker M, Koidl S, et al. The Tie-2 ligand angiopoietin-2 is stored in and rapidly released upon stimulation from endothelial cell Weibel-Palade bodies. Blood 2004;103(11):4150–6.

50. Mandriota SJ, Pepper MS. Regulation of angiopoietin-2 mRNA levels in bovine microvascular endothelial cells by cytokines and hypoxia. Circ Res 1998;83(8): 852–9.

51. Oh H, Takagi H, Suzuma K, et al. Hypoxia and vascular endothelial growth factor selectively up-regulate angiopoietin-2 in bovine microvascular endothelial cells. J Biol Chem 1999;274(22):15732–9.

52. Goettsch W, Gryczka C, Korff T, et al. Flow-dependent regulation of angiopoietin-2. J Cell Physiol 2008;214(2):491–503.

53. Tressel SL, Huang R-P, Tomsen N, et al. Laminar shear inhibits tubule formation and migration of endothelial cells by an angiopoietin-2–dependent mechanism. Arterioscler Thromb Vasc Biol 2007;27(10):2150–6.

54. Dixit M, Bess E, Fisslthaler B, et al. Shear stress-induced activation of the AMP-activated protein kinase regulates FoxO1a and angiopoietin-2 in endothelial cells. Cardiovasc Res 2007;77(1):160–8.

55. Daly C, Wong V, Burova E, et al. Angiopoietin-1 modulates endothelial cell function and gene expression via the transcription factor FKHR (FOXO1). Genes Dev 2004;18(9):1060–71.

56. Puri MC, Partanen J, Rossant J, et al. Interaction of the TEK and TIE receptor tyrosine kinases during cardiovascular development. Development 1999;126:4569–80.

57. Felcht M, Luck R, Schering A, et al. Angiopoietin-2 differentially regulates angiogenesis through TIE2 and integrin signaling. J Clin Invest 2012;122(6): 1991–2005.

58. Ghosh CC, David S, Zhang R, et al. Gene control of tyrosine kinase TIE2 and vascular manifestations of infections. Proc Natl Acad Sci U S A 2016;113(9): 2472–7.

59. Ghosh CC, Thamm K, Berghelli AV, et al. Drug repurposing screen identifies Foxo1-dependent angiopoietin-2 regulation in sepsis. Crit Care Med 2015; 43(7):e230–40.

60. Mammoto T, Parikh SM, Mammoto A, et al. Angiopoietin-1 requires p190 Rho-GAP to protect against vascular leakage in vivo. J Biol Chem 2007;282(33): 23910–8.

61. Cascone I, Audero E, Giraudo E, et al. Tie-2–dependent activation of RhoA and Rac1 participates in endothelial cell motility triggered by angiopoietin-1. Blood 2003;102(7):2482–90.

62. Alfieri A, Ong ACM, Kammerer RA, et al. Angiopoietin-1 regulates microvascular reactivity and protects the microcirculation during acute endothelial dysfunction: role of eNOS and VE-cadherin. Pharmacol Res 2014;80:43–51.

63. Kim I, Moon SO, Park SK, et al. Angiopoietin-1 reduces VEGF-stimulated leuko-cyte adhesion to endothelial cells by reducing ICAM-1, VCAM-1, and E-selectin expression. Circ Res 2001;89(6):477–9.

64. Wehrle C, Van Slyke P, Dumont DJ. Angiopoietin-1-induced ubiquitylation of Tie2 by c-Cbl is required for internalization and degradation. Biochem J 2009;423(3): 375–80.

65. Bogdanovic E, Nguyen VPKH, Dumont DJ. Activation of Tie2 by angiopoietin-1 and angiopoietin-2 results in their release and receptor internalization. J Cell Sci 2006;119(17):3551–60.

66. Findley CM, Cudmore MJ, Ahmed A, et al. VEGF induces Tie2 shedding via a phosphoinositide 3-kinase/Akt–dependent pathway to modulate Tie2 signaling. Arterioscler Thromb Vasc Biol 2007;27(12):2619–26.

67. Reusch P, Barleon B, Weindel K, et al. Identification of a soluble form of the an-giopoietin receptor TIE-2 released from endothelial cells and present in human blood. Angiogenesis 2001;4(2):123–31.

68. Puri MC, Rossant J, Alitalo K, et al. The receptor tyrosine kinase TIE is required for integrity and survival of vascular endothelial cells. EMBO J 1995;14(23): 5884–91.

69. Marron MB, Singh H, Tahir TA, et al. Regulated proteolytic processing of Tie1 modulates ligand responsiveness of the receptor-tyrosine kinase Tie2. J Biol Chem 2007;282(42):30509–17.

70. Fachinger G, Deutsch U, Risau W. Functional interaction of vascular endothelial-protein-tyrosine phosphatase with the angiopoietin receptor Tie-2. Oncogene 1999;18(43):5948–53.

71. Nawroth R, Poell G, Ranft A, et al. VE-PTP and VE-cadherin ectodomains interact to facilitate regulation of phosphorylation and cell contacts. EMBO J 2002;21(18):4885–95.

72. Hayashi M, Majumdar A, Li X, et al. VE-PTP regulates VEGFR2 activity in stalk cells to establish endothelial cell polarity and lumen formation. Nat Commun 2013;4:1672.

73. Dominguez MG, Hughes VC, Pan L, et al. Vascular endothelial tyrosine phos-phatase (VE-PTP)-null mice undergo vasculogenesis but die embryonically because of defects in angiogenesis. Proc Natl Acad Sci U S A 2007;104(9): 3243–8.

74. Shen J, Frye M, Lee BL, et al. Targeting VE-PTP activates TIE2 and stabilizes the ocular vasculature. J Clin Invest 2014;124(10):4564–76.

75. Campochiaro PA, Sophie R, Tolentino M, et al. Treatment of diabetic macular edema with an inhibitor of vascular endothelial-protein tyrosine phosphatase that activates Tie2. Ophthalmology 2015;122(3):545–54.

76. Witzenbichler B, Westermann D, Knueppel S, et al. Protective role of angiopoietin-1 in endotoxic shock. Circulation 2005;111(1):97–105.

77. Ghosh CC, Mukherjee A, David S, et al. Angiopoietin-1 requires oxidant signaling through p47phox to promote endothelial barrier defense. PLoS One 2015;10(3):e0119577.

78. David S, Park J-K, Meurs MV, et al. Acute administration of recombinant Angiopoietin-1 ameliorates multiple-organ dysfunction syndrome and improves survival in murine sepsis. Cytokine 2011;55(2):251–9.

79. Ziegler T, Horstkotte J, Schwab C, et al. Angiopoietin 2 mediates microvascular and hemodynamic alterations in sepsis. J Clin Invest 2013;123(8):3436–45.

80. Stiehl T, Thamm K, Kaufmann J, et al. Lung-targeted RNA interference against angiopoietin-2 ameliorates multiple organ dysfunction and death in sepsis. Crit Care Med 2014;42(10):e654–62.
81. Han S, Lee SJ, Kim KE, et al. Amelioration of sepsis by TIE2 activation-induced vascular protection. Sci Transl Med 2016;20:335–55.
82. McCarter SD, Mei SHJ, Lai PFH, et al. Cell-based angiopoietin-1 gene therapy for acute lung injury. Am J Respir Crit Care Med 2007;175(10):1014–26.
83. Kumpers P, Gueler F, David S, et al. The synthetic Tie2 agonist peptide vasculo-tide protects against vascular leakage and reduces mortality in murine abdom-inal sepsis. Crit Care 2011;15(5):R261.
84. Bhandari V, Choo-Wing R, Lee CG, et al. Hyperoxia causes angiopoietin 2-medi-ated acute lung injury and necrotic cell death. Nat Med 2006;12(11):1286–93.
85. Shen J, Wang J, Shao Y-R, et al. Adenovirus-delivered angiopoietin-1 treatment for phosgene-induced acute lung injury. Inhal Toxicol 2013;25(5):272–9.
86. Shao Y, Shen J, Zhou F, et al. Mesenchymal stem cells overexpressing Ang1 at-tenuates phosgene-induced acute lung injury in rats. Inhal Toxicol 2018;30(7–8): 313–20.
87. Kugathasan L, Ray JB, Deng Y, et al. The angiopietin-1-Tie2 pathway prevents rather than promotes pulmonary arterial hypertension in transgenic mice. J Exp Med 2009;206(10):2221–34.
88. Zhao YD, Campbell AIM, Robb M, et al. Protective role of angiopoietin-1 in experimental pulmonary hypertension. Circ Res 2003;92(9):984–91.
89. Kim W, Moon SO, Lee SY, et al. COMP-angiopoietin-1 ameliorates renal fibrosis in a unilateral ureteral obstruction model. J Am Soc Nephrol 2006;17(9): 2474–83.
90. Lee S, Kim W, Kim DH, et al. Protective effect of COMP-angiopoietin-1 on cyclosporine-induced renal injury in mice. Nephrol Dial Transplant 2008;23(9): 2784–94.
91. Tabruyn SP, Colton K, Morisada T, et al. Angiopoietin-2-driven vascular remod-eling in airway inflammation. Am J Pathol 2010;177(6):3233–44.
92. Gavrilovskaya IN, Gorbunova EE, Mackow NA, et al. Hantaviruses direct endo-thelial cell permeability by sensitizing cells to the vascular permeability factor VEGF, while angiopoietin 1 and sphingosine 1-phosphate inhibit hantavirus-directed permeability. J Virol 2008;82(12):5797–806.
93. Rasmussen AL, Okumura A, Ferris MT, et al. Host genetic diversity enables Ebola hemorrhagic fever pathogenesis and resistance. Science 2014; 346(6212):987–91.
94. Phanthanawiboon S, Limkittikul K, Sakai Y, et al. Acute systemic infection with dengue virus leads to vascular leakage and death through tumor necrosis fac-tor-α and Tie2/angiopoietin signaling in mice lacking type I and II interferon re-ceptors. PLoS One 2016;11:e0148564.
95. Higgins SJ, Purcell LA, Silver KL, et al. Dysregulation of angiopoietin-1 plays a mechanistic role in the pathogenesis of cerebral malaria. Sci Transl Med 2016; 8(358):358ra128.
96. Ghosh CC, Mukherjee A, David S, et al. Impaired function of the Tie-2 receptor contributes to vascular leakage and lethality in anthrax. Proc Natl Acad Sci U S A 2012;109(25):10024–9.
97. Orfanos SE, Kotanidou A, Glynos C, et al. Angiopoietin-2 is increased in severe sepsis: correlation with inflammatory mediators. Crit Care Med 2007;35(1): 199–206.

98. Ong T, McClintock DE, Kallet RH, et al. Ratio of angiopoietin-2 to angiopoietin-1 as a predictor of mortality in acute lung injury patients. Crit Care Med 2010; 38(9):1845–51.
99. Kumpers P, van Meurs M, David S, et al. Time course of angiopoietin-2 release during experimental human endotoxemia and sepsis. Crit Care 2009;13(3):R64.
100. Giuliano JS Jr, Lahni PM, Harmon K, et al. Admission angiopoietin levels in children with septic shock. Shock 2007;28:650–4.
101. Ganter MT, Cohen MJ, Brohi K, et al. Angiopoietin-2, marker and mediator of endothelial activation with prognostic significance early after trauma? Ann Surg 2008;247(2):320–6.
102. Fremont RD, Koyama T, Calfee CS, et al. Acute lung injury in patients with traumatic injuries: utility of a panel of biomarkers for diagnosis and pathogenesis. J Trauma 2010;68(5):1121–7.
103. Meyer NJ, Li M, Feng R, et al. ANGPT2 genetic variant is associated with trauma-associated acute lung injury and altered plasma angiopoietin-2 isoform ratio. Am J Respir Crit Care Med 2011;183(10):1344–53.
104. Su L, Zhai R, Sheu CC, et al. Genetic variants in the angiopoietin-2 gene are associated with increased risk of ARDS. Intensive Care Med 2009;35(6):1024–30.
105. Clajus C, Lukasz A, David S, et al. Angiopoietin-2 is a potential mediator of endothelial barrier dysfunction following cardiopulmonary bypass. Cytokine 2012;60(2):352–9.
106. Sporek M, Dumnicka P, Gala-Bladzinska A, et al. Angiopoietin-2 is an early indicator of acute pancreatic-renal syndrome in patients with acute pancreatitis. Mediators Inflamm 2016;2016:5780903.
107. Nusshag C, Osberghaus A, Baumann A, et al. Deregulation of levels of angiopoietin-1 and angiopoietin-2 is associated with severe courses of hantavirus infection. J Clin Virol 2017;94:33–6.
108. Sancakdar E, Guven AS, Uysal EB, et al. Important of angiopoietic system in evaluation of endothelial damage in children with Crimean-Congo hemorrhagic fever. Pediatr Infect Dis J 2015;34(8):e200–5.
109. van de Weg CAM, Pannuti CS, van den Ham H-J, et al. Serum angiopoietin-2 and soluble VEGF receptor 2 are surrogate markers for plasma leakage in patients with acute dengue virus infection. J Clin Virol 2014;60(4):328–35.
110. Xie Z, Ghosh CC, Patel R, et al. Vascular endothelial hyperpermeability induces the clinical symptoms of Clarkson disease (the systemic capillary leak syndrome). Blood 2012;119(18):4321–32.
111. Druey KM, Parikh SM. Idiopathic systemic capillary leak syndrome (Clarkson disease). J Allergy Clin Immunol 2017;140(3):663–70.
112. Yeo TW, Lampah DA, Gitawati R, et al. Angiopoietin-2 is associated with decreased endothelial nitric oxide and poor clinical outcome in severe falciparum malaria. Proc Natl Acad Sci U S A 2008;105(44):17097–102.
113. Papadopoulos KP, Kelley RK, Tolcher AW, et al. A phase I first-in-human study of nesvacumab (REGN910), a fully human anti-angiopoietin-2 (Ang2) monoclonal antibody, in patients with advanced solid tumors. Clin Cancer Res 2016;22(6): 1348–55.
114. Matthay MA, Calfee CS, Zhuo H, et al. Treatment with allogeneic mesenchymal stromal cells for moderate to severe acute respiratory distress syndrome (START study): a randomised phase 2a safety trial. Lancet Respir Med 2019;7(2):154–62.
115. Campochiaro PA, Khanani A, Singer M, et al. Enhanced benefit in diabetic macular edema from AKB-9778 Tie2 activation combined with vascular endothelial growth factor suppression. Ophthalmology 2016;123(8):1722–30.

Endothelial Glycocalyx

Jan Jedlicka, MD[a], Bernhard F. Becker, MD, PhD[b],
Daniel Chappell, MD, PhD[c],*

KEYWORDS

- Endothelial glycocalyx • Shedding • Septic injury • Organ dysfunction • ARDS • AKI
- Trauma

KEY POINTS

- The endothelial glycocalyx is the most inner stratum of the vessel wall. Shedding of the endothelial glycocalyx plays a crucial role in a large number of critical illnesses.
- Shedding of the endothelial glycocalyx can be caused by trauma, inflammation, infection, or numerous iatrogenic interventions like fluid therapy or major surgery. The level of endothelial glycocalyx shedding correlates with morbidity and mortality.
- Ameliorating the shedding and the restitution of the endothelial glycocalyx could be a beneficial supportive therapeutic goal in the treatment of critical diseases.

INTRODUCTION

The endothelial glycocalyx (EG) is the most luminal layer of the blood vessel, growing on and within the vascular wall. It is mainly composed of a variety of proteoglycans and glycosaminoglycans. By attaching circulating plasma proteins, such as albumin, the so-called "endothelial surface layer" (ESL) is formed. The ESL is crucial for the maintenance and functioning of the vascular barrier, microcirculation, and organ perfusion alike. Accordingly, shedding or deterioration of this structure plays a central role in the pathophysiology of numerous critical illnesses. Degradation of the EG is associated with increased morbidity and mortality and is probably a common final pathway in diverse pathologies, including sepsis, acute respiratory distress syndrome (ARDS), trauma, and ischemia/reperfusion injury. Not only certain illnesses, foremost diabetes and arterial hypertension, can cause degradation of the EG, but also several iatrogenic interventions, such as major surgery or hypervolemia. Common problems of critically ill patients are hyperglycemia and hypernatremia, which are well known to have negative effects on outcome. During hyperglycemic or hypernatremic

The authors declare to have no conflict of interest in writing this article.
[a] Department of Anaesthesiology, University Hospital of Munich (LMU), Nussbaumstr. 20, Munich 80336, Germany; [b] Walter-Brendel-Centre of Experimental Medicine, Ludwig-Maximilians-University, Marchioninistr. 27, Munich 81377, Germany; [c] Department of Anaesthesiology, University Hospital of Munich (LMU), Marchioninistr. 15, Munich 81377, Germany
* Corresponding author.
E-mail address: Daniel.chappell@med.uni-muenchen.de

Crit Care Clin 36 (2020) 217–232
https://doi.org/10.1016/j.ccc.2019.12.007
0749-0704/20/© 2020 Elsevier Inc. All rights reserved.

phases, the EG has been shown to suffer degradation. However, the mechanistic insights into the underlying complex pathophysiology remain unclear. It is also not known whether restitution of the EG as a therapeutic goal promotes the survival of the patient or not. First trials that focus on the reorganization and/or restitution of the EG via immunomodulation or substitution in the treatment of critical diseases seem quite promising. Nevertheless the step "from bench to bedside" is still a big one.

COMPOSITION AND FUNCTION OF THE ENDOTHELIAL GLYCOCALYX

Typically, the vessel wall is described as a construct composed of 3 layers. The outermost layer consists of a network of connective tissue and, in larger vessels, contains the "vasa et nervi privata" of the vessel (tunica adventitia). It is followed by the "tunica media," which contains mostly vascular myocytes. Naturally this layer is more prominent in arteries of the muscular type and in larger veins. The innermost part of the vessel wall is called "tunica intima" and is composed of endothelial cells that are connected to each other, generally through tight junctions in most vascular proveniences, but also with fenestrae and gaps in some segments, especially venular, kidney, and liver microvessels. Furthermore, this layer contains the subendothelial space and the "membrana elastica interna." For a long time, the endothelial cells of the "tunica intima" were believed to be the part of the vessel wall in direct contact with the streaming blood. The fact that circulating blood cells seen through an intravital microscope practically never touch the vessel wall was explained by the Fåhraeus-Lindquist effect. By improving fixation techniques for electron microscopy and the introduction of confocal microscopy, it became obvious that there is a fourth layer of the vessel wall forming the final border toward the vascular lumen. The existence of this most inner stratum of the vessel, now called the EG, was discerned more than 70 years ago. Initially, it was believed to be insignificant due to an assumed small dimension of less than 10 nm. The EG actually has a thickness ranging from 0.2 μm to 2 μm, therefore being as thick as the endothelial cell itself. Interestingly, composition and thickness vary with vessel type and location of the vessel in the organism.

Proteoglycans (syndecans and glypicans) form the backbone of the EG. Sulfated glycosaminoglycans (heparan, chondroitin, dermatan, and keratan sulfates) are connected to the proteoglycans via negatively charged polysaccharide sidechains. Another major constituent, the polysaccharide hyaluronic acid, is embedded in the EG via connection to the CD44 receptor on the endothelial cell membrane.[1] Albumin and many other proteinaceous plasma components are intercalated into the EG, mainly via electrostatic interaction (**Fig. 1**),[2] thus forming the ESL. Somewhat unexpectedly, the ESL has proved to be a main component of the vascular barrier. Although this barrier is permeable for small molecules and electrolytes, larger molecules like albumin or other proteins are held back in the vascular lumen by the EG. That means the EG is crucial for the maintenance of the intravascular oncotic pressure. It is also important for both microvascular homeostasis and organ perfusion.[3] The EG undergoes continuous turnover, shedding caused by, for example, sheer-stress and enzymatic degradation, and reconstruction by de novo synthesis of constituent molecules. The entire ESL has to be thought of as a highly dynamic construct with a high variability in form and structure, constantly renewing itself.[4] In general, alterations in ESL can be considered as synonymous with changes in EG, and vice versa.

The high-grade sulfation of heparans, dermatans, keratans, and chondroitin, together with the carboxyl groups of the hyaluronic acid, cause the mainly negative charge of the EG. That negative charge is essential for the homeostasis of the vascular system. The EG harbors and contains adhesion molecules (ICAM/VCAM), von

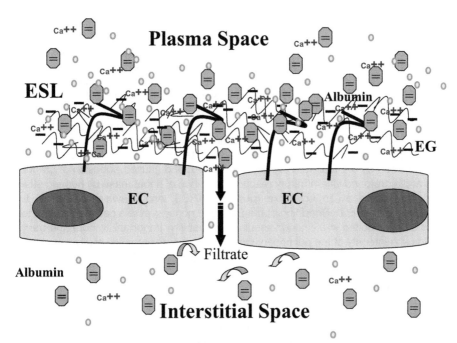

Fig. 1. Schematic representation of the ESL. The ESL consists primarily of the following: (1) the EG in its strictest sense, indicated by the thick and thin black lines denoting membrane-anchored glycosaminoglycans and their highly negatively charged side chains; (2) a zone enriched with cations from the plasma space (of special importance are the divalent cation Ca^{++} (in *red*), because of its charge density, and Na^+ (*yellow circles*), because of its high concentration); and (3) the intercalated plasma proteins such as albumin (*green symbols*). It is the high concentration of cations in the border zone that allows the negatively charged plasma protein molecules to approach into the EG, despite the negative sulfate and carboxylate groups located there. The dependence on the cation-dominated border zone explains why the ESL is so sensitive to changes in plasma electrolytes and plasma pH. Not included in this scheme are endothelial cell membrane ecto-molecules, such as receptors, adhesion molecules, and channel proteins, or plasma electrolytes, such as Mg^{++}, K^+, and Cl^-. With respect to the latter, one must expect a certain degree of exclusion from the ESL, a situation akin to the Donnan distribution for Cl^- across the membrane of the red blood cell. For further details, see Refs.[2,60]

Willebrand factor, antithrombin, tissue factor pathway inhibitor, the NO-synthase (NOS), and the extracellular superoxide dismutase, just to mention a few. Shedding of the EG and, thus, activation or liberation of the aforementioned molecules, can be caused by different pathologic situations like inflammation, ischemia, or trauma. Furthermore, shedding of the EG causes an endothelial dysfunction impairing the vascular barrier function. The plasmatic coagulation is activated, as are adhesion and aggregation of platelets. Leukocyte adhesion and migration are likewise promoted.[5] It seems obvious today that the EG plays a key role in various diseases, especially in critically ill patients.

ENDOTHELIAL GLYCOCALYX AND ACUTE RESPIRATORY DISTRESS SYNDROME

The "acute respiratory distress syndrome" (ARDS) has a high mortality. The incidence of ARDS in Europe is approximately 3 to 7 cases per 100,000 inhabitants.[6] ARDS can be caused by a large variety of pulmonary (eg, infection of the lungs, aspiration, contusion of the lungs) and extrapulmonary diseases (eg, sepsis, polytrauma, traumatic brain injury, pancreatitis, burns). What these different triggers for ARDS have in common is that they cause a dysfunction of the alveolo-capillary barrier, leading to edema of the lung and a massive immunologic-inflammatory reaction.[7] It seems likely that shedding of the EG plays a role in the pathophysiology of ARDS, because dysfunction of the vascular barrier is a crucial aspect in the development of the disease. Furthermore, it seems that all the different causes for ARDS have a common final pathway. Schmidt and colleagues[8] demonstrated a rapid shedding of the EG in pulmonary vessels in the course of endotoxemia. Endothelial heparanase was activated by tumor necrosis factor (TNF)-α and led to shedding of heparan sulfate from the EG. Adhesion molecules once harbored by the EG were exposed, activated, and caused adhesion of granulocytes and a profound inflammatory reaction. Inhibition of heparanase by heparin attenuated the course of an endotoxin-mediated ARDS, and likewise attenuated the degradation of the EG.[8] Shedding of the EG in pulmonary vessels caused by a hemorrhagic shock resulted in elevated vascular permeability. Important to note, the barrier function and integrity of the pulmonary vascular EG can be reconstituted by the administration of plasma products. Cellular expression of syndecan-1 seems to be crucial for that mechanism, as without syndecan-1 expression, plasma products do not have any protective effect on the pulmonary EG.[9]

Alternative therapies aiming for restitution of the EG during ARDS are currently under investigation and could point out key elements of the pathophysiology of ARDS. For instance, the course of ARDS can be attenuated by the administration of neferine, an alkaloid derived from the Indian lotus flower. Neferine significantly lowered the expression of interleukins (IL-1β, IL-6, IL-10) and TNF-α in an animal model of the lipopolysaccharide-induced ARDS.[10] Translocation of nuclear factor-κB was reduced by neferine as well as the mitochondrial reactive oxygen species–mediated degradation of pulmonary vascular EG. Restitution of the EG was eased by neferine. The results of this trial emphasize the immunologic-inflammatory genesis of ARDS and show that the course can be attenuated by immunomodulation. Unfortunately, tangible recommendations for clinical practice cannot be drawn from this study.

Immunomodulation can be achieved by the administration of hydrocortisone during septic shock, significantly lowering levels of IL-6 and IL-8 and, thus, improving organ function.[11] However, this has not been found to work as well for treatment of ARDS. The function of the lungs was improved by the application of hydrocortisone, but a benefit in survival could not be shown.[12] A more specialized immunomodulatory approach other than the application of hydrocortisone, one not causing hypernatremia and hyperglycemia, might be beneficial.

ENDOTHELIAL GLYCOCALYX AND TRAUMA

A frequently occurring facet of trauma is a concomitant microvascular disorder. Shedding of the EG is one of the key elements of the so-called "endotheliopathy of trauma." Almost immediately after trauma, raised levels of syndecan-1 and thrombomodulin can be measured in the patient. The height of the respective blood levels correlates positively with the severity of organ dysfunction.[13] Patients suffering from trauma with increased levels of syndecan-1 usually also have higher levels of IL-6, IL-10, thrombomodulin, and tissue plasminogen activator, and lower levels of protein C. Trauma patients with that constellation have a remarkably higher mortality.[14] Although the release of tissue plasminogen activator is increased, the activity of plasminogen activator inhibitor is reduced, a combination causing hyperfibrinolysis. This constellation is associated with a worse outcome as well.[15] During the CRASH-2 trial, traumatized patients received tranexamic acid to prevent exsanguination. CRASH-2 demonstrated in a remarkable way an improved survival of trauma patients who received tranexamic acid.[16] It is important to note that there was no correlation between receiving tranexamic acid or placebo, and the syndecan-1 blood level (as marker of EG shedding) in the trauma patients. Although at first sight this aspect seems unexpected, it is actually quite logical and explainable. Although tranexamic acid cannot restore the integrity of the EG, it still can ameliorate the hyperfibrinolysis caused by EG shedding.[16]

The blood loss during trauma not only reduces preload and the amount of oxygen carriers, it also lowers the level of circulating plasma proteins. These plasma proteins are crucial for the health and vitality of the EG/ESL. Appropriately, administering "fresh frozen plasma" in an animal trauma model restored the integrity of the EG. Even posttraumatic ARDS was ameliorated by this means.[17] Besides fresh frozen plasma, factor concentrates (eg, prothrombin complex concentrate) seem to have the capability to rebuild the EG. This effect is most likely not caused by the contained blood clotting factors but by the additional plasma proteins contained in the preparation.[18] This affirms the usual procedure of administering packed red blood cells plus plasma proteins when treating mass bleeding. Tissue oxygenation is optimized by this dual intervention, and the likelihood of restitution of the EG/ESL is raised.

ENDOTHELIAL GLYCOCALYX AND HYPERVOLEMIA

Hypervolemia caused by excessive fluid administration or impaired fluid excretion is a relevant problem of critical care medicine. For example, when only crystalloid fluids are used for fluid and volume therapy during treatment of septic shock, approximately 67% of the patients will show signs of hypervolemia on day 1 of the treatment period.[19] Interstitial edema occurs and worsens the preexisting microcirculatory disorder.[20] This further impairs tissue oxygenation, leading to organ dysfunction. Hypervolemia causes edema of various tissues and organs, especially of the lungs or the gastrointestinal system. Consequences are pulmonary edema and edema of the bowel wall, the latter potentially leading to paralytic ileus, malabsorption, and anastomotic leakage. Nowadays there is strong evidence that hypervolemia alone has a negative impact on patient outcome. For instance, in patients with acute kidney injury, hypervolemia increased mortality and further impaired renal function.[21] In colorectal surgery, a positive fluid balance of 3 L led to impaired bowel motility and prolonged stomach and bowel transit.[22] In addition, hypervolemia caused myocardial edema with impairment of conduction, contractility, and diastolic function.[20] The rate of cardiac complications is consequently increased. The oxygen transport capability and compliance of the lungs is impaired by hypervolemia and the duration of assisted/mandatory ventilation is prolonged. Neurologic disorders can occur, because brain edema can induce neurologic failure and cognitive impairment. Dysfunction of the liver can occur due to hypervolemia. Last but not least, hypervolemia impairs wound healing and promotes ulcers and wound infection. Length of hospital and intensive care unit (ICU) stay, duration of ventilation, infection rates, morbidity, and mortality, as well as overall hospital treatment costs are increased in hypervolemic patients.[20,22–25] All in all, hypervolemia seems to be as dangerous as hypovolemia, a condition in which it is well known that organ perfusion is impaired and organ failure promoted.

Volume overload induces atrial stretching, which triggers the release of atrial natriuretic peptide (ANP). ANP activates metalloproteinases and mediates quick extravasation of fluid from the vessel lumen into the interstitial space, thus causing tissue edema. The main mechanism is the creation of "holes" in the EG, so that the permeability of the vessel wall is increased in distinct areas.[26] During aorto-coronary bypass surgery, a significant rise of ANP levels can be measured, followed by shedding of the EG.[27] Patients who received a preoperative "volume load" with 20 mL per kg body weight of an iso-oncotic colloid to lower intraoperative blood loss showed a significant rise of ANP followed by a significant rise of syndecan-1 and hyaluronan in plasma, indicating shedding of the EG. The occurrence of this phenomenon can be prevented by keeping the patient in an euvolemic state through acute normovolemic hemodilution (ANH). During ANH, the removed blood is replaced simultaneously by an iso-oncotic colloid to keep the patient euvolemic at all times.[28] Release of ANP is not only a surrogate of volume (over)load, but it directly interacts with the EG: an animal model suggested that ANP itself is a relevant factor when it comes to shedding of the EG. An infusion of ANP without a concomitant volume load leads to a rise of syndecan-1 levels and degradation of the EG assessed using electron microscopy.[26]

Every experienced critical care physician knows of the difficulties encountered when it comes to the evaluation of the functional volume status of a critically ill patient. These patients often suffer from peripheral edema despite signs of intravascular hypovolemia, assessed by ultrasonography of the inferior vena cava or the left ventricle. However, a key factor in the treatment of septic shock is to keep the patients in a euvolemic state during hemodynamic resuscitation. It is important to keep the balance between volume resuscitation and catecholamine therapy to prevent further harm ensuing from the treatment itself. Especially high doses of vasopressors in hypovolemic patients have been shown to impair the microcirculation and cause organ failure. It is, thus, important to perform extended hemodynamic monitoring for guidance of the treatment and to try to normalize blood volume before initiating vasoactive treatment. In the near future, bedside monitoring of the microcirculation might offer an improved diagnostic target and help in therapeutic decisions.[29] It will also be necessary to overcome the false idea that by treating the macrocirculatory dysfunction the microcirculatory dysfunction will automatically be improved.[30]

ENDOTHELIAL GLYCOCALYX AND ISCHEMIA/REPERFUSION

Reperfusion after local or total ischemia aggravates tissue damage caused by ischemia. A drastic rise in syndecan-1 and heparan sulfate levels has been measured in the blood of patients after partial or local ischemia, suggesting major destruction of the EG.[31] A core element of the pathophysiology of ischemia/reperfusion (I/R) is microvascular dysfunction.[32] During the course of I/R, endothelial cells start swelling[33] and, after a period of time that is tissue-specific, degradation of the EG promotes vascular permeability as well as adhesion and migration of leukocytes.[34–36] These alterations result in tissue edema. Administration of hydrocortisone or antithrombin III before I/R has the potential to attenuate EG degradation.[37–39] The underlying mechanism of protection mediated through hydrocortisone seems to be multifactorial. Mast cell stabilization and the blockade of synthesis of cytokines, chemokines, and serine-proteases seem to be the essential interventions shown in animal models.[33,36] Antithrombin, by nature, is an inhibitor of serine-proteases, thus acting in an anti-inflammatory manner.[40] Preconditioning via the application of sevoflurane has also been shown to reduce damage to the EG caused by I/R. Sevoflurane significantly lowered the levels of TNF-α, IL-1, lipid-hydroperoxidase, and myeloperoxidase.[41] Also, the plasma levels of syndecan-1 and heparan sulfate were significantly lower in an I/R animal model after preconditioning with sevoflurane.[20,42]

ENDOTHELIAL GLYCOCALYX AND HYPERNATREMIA/HYPERGLYCEMIA

Dysregulations of blood sodium level are common and relevant problems of critically ill patients. Approximately 7% to 16% of all critically ill patients present with hypernatremia on admission to the ICU. In addition, approximately 25% of all critically ill patients will develop hypernatremia during their stay in the ICU.[43] Critically ill patients with hypernatremia have a more than doubled risk of mortality compared with patients with normal sodium levels (16% vs 34%).[44] Hypernatremia is usually accompanied by hyperosmolarity, thus leading to a shift of water from the intracellular to the extracellular space. This results in the formation of interstitial edema, dehydration causing adjacent cells to shrink. Especially the susceptible cells of the central nervous system can suffer permanent damage through this mechanism. Furthermore, hypernatremia can cause muscle cramps and rhabdomyolysis. Glucose utilization is impaired as well as gluconeogenesis. Hypernatremia lowers the contractility of cardiomyocytes, lowers the peripheral vascular resistance, and impairs the lactate clearance of the liver.[45]

A relevant part of hypernatremia is caused iatrogenically by exogenous administration of sodium-containing fluids or drugs. The infusion of 0.9% saline in particular not only raises the serum sodium level but predominantly increases serum chloride, resulting in metabolic acidosis. Approximately one-third of all instances of metabolic acidosis seen during the course of sepsis are caused by the use of intravenous saline for fluid therapy.[46] Hyperchloremic load activates the tubuloglomerular feedback, thus lowering the glomerular filtration rate. This is a powerful mechanism, because saline infusion does not only affect the critically ill: the infusion of 2 L of saline to healthy volunteers caused a relevant decline of the renal blood flow, eliciting a decline of the glomerular filtration rate.[47] During sepsis, in which elimination of protons and avoidance of fluid overload are relevant therapeutic goals, this mechanism is derogatory.

Besides the negative effects of hypernatremia on almost all organ systems, it seems that hypernatremia has direct toxic effects on the EG. A recent experimental study has pointed in that direction. Human endothelial cells derived from the umbilical cord cultured in microfluidic channels were exposed to I/R to simulate shock injury. During the course of reperfusion, all subgroups showed increased levels of syndecan-1 and hyaluronic acid, suggesting shedding of the EG. However, the levels of syndecan-1 and hyaluronic acid were highest in the subgroup in which hypertonic saline was used for reperfusion. All groups showed signs of endothelial activation expressed by raised thrombomodulin levels. Besides that, the levels of tissue plasminogen activator were higher than normal and were accompanied by low levels of plasminogen activator inhibitor-1, suggestive of a state of pro-fibrinolytic coagulopathy. On top of these molecular effects, the thickness of the EG was halved by the infusion of hypertonic saline. It was further reduced to only a third of the normal thickness by inducing I/R and treating with epinephrine.[48] The conclusion one may draw from this particular study is that hypernatremia leads to shedding of the EG, aggravating the symptoms of shock. Of course the presented data were derived from a highly experimental study setting, questioning any extrapolation to the whole human organism.

It remains unclear what role ANP plays in the context of hypernatremia and shedding of the EG, although it is likely that ANP has a relevant role in that setting. Nonetheless, the currently available data clearly support the recent grade A recommendations of the German S3 "guidelines for intravascular volume therapy in adults"; that is, not to use saline for fluid replacement therapy in critically ill patients.[49]

Beside hypernatremia, stress-induced hyperglycemia is a typical problem of critically ill patients. Hyperglycemia is associated with both raised mortality and elevated rate of infection.[50] Shedding of the EG is promoted by hyperglycemia, especially in combination with an inflammatory state of the organism. Hyperglycemia leads to increased inducible nitric oxide synthase activity, through the activation of diacylglycerol and protein kinase C, which in turn leads to the generation of reactive oxygen species engendering endothelial dysfunction.[51] An insulin regimen aiming for blood glucose levels between 120 and 150 mg/dL might be beneficial regarding survival,[52] but remains a controversial topic in the critical care literature.

ENDOTHELIAL GLYCOCALYX, MICROCIRCULATION, AND VOLUME THERAPY

During sepsis or severe trauma, dissociation occurs between the macrocirculatory and microcirculatory systems.[29,53] The so-called hemodynamic coherence is abolished.[30] Nowadays, monitoring focuses on the macrocirculation when defining therapeutic goals. Although such data certainly are important and helpful for therapy guidance, information on the microcirculation remains scarce. Recent publications have shown that the microcirculation seems to play a key role in treating sepsis.[54,55] In this context, one would perhaps expect that the levels of EG shedding and microcirculatory disorder almost coincide. A recently published study suggested that this might not always be the case. In septic patients, there is an increase of the "perfused boundary region" (PBR), an inverse marker for EG thickness measured sublingually, compared with healthy volunteers. PBR and markers of microcirculatory dysfunction correlated well with markers of critical illness, but not with each other, suggesting that EG shedding might occur without microcirculatory disturbance.[56] However, the capacity to detect or diagnose microcirculatory disturbances may be limited by the shortcomings of current monitoring devices. Microcirculatory flow assessment relies on quantification of blood flow in a subjective manner, and, thus, more subtle disturbances may remain undetected by physicians. These disturbances can also be too subtle for current monitoring devices to identify.

Because there seem to be dissociations among macrocirculation, microcirculation, and EG shedding, the identification of effective therapies remains elusive. It does not come as a surprise that, in this context, therapeutic interventions can potentially be harmful, as they do not address the right target. There is strong evidence that during the treatment of sepsis the infused fluids can cause a rise of biomarkers suggestive of shedding of the EG. A recent study derived from the ProCESS-trial showed a consistent rise of heparan sulfate for each liter of intravenous fluid delivered. This suggests that iatrogenic "collateral" damage to the endothelium occurs as a result of fluid resuscitation.[57] Because in this study the nonspecific term "fluid" was used throughout, one may be led to believe that all sorts of fluids cause the same sort of damage. However, there is evidence that some intravenous fluids are better than others regarding patient survival, homeostasis, and protection of the EG.[58] There is an interesting, very important distinction: with an intact vascular barrier, the capacity of volume expansion of iso-oncotic colloids is approximately 90% to 100%, whereas crystalloid fluids are far less effective, forcing one to infuse 3 to 4 L for every liter of blood lost. On the other hand, in critically ill patients, in whom the vascular barrier is perturbed (capillary leak), the volume effect of both sorts of fluids lie much closer together. The capacity of fluids to expand the intravascular volume is obviously dependent on the integrity of the vascular barrier and, therefore, on the integrity of the EG. The more shedding of the EG, the lower the volume expansion effect of colloids will be. It is an important aspect that neither iso-oncotic nor isotonic fluids can reverse existing tissue edema.[58]

Human albumin seems to have protective effects when it comes to preservation and restoration of the EG.[59,60] This result is not unequivocal. Especially when compared with fresh frozen plasma, experimental trials show contradictory results regarding human albumin.[18,61] Fresh frozen plasma itself seems to have strong protective and restorative effects on the EG,[62] whereas packed red blood cells have none.[63] Furthermore, there is evidence to suggest that platelets might have protective effects.[64] Conversely, crystalloids have no effect on the EG and are probably even deleterious. Synthetic colloids seem to have inferior protective effects compared with albumin and plasma. However, their use, especially that of hydroxyethyl starch, is no longer recommended in critically ill patients.[60,65,66]

ENDOTHELIAL GLYCOCALYX, SEPSIS, AND ACUTE KIDNEY INJURY

Approximately 40% of all patients suffering from severe sepsis or septic shock develop acute kidney injury. During systemic hypotension, reflex vessel constriction occurs leading to a decline of renal perfusion and, finally, ischemia of renal tissue.[67] Perfusion of the renal cortex, the site of filtration, is the first to decline. Second, perfusion of the medulla, the place of urine generation, declines as well. Besides hypotension causing a decline of renal perfusion, a concomitant disorder of the microcirculation causes a shift from aerobic to anaerobic metabolism. Again, this happens first in the renal cortex and second in the renal medulla.[68] Hypotension leading to a lowered filtration pressure in the glomeruli also results in a lowered sodium reabsorption in the tubular system of the renal medulla.[69] Because sodium reabsorption accounts for the largest part of oxygen consumption in the renal medulla, this explains the time shift between cortex and medulla regarding the shift from aerobic to anaerobic metabolism.[70] Finally, all described mechanisms can lead to apoptosis of the tubuli. Apoptosis or necrosis of renal tubular cells is a rare (5%) finding even at late stages of sepsis.[71] Tubuli that are damaged in the course of microcirculatory disorder or inflammation are capable of increasing secretion of the proinflammatory cytokines IL-6, IL-1β, and monocyte chemotactic peptide-1 by paracrine secretion of the Toll-like receptor-4 ligand HMGB 1. Thus, regional inflammation is enforced and kidney injury promoted.[72] Amelioration of tubular damage can probably ameliorate or even stop the damaging spiral of ischemia and inflammation. Development of acute tubular necrosis seems to be dependent on loss of cardiocirculatory stability and ensuing infringement of renal blood flow. Indeed, keeping cardiac output, cardiac index, and renal blood flow (RBF) within or above the normal physiologic range prevents development of acute tubular necrosis.[65] However, this is not a therapeutic goal physicians would strive to attain during treatment of sepsis. It is important to mention here that not acute tubular necrosis but acute tubular apoptosis (92.9%) is the typical finding in septic kidney injury, when changes occur.[73]

The pathophysiology of septic acute kidney injury is far more complex than described in the preceding paragraph, and the contribution of circulatory depression and vasoconstriction to kidney injury is just a small piece of a great puzzle. This is shown best by the fact that a declined RBF is not a *conditio sine qua non* when it comes to the development of kidney injury during sepsis.[74] Besides oxidative stress and ATP depletion in tubular cells, inflammation is a further promoter. There is a significant association between the levels of cytokines (IL-6, IL-10, macrophage migration inhibitory factor) and the development of septic kidney injury.[75] Not only can cells of the immune system be activated through endogenous or exogenous mediators (the damage-associated and pathogen-associated molecular patterns or DAMPs and PAMPs) via pattern recognition receptors, but also epithelial and parenchymal cells. Because the kidneys receive approximately 20% of the cardiac output and filter approximately 120 to 150 mL plasma per minute, the kidneys are naturally more exposed to endogenous or exogenous inflammatory mediators than most other organs. Moreover, renal tubular cells seem to be very susceptible to damage in an inflammatory setting.[74] Proinflammatory mediators activate leukocytes, thrombocytes, and endothelial cells. Subsequent microcirculatory dysfunction and disturbed vascular barrier functioning lead to regional hypoxia and tissue edema. Furthermore, the microcirculatory dysfunction prolongs passage of leukocytes, thus extending time for interaction and exchange of inflammatory mediators between leukocytes and renal dendritic cells.[76]

Every single entity of the complex chorus of inflammation, cardiovascular instability, disorders of electrolytes, and the acid-base-balance can cause acute kidney injury as well as disruption of the ESL, going all the way to shedding of the EG (see **Fig. 1**). Nowadays it is suspected that the EG itself seems to contribute to development and progress of acute kidney injury. Endothelial cells of the glomerulus have an EG on their luminal side.[77] Enzymes like heparanase are able to cause EG shedding, leading to an increased permeability of the glomerular filter.[78] It is well known that proteins larger than the physiologic filter size of the glomerular apparatus, for example, albumin, cause interstitial inflammation on tubular resorption, thus leading to impaired renal function. Of course, this also applies to all those inflammatory proteins summarized as DAMPs and PAMPs.[74] Interstitial inflammation, just like shedding of the EG, seems to be part of a common pathophysiologic pathway in a variety of conditions promoting acute and chronic kidney disease.[79] EG shedding itself can contribute to progression from acute kidney injury to chronic kidney disease and, by the same token, may also be a motor of systemic inflammation.[80] In this context, it is noteworthy that urinary glycosaminoglycans can be measured and used as a predictor for acute kidney injury and even mortality in patients with sepsis.[81] This is further evidence suggesting a crucial pathophysiological role of EG shedding. Several perioperative studies even hint that measurement of plasma or urinary syndecan-1 can accurately predict acute kidney injury.[82,83]

Mortality in patients with septic shock is much higher when associated with acute kidney injury than in the absence of kidney injury (67% vs 43%).[84] It is logical therefore to submit that one of the therapeutic goals in the treatment of sepsis must be the prevention of acute kidney injury.

Today we have a fundamental problem regarding treatment or prevention of acute kidney injury (AKI): it is mostly diagnosed too late. AKIN criteria are based on urine output and variations in serum creatinine. Especially urinary production is not a reliable marker in the perioperative setting.[85] The other commonly measured surrogate parameters, such as serum creatinine, creatinine clearance, or glomerular filtration rate, unfortunately only show that acute kidney injury and functional impairment have already occurred. In the field of cardiology by comparison, the measurement of troponin can detect an active cardiac condition before it is functionally relevant. By using troponin, it has become possible to set the starting point and indication for invasive therapy earlier, thereby, for example, halving the mortality of a non-ST elevation myocardial infarction.[86,87] There is an urgent need for a comparable marker that detects structural damage of the kidney before kidney function is impaired and the vicious circle of inflammation, microcirculatory disorder, and regional ischemia is started.

There are novel biomarkers with the potential to overcome the limitations of creatinine measurement. As an example, cystatin C is suited to detect renal impairment in the so-called creatinine blind range. It is also not as strongly influenced by muscle mass, age, or race. Rise of cystatin C starts 24 to 48 hours after acute kidney injury, a response much faster than that of creatinine (rise 2–7 days after acute kidney injury, depending on preexisting renal impairment), but still quite slow.[88,89] Another marker is neutrophil gelatinase-associated lipocalin (NGAL). Its dynamic properties are comparable to those of troponin, with a maximum rise 6 hours after onset of acute kidney injury. It is a reliable predictor for acute kidney injury in critically ill patients.[90] Even in the presence of sepsis, where NGAL measurement is confounded due to its partial origin in neutrophilic granulocytes, cutoff values have been established.[91]

Although these new markers can probably help to find the right time point for starting treatment against kidney damage, they do not tell us what to do. In truth, there is no working therapeutic concept for prevention of acute kidney injury available. Possibly implications from other fields like in the treatment of ARDS, where the importance of the EG was implemented in the development of an experimental therapy regimen, could help to improve outcome in critically ill patients suffering from acute kidney injury. It is most unsatisfactory that the only proven point in the treatment of acute kidney injury is that of the time point of when to start dialysis.[92]

DISCLOSURE

All authors have nothing to disclose.

REFERENCES

1. Wiesinger A, Peters W, Chappell D, et al. Nanomechanics of the endothelial glycocalyx in experimental sepsis. PLoS One 2013;8(11):e80905.
2. Becker BF, Jacob M, Leipert S, et al. Degradation of the endothelial glycocalyx in clinical settings: searching for the sheddases. Br J Clin Pharmacol 2015;80(3): 389–402.
3. Becker BF, Chappell D, Jacob M. Endothelial glycocalyx and coronary vascular permeability: the fringe benefit. Basic Res Cardiol 2010;105(6):687–701.
4. Chappell D, Jacob M, Becker BF, et al. Expedition glycocalyx. A newly discovered "Great Barrier Reef". Anaesthesist 2008;57(10):959–69 [in German].
5. Nieuwdorp M, Meuwese MC, Vink H, et al. The endothelial glycocalyx: a potential barrier between health and vascular disease. Curr Opin Lipidol 2005;16(5): 507–11.
6. Taylor BE, McClave SA, Martindale RG, et al. Guidelines for the provision and assessment of nutrition support therapy in the adult critically ill patient: Society of Critical Care Medicine (SCCM) and American Society for Parenteral and Enteral Nutrition (A.S.P.E.N.). Crit Care Med 2016;44(2):390–438.
7. Gottschaldt U, Reske AW. Pathophysiologie des Lungenversagens. Anästh Intensivmed 2018;59:249–64.
8. Schmidt EP, Yang Y, Janssen WJ, et al. The pulmonary endothelial glycocalyx regulates neutrophil adhesion and lung injury during experimental sepsis. Nat Med 2012;18(8):1217–23.
9. Wu F, Peng Z, Park PW, et al. Loss of syndecan-1 abrogates the pulmonary protective phenotype induced by plasma after hemorrhagic shock. Shock 2017; 48(3):340–5.
10. Liu XY, Xu HX, Li JK, et al. Neferine protects endothelial glycocalyx via mitochondrial ROS in lipopolysaccharide-induced acute respiratory distress syndrome. Front Physiol 2018;9:102.
11. Briegel J, Jochum M, Gippner-Steppert C, et al. Immunomodulation in septic shock: hydrocortisone differentially regulates cytokine responses. J Am Soc Nephrol 2001;12(Suppl 17):S70–4.

12. Tongyoo S, Permpikul C, Mongkolpun W, et al. Hydrocortisone treatment in early sepsis-associated acute respiratory distress syndrome: results of a randomized controlled trial. Crit Care 2016;20(1):329.
13. Naumann DN, Hazeldine J, Davies DJ, et al. Endotheliopathy of trauma is an on-scene phenomenon, and is associated with multiple organ dysfunction syndrome: a prospective observational study. Shock 2018;49(4):420–8.
14. Johansson PI, Stensballe J, Rasmussen LS, et al. A high admission syndecan-1 level, a marker of endothelial glycocalyx degradation, is associated with inflammation, protein C depletion, fibrinolysis, and increased mortality in trauma patients. Ann Surg 2011;254(2):194–200.
15. Cardenas JC, Matijevic N, Baer LA, et al. Elevated tissue plasminogen activator and reduced plasminogen activator inhibitor promote hyperfibrinolysis in trauma patients. Shock 2014;41(6):514–21.
16. CRASH-2 trial collaborators, Shakur H, Roberts I, Bautista R, et al. Effects of tranexamic acid on death, vascular occlusive events, and blood transfusion in trauma patients with significant haemorrhage (CRASH-2): a randomised, placebo-controlled trial. Lancet 2010;376(9734):23–32.
17. Kozar RA, Peng Z, Zhang R, et al. Plasma restoration of endothelial glycocalyx in a rodent model of hemorrhagic shock. Anesth Analg 2011;112(6):1289–95.
18. Pati S, Potter DR, Baimukanova G, et al. Modulating the endotheliopathy of trauma: factor concentrate versus fresh frozen plasma. J Trauma Acute Care Surg 2016;80(4):576–84 [discussion: 584–5].
19. Kelm DJ, Perrin JT, Cartin-Ceba R, et al. Fluid overload in patients with severe sepsis and septic shock treated with early goal-directed therapy is associated with increased acute need for fluid-related medical interventions and hospital death. Shock 2015;43(1):68–73.
20. Claure-Del Granado R, Mehta RL. Fluid overload in the ICU: evaluation and management. BMC Nephrol 2016;17(1):109.
21. Zhang L, Chen Z, Diao Y, et al. Associations of fluid overload with mortality and kidney recovery in patients with acute kidney injury: a systematic review and meta-analysis. J Crit Care 2015;30(4):860.e7-13.
22. Nisanevich V, Felsenstein I, Almogy G, et al. Effect of intraoperative fluid management on outcome after intraabdominal surgery. Anesthesiology 2005;103(1):25–32.
23. Lobo DN, Bostock KA, Neal KR, et al. Effect of salt and water balance on recovery of gastrointestinal function after elective colonic resection: a randomised controlled trial. Lancet 2002;359(9320):1812–8.
24. Brandstrup B, Tønnesen H, Beier-Holgersen R, et al. Effects of intravenous fluid restriction on postoperative complications: comparison of two perioperative fluid regimens: a randomized assessor-blinded multicenter trial. Ann Surg 2003;238(5):641–8.
25. Thacker JK, Mountford WK, Ernst FR, et al. Perioperative fluid utilization variability and association with outcomes: considerations for enhanced recovery efforts in sample US surgical populations. Ann Surg 2016;263(3):502–10.
26. Bruegger D, Jacob M, Rehm M, et al. Atrial natriuretic peptide induces shedding of endothelial glycocalyx in coronary vascular bed of Guinea pig hearts. Am J Physiol Heart Circ Physiol 2005;289(5):H1993–9.
27. Bruegger D, Schwartz L, Chappell D, et al. Release of atrial natriuretic peptide precedes shedding of the endothelial glycocalyx equally in patients undergoing on- and off-pump coronary artery bypass surgery. Basic Res Cardiol 2011;106(6):1111–21.

28. Chappell D, Bruegger D, Potzel J, et al. Hypervolemia increases release of atrial natriuretic peptide and shedding of the endothelial glycocalyx. Crit Care 2014; 18(5):538.
29. Tachon G, Harrois A, Tanaka S, et al. Microcirculatory alterations in traumatic hemorrhagic shock. Crit Care Med 2014;42(6):1433–41.
30. Ince C. Hemodynamic coherence and the rationale for monitoring the microcirculation. Crit Care 2015;19(Suppl 3):S8.
31. Rehm M, Bruegger D, Christ F, et al. Shedding of the endothelial glycocalyx in patients undergoing major vascular surgery with global and regional ischemia. Circulation 2007;116(17):1896–906.
32. Seal JB, Gewertz BL. Vascular dysfunction in ischemia-reperfusion injury. Ann Vasc Surg 2005;19(4):572–84.
33. Oliver MG, Specian RD, Perry MA, et al. Morphologic assessment of leukocyte-endothelial cell interactions in mesenteric venules subjected to ischemia and re-perfusion. Inflammation 1991;15(5):331–46.
34. Chappell D, Jacob M, Hofmann-Kiefer K, et al. Hydrocortisone preserves the vascular barrier by protecting the endothelial glycocalyx. Anesthesiology 2007; 107(5):776–84.
35. Rehm M, Zahler S, Lötsch M, et al. Endothelial glycocalyx as an additional barrier determining extravasation of 6% hydroxyethyl starch or 5% albumin solutions in the coronary vascular bed. Anesthesiology 2004;100(5):1211–23.
36. Vollmar B, Glasz J, Menger MD, et al. Leukocytes contribute to hepatic ischemia/reperfusion injury via intercellular adhesion molecule-1-mediated venular adherence. Surgery 1995;117(2):195–200.
37. Brettner F, Chappell D, Nebelsiek T, et al. Preinterventional hydrocortisone sustains the endothelial glycocalyx in cardiac surgery. Clin Hemorheol Microcirc 2019;71(1):59–70.
38. Chappell D, Jacob M, Hofmann-Kiefer K, et al. Antithrombin reduces shedding of the endothelial glycocalyx following ischaemia/reperfusion. Cardiovasc Res 2009;83(2):388–96.
39. Lopez E, Peng Z, Kozar RA, et al. Antithrombin III contributes to the protective effects of fresh frozen plasma following hemorrhagic shock by preventing syndecan-1 shedding and endothelial barrier disruption. Shock 2019. https://doi.org/10.1097/SHK.0000000000001432.
40. Chappell D, Dörfler N, Jacob M, et al. Glycocalyx protection reduces leukocyte adhesion after ischemia/reperfusion. Shock 2010;34(2):133–9.
41. Casanova J, Garutti I, Simon C, et al. The effects of anesthetic preconditioning with sevoflurane in an experimental lung autotransplant model in pigs. Anesth Analg 2011;113(4):742–8.
42. Casanova J, Simon C, Vara E, et al. Sevoflurane anesthetic preconditioning protects the lung endothelial glycocalyx from ischemia reperfusion injury in an experimental lung autotransplant model. J Anesth 2016;30(5):755–62.
43. Arora SK. Hypernatremic disorders in the intensive care unit. J Intensive Care Med 2013;28(1):37–45.
44. Stelfox HT, Ahmed SB, Khandwala F, et al. The epidemiology of intensive care unit-acquired hyponatraemia and hypernatraemia in medical-surgical intensive care units. Crit Care 2008;12(6):R162.
45. Lindner G, Funk GC. Hypernatremia in critically ill patients. J Crit Care 2013; 28(2):216.e11-20.
46. Kellum JA, Bellomo R, Kramer DJ, et al. Etiology of metabolic acidosis during saline resuscitation in endotoxemia. Shock 1998;9(5):364–8.

47. Chowdhury AH, Cox EF, Francis ST, et al. A randomized, controlled, double-blind crossover study on the effects of 2-L infusions of 0.9% saline and plasma-lyte(R) 148 on renal blood flow velocity and renal cortical tissue perfusion in healthy volunteers. Ann Surg 2012;256(1):18–24.

48. Martin JV, Liberati DM, Diebel LN. Excess sodium is deleterious on endothelial and glycocalyx barrier function: a microfluidic study. J Trauma Acute Care Surg 2018;85(Jul):128–34.

49. Marx G, Schindler AW, Mosch C, et al. Intravascular volume therapy in adults: guidelines from the Association of the Scientific Medical Societies in Germany. Eur J Anaesthesiol 2016;33(7):488–521.

50. Laird AM, Miller PR, Kilgo PD, et al. Relationship of early hyperglycemia to mortality in trauma patients. J Trauma 2004;56(5):1058–62.

51. Diebel ME, Diebel ME, Martin JV, et al. Acute hyperglycemia exacerbates trauma induced endothelial and glycocalyx injury: an in vitro model. J Trauma Acute Care Surg 2018;85(5):960–7.

52. Eakins J. Blood glucose control in the trauma patient. J Diabetes Sci Technol 2009;3(6):1373–6.

53. De Backer D, Donadello K, Sakr Y, et al. Microcirculatory alterations in patients with severe sepsis: impact of time of assessment and relationship with outcome. Crit Care Med 2013;41(3):791–9.

54. Legrand M, De Backer D, Dépret F, et al. Recruiting the microcirculation in septic shock. Ann Intensive Care 2019;9(1):102.

55. Montomoli J, Donati A, Ince C. Acute kidney injury and fluid resuscitation in septic patients: are we protecting the kidney? Nephron 2019;143(3):170–3.

56. Rovas A, Seidel LM, Vink H, et al. Association of sublingual microcirculation parameters and endothelial glycocalyx dimensions in resuscitated sepsis. Crit Care 2019;23(1):260.

57. Hippensteel JA, Uchimido R, Tyler PD, et al. Intravenous fluid resuscitation is associated with septic endothelial glycocalyx degradation. Crit Care 2019;23(1):259.

58. Milford EM, Reade MC. Resuscitation fluid choices to preserve the endothelial glycocalyx. Crit Care 2019;23(1):77.

59. Jacob M, Rehm M, Loetsch M, et al. The endothelial glycocalyx prefers albumin for evoking shear stress-induced, nitric oxide-mediated coronary dilatation. J Vasc Res 2007;44(6):435–43.

60. Jacob M, Bruegger D, Rehm M, et al. The endothelial glycocalyx affords compatibility of Starling's principle and high cardiac interstitial albumin levels. Cardiovasc Res 2007;73(3):575–86.

61. Torres LN, Chung KK, Salgado C, et al. Low-volume resuscitation with normal saline is associated with microvascular endothelial dysfunction after hemorrhage in rats, compared to colloids and balanced crystalloids. Crit Care 2017;21(1):160.

62. Barelli S, Alberio L. The role of plasma transfusion in massive bleeding: protecting the endothelial glycocalyx? Front Med (Lausanne) 2018;5:91.

63. Torres LN, Sondeen JL, Dubick MA, et al. Systemic and microvascular effects of resuscitation with blood products after severe hemorrhage in rats. J Trauma Acute Care Surg 2014;77(5):716–23.

64. Baimukanova G, Miyazawa B, Potter DR, et al. Platelets regulate vascular endothelial stability: assessing the storage lesion and donor variability of apheresis platelets. Transfusion 2016;56(Suppl 1):S65–75.

65. Straat M, Müller MC, Meijers JC, et al. Effect of transfusion of fresh frozen plasma on parameters of endothelial condition and inflammatory status in non-bleeding

critically ill patients: a prospective substudy of a randomized trial. Crit Care 2015; 19:163.

66. Jacob M, Bruegger D, Rehm M, et al. Contrasting effects of colloid and crystal-loid resuscitation fluids on cardiac vascular permeability. Anesthesiology 2006; 104(6):1223–31.

67. Ishikawa K, May CN, Gobe G, et al. Pathophysiology of septic acute kidney injury: a different view of tubular injury. Contrib Nephrol 2010;165:18–27.

68. Post EH, Su F, Hosokawa K, et al. Changes in kidney perfusion and renal cortex metabolism in septic shock: an experimental study. J Surg Res 2017;207:145–54.

69. Thurau K, Boylan JW. Acute renal success. The unexpected logic of oliguria in acute renal failure. Am J Med 1976;61(3):308–15.

70. Ricksten SE, Bragadottir G, Redfors B. Renal oxygenation in clinical acute kidney injury. Crit Care 2013;17(2):221.

71. Takasu O, Gaut JP, Watanabe E, et al. Mechanisms of cardiac and renal dysfunc-tion in patients dying of sepsis. Am J Respir Crit Care Med 2013;187(5):509–17.

72. Kruger B, Krick S, Dhillon N, et al. Donor Toll-like receptor 4 contributes to ischemia and reperfusion injury following human kidney transplantation. Proc Natl Acad Sci U S A 2009;106(9):3390–5.

73. Kosaka J, Lankadeva YR, May CN, et al. Histopathology of septic acute kidney injury: a systematic review of experimental data. Crit Care Med 2016;44(9): e897–903.

74. Gomez H, Ince C, De Backer D, et al. A unified theory of sepsis-induced acute kidney injury: inflammation, microcirculatory dysfunction, bioenergetics, and the tubular cell adaptation to injury. Shock 2014;41(1):3–11.

75. Payen D, Lukaszewicz AC, Legrand M, et al. A multicentre study of acute kidney injury in severe sepsis and septic shock: association with inflammatory pheno-type and HLA genotype. PLoS One 2012;7(6):e35838.

76. Wu L, Tiwari MM, Messer KJ, et al. Peritubular capillary dysfunction and renal tubular epithelial cell stress following lipopolysaccharide administration in mice. Am J Physiol Renal Physiol 2007;292(1):F261–8.

77. Li L, Bonventre JV. Endothelial glycocalyx: not just a sugar coat. Am J Respir Crit Care Med 2016;194(4):390–3.

78. Singh A, Satchell SC, Neal CR, et al. Glomerular endothelial glycocalyx consti-tutes a barrier to protein permeability. J Am Soc Nephrol 2007;18(11):2885–93.

79. Jedlicka J, Soleiman A, Draganovici D, et al. Interstitial inflammation in Alport syn-drome. Hum Pathol 2010;41(4):582–93.

80. Garsen M, Rops AL, Rabelink TJ, et al. The role of heparanase and the endothe-lial glycocalyx in the development of proteinuria. Nephrol Dial Transplant 2014; 29(1):49–55.

81. Schmidt EP, Overdier KH, Sun X, et al. Urinary glycosaminoglycans predict out-comes in septic shock and acute respiratory distress syndrome. Am J Respir Crit Care Med 2016;194(4):439–49.

82. Ferrer NMB, de Melo Bezerra Cavalcante CT, Branco KMC, et al. Urinary syndecan-1 and acute kidney injury after pediatric cardiac surgery. Clin Chim Acta 2018;485:205–9.

83. de Melo Bezerra Cavalcante CT, Castelo Branco KM, Pinto Júnior VC, et al. Syn-decan-1 improves severe acute kidney injury prediction after pediatric cardiac surgery. J Thorac Cardiovasc Surg 2016;152(1):178–86.e2.

84. Briegel J. SIRS, sepsis und multiorganversagen. In: Roissant W, Zwißler B, edi-tors. Die Anästhesiologie. Germany: Springer Medizin; 2012. p. 1578–92.

85. Kheterpal S, Tremper KK, Englesbe MJ, et al. Predictors of postoperative acute renal failure after noncardiac surgery in patients with previously normal renal function. Anesthesiology 2007;107(6):892–902.

86. Roffi M, Patrono C, Collet JP, et al. 2015 ESC Guidelines for the management of acute coronary syndromes in patients presenting without persistent ST-segment elevation: task force for the management of acute coronary syndromes in patients presenting without persistent ST-segment elevation of the European Society of Cardiology (ESC). Eur Heart J 2016;37(3):267–315.

87. Morrow DA, Cannon CP, Rifai N, et al. Ability of minor elevations of troponins I and T to predict benefit from an early invasive strategy in patients with unstable angina and non-ST elevation myocardial infarction: results from a randomized trial. JAMA 2001;286(19):2405–12.

88. Waikar SS, Bonventre JV. Creatinine kinetics and the definition of acute kidney injury. J Am Soc Nephrol 2009;20(3):672–9.

89. Rickli H, Benou K, Ammann P, et al. Time course of serial cystatin C levels in comparison with serum creatinine after application of radiocontrast media. Clin Nephrol 2004;61(2):98–102.

90. Haase-Fielitz A, Haase M, Devarajan P. Neutrophil gelatinase-associated lipocalin as a biomarker of acute kidney injury: a critical evaluation of current status. Ann Clin Biochem 2014;51(Pt 3):335–51.

91. Tecson KM, Erhardtsen E, Eriksen PM, et al. Optimal cut points of plasma and urine neutrophil gelatinase-associated lipocalin for the prediction of acute kidney injury among critically ill adults: retrospective determination and clinical validation of a prospective multicentre study. BMJ Open 2017;7(7):e016028.

92. Barbar SD, Clere-Jehl R, Bourredjem A, et al. Timing of renal-replacement therapy in patients with acute kidney injury and sepsis. N Engl J Med 2018; 379(15):1431–42.

Platelet Activation and Endothelial Cell Dysfunction

Tom van der Poll, MD, PhD[a], Robert I. Parker, MD[b],*

KEYWORDS

- Platelets • Endothelial cells • Inflammation • Complement • Hemostasis

KEY POINTS

- Activated platelets can enhance inflammation through activation of the complement system either directly or indirectly through interaction with other cell types.
- Through the process of NET formation and NETosis, activated platelets play a role in the clearance of pathogens from circulation.
- Proinflammatory stimulation of Endothelial cells induces expression of tissue factor and links and modulates the processes of hemostasis/coagulation and inflammation.
- Inflammation can lead to disruption of endothelial barrier function with resultant tissue edema and activation of coagulation through exposure of pro-hemostatic proteins (eg, von Willebrand factor) in the adventitia.
- The endothelial cell glycocalyx plays an important role in regulating the local hemostasis and the prevention of microvascular thrombosis.

INTRODUCTION

It is well recognized that in sepsis, coagulation is activated and there is an increased risk of developing a consumptive coagulopathy (eg, DIC [disseminated intravascular coagulation]) with an attendant increase in mortality.[1] Although we often think of hemostasis/coagulation and inflammation as being separate entities, there is considerable evidence that the processes that regulate hemostasis evolved as a component of the inflammatory response to infection. Many of these points of interaction occur on the endothelial cell surface linking these 2 cell types in the initiation and regulation of hemostasis and inflammation.[2–5] Consequently, it is not surprising that inflammation has been shown to stimulate both platelets and endothelial cells in ways that affect both hemostasis and the immune response. In addition, platelets have been shown to be a prime driver of the inflammatory response. This article discusses the

[a] Amsterdam University Medical Centers, Location Academic Medical Center, University of Amsterdam, Center of Experimental and Molecular Medicine & Division of Infectious Diseases, Meibergdreef 9, Room G2-130, Amsterdam 1105AZ, the Netherlands; [b] Department of Pediatrics, Pediatric Hematology/Oncology, Renaissance School of Medicine, Stony Brook University, Stony Brook, NY 11794-8111, USA
* Corresponding author.
E-mail address: robert.parker@stonybrookmedicine.edu

Crit Care Clin 36 (2020) 233–253
https://doi.org/10.1016/j.ccc.2019.11.002
0749-0704/20/© 2019 Elsevier Inc. All rights reserved.

more important pathways wherein inflammation serves to regulate platelet and endothelial cell function.

OVERVIEW OF PLATELET FUNCTION AND ACTIVATION

Although platelets are most connected to hemostasis, they have multiple other functions, including participation in inflammation via complement activation interaction with leukocytes and monocytes, participation in host defenses against infection, regulation of vascular tone, and playing a role, as yet poorly defined, in tumor biology (**Table 1**).

Platelets are anuclear cells derived through demarcation and shedding of megakaryocyte cytoplasm. As such, they contain cytoplasmic organelle (granules, mitochondria) and proteins, and a complex internal membrane network, the open canalicular system (OCS), that allows communication with the external plasma environment. Although platelets are anuclear, they do contain mitochondria and remnants of megakaryocytic RNA and consequently have a limited capacity to synthesize new protein, and platelets have been shown to be able to supply RNA fragments to other cells, thereby affecting their function[6,7] (**Table 2**). There are 3 types of granules in platelets: α-granules, δ-granules (dense bodies), and lysosomes (**Table 3**). The most numerous platelet granules are the α-granules, which contain proteins that help promote the hemostatic function of platelets (fibrinogen, von Willebrand factor [vWf], clotting factor V [F.V], thrombospondin, fibronectin), growth factors, and other proteins important in the biology of platelets, including platelet-derived growth factor (PDGF), insulinlike growth factor-1 (IGF-1), transforming growth factor-β1, platelet factor-4 (a heparin-binding protein), and the cytoadhesion molecules p-selectin, CD40L, and CD63. Dense bodies (δ-granules) contain proteins/peptides that accelerate platelet activation (such as ADP, serotonin [5HT], ATP, Ca++, pyrophosphate), and lysosomes contain proteolytic and hydrolytic enzymes needed for clot degradation.

Table 1
Platelet functions

Hemostasis	Inflammation	Host Defenses	Vascular Tone	Tumor Biology
Adhesion	Complement activation	Internalization of bacteria and viruses by phagocytes	Serotonin reuptake	Tumor growth
Aggregation	Platelet-leukocyte interactions	Bacterial killing	Secretion of serotonin, thromboxane, and prostaglandins	Tumor killing
Spreading	Chemotaxis	Platelet-derived microbacteriocidal proteins		Tumor metastases
Granule secretion	Allergy	Superoxide generation		
Procoagulant activation				
Clot retraction				
Tissue repair				

Table 2
Proteins synthesized by platelets

Signal-Dependent Synthesis	Synthesis Not Signal-Dependent
IL-1β	Actin
Tissue factor	Albumin
Bcl-3	Factor XIIIa
Plasminogen activator inhibitor-1	Fibrinogen
Tetrahydrobiopterin	Glutathione-dependent peroxidase
Sodium-dependent vitamin C transporter 2	GPIb
COX-1	GPIIb
Nitric oxide synthase	GPIIIa
CXCL12	HLA
Orai1	Receptor CK protein
Glucocorticoid-inducible kinase-1	RhoGDIa
	RhoGDIb
	Thrombospondin
	Thrombothemin von Willebrand factor

Abbreviations: Bcl-3, B-cell lymphoma-3; COX-1, cyclooxygenase-1; CXCL12, C-X-C motif chemokine ligand 12; GP, glycoprotein; HLA, human leukocyte antigen; IL, interleukin.

On stimulation, platelets undergo shape change during which the platelet shape morphs to increase its surface area by exposing regions of the OCS that were effectively shielded from plasma proteins and endothelial receptors by invagination of the membrane (**Figs. 1** and **2**). In addition, platelets possess a cytoskeletal system that determines cell shape, and an internal membrane system analogous to the sarcoplasmic reticulum of cardiac myocytes, the dense tubular system (DTS), that contains a pool of calcium that is released into the cytoplasm on stimulation promoting

Table 3
Platelet granules

Alpha Granule	Dense Body	Lysosome
Clotting proteins (factor V, factor XIII, protein S, plasminogen, kininogen)	Serotonin (5HT)	Hydrolases
Adhesive glycoproteins (fibrinogen, vWf, thrombospondin, fibronectin, vitronectin)	ADP	Proteases
Cytokine, chemokines, mediators (CXCL4 [platelet factor-4], CXCL12, CCL5 [RANTES], chondroitin sulfate A)	ATP	
Proteoglycans (histidine-rich glycoprotein, serglycan)	Ca++	
Protease inhibitors (TFPI, PAI-1, C$_1$-esterase inhibitor, α2PI, α$_2$antitrypsin, α$_2$Macroglobulin, α$_1$protease inhibitor)	Pyrophosphate	
Growth factors (PDGF, TGFβ, IGF-1, VEGF, epidermal growth factor, endothelial growth factor, vascular permeability factor)		
Membrane (CD63, GPIIb/IIIa, GPIb/IX, GPIV, PECAM, P-selectin, GMP33, GLUT3)		

Abbreviations: CCL5, chemokine ligand 5; CXCL, C-X-C motif chemokine ligand; GLUT3, glucose transporter 3; GP, glycoprotein; IGF, insulinlike growth factor; PAI-1, plasminogen activator inhibitor-1; PDGF, platelet-derived growth factor; PECAM, platelet endothelial cell adhesion molecule; TFPI, tissue factor pathway inhibitor; TGFβ, transforming growth factor β; VEGF, vascular endothelial growth factor; vWf, von Willebrand factor.

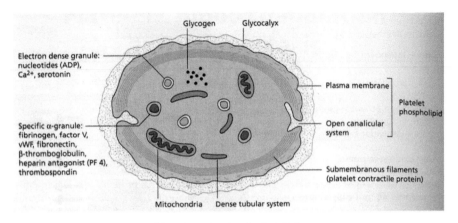

ultrastructure of platelet

Fig. 1. Platelet ultrastructure.

activation of biochemical pathways initiated via binding of platelet agonists to specific surface receptors.

Platelets possess several different activation pathways with each being initiated by binding of agonists to specific surface receptors (**Fig. 3**) (**Table 4**).[8–11] Thrombin generated on activation of the coagulation cascade by cleavage of prothrombin by clotting factor complex consisting of Xa/Va and negatively charged phospholipids (the "prothrombinase" complex) binds to one of the platelets' g-protein linked protease activated receptors (PARs) to activate platelets, which in turn initiates myriad internal and membrane changes in the platelet. Two important cytoadhesion receptors play critical roles in the hemostatic function of platelets. The most abundant

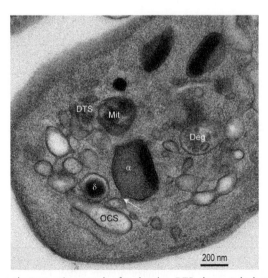

Fig. 2. Transmission electron micrograph of a platelet. DTS, dense tubular system; OCS, open canalicular system; α, alpha granule; δ, dense granule (dense body); Mit, mitochondria; Deg, degraded material contained within a lysosome.

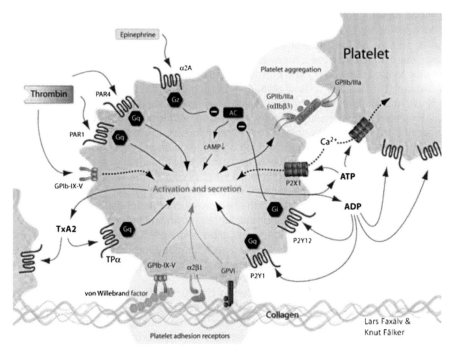

Fig. 3. Various receptors expressed on the platelet surface.

Table 4 Platelet receptors			
Receptor	**Ligand**	**Pathway**	**Function**
GPIIb/IIIa (αIIb/β3)	Fibrin(ogen), vWf, Mac-1		H
GPIb/IX/V	vWf, thrombin		H
GPVI	Collagen		H, I
α2β1	Collagen		H
PAR1, PAR4	Thrombin		H, I, V
P2Y$_{12}$, PG2Y$_1$	ADP		H, I
α2A	Epinephrine		H
5HT$_{2A}$	5HT		H, V
TPα	Thromboxane A2	src	H, I, V
EP3, EP4, DP1	Prostaglandins, prostanoids		H, I
FcγRIIa	CD40L	PI3K, AKT	I
C-type Lectin 2 (CLEC-2)	Podolanin	TLR	I, T
Complement receptors	C1q, C3a, C3b		I
PSGL-1	P-selectin		I
P-selectin	PSGL-1		I

Abbreviations: GP, glycoprotein; H, hemostatic; I, immunomodulatory and/or inflammatory; PAR, protease activated receptor; PSGL-1, P-selectin glycoprotein ligand-1; T, tumor biology; V, regulation of vascular tone and vascular endothelium; vWf, von Willebrand factor.

of these platelet surface receptors is glycoprotein IIb/IIIa (GPIIb/IIIa), which binds fibrinogen and vWf. GPIIb/IIIa belongs to the integrin family of cytoadhesion receptors and is present on the platelet surface in a "nonactivated" conformation. Following stimulation of platelets, the 2 subunits associate to an "active" conformation in which it is able to bind fibrin(ogen) and promote platelet aggregation (the binding of platelet-to-platelet). Under conditions of platelet activation by thrombin, GPIIb/IIIa is also able to bind vWf and enhance platelet adhesion (binding of platelets to nonplatelets). Under nonstimulated conditions, the primary receptor for vWf is the GPIb/IX/V complex. This cytoadhesion receptor, in contrast to GPIIb/IIIa, is able to bind vWf in the absence of platelet activation and does not change conformation on activation. Under conditions of high shear stress, vWf undergoes a conformational change that allows it binding to the GPIb/IX/V complex. Once sufficient vWf is bound to the GPIb/IX/V complex, a transmembrane signal may be generated with consequent platelet activation. Platelet activation also results in exposure of the negatively charged phospholipid phosphatidylserine on the outer platelet membrane, further enhancing the prothrombotic phenotype of activated platelets. In addition, expression of phosphatidylserine on the platelet surface under conditions that promote antibody formation may result in the formation of anti-phospholipid antibodies specific for phosphatidylserine, which are strongly associated with increased thrombotic risk.[12,13]

Although platelets have been identified as being important in thrombus formation, platelet activation does not always result in generating a prothrombotic environment. Recent experimental evidence has demonstrated that platelet responses to agonists are more varied and complex, with the platelet phenotype produced by ligand interaction with its receptor dependent on the ligand, the amount of ligand, and/or the specific downstream pathways linked to the receptor.[14,15] It is important to note that hemostatically linked and immunomodulatory responses have been shown to occur independent of each other.[16]

OVERVIEW OF ENDOTHELIAL CELL FUNCTION

The vascular endothelium forms the interface between blood and the parenchyma and is essential for hemostasis and regulation of the movement of water, solutes, gases, macromolecules, and cells (**Table 5**). We here first discuss endothelial cell function in its normal quiescent state. In a separate section that follows, pathologic alterations in endothelial function are discussed, together with potential underlying mechanisms.

HEMOSTASIS

The endothelium plays a crucial role in the regulation of hemostasis.[17] Under physiologic conditions, the anatomically and functionally intact endothelium is essential for the prevention of microvascular thrombosis. Activation of coagulation is prevented by 3 main anticoagulant mechanisms: the protein C system, tissue factor pathway

Table 5
Role of endothelial glycocalyx

Endothelial Function	Permeability	Hemostasis	Inflammation
• Shear-induced • NO-synthesis • Superoxide dismutase	• Sieving	• Inhibition of platelet adhesion • Modulation of coagulation	• Modulation of leukocyte adhesion

inhibitor (TFPI), and by antithrombin; the endothelial cell regulates the activity of all 3 systems.[1,17] The protein C system inhibits via proteolytic inactivation of the coagulation cofactors Va and VIIIa by activated protein C (APC). APC is formed at the surface of the endothelium from protein C when thrombin binds to the endothelial cell receptor thrombomodulin.[1,18] As such, the protein C system makes use of a classic feedback mechanism wherein the interaction between thrombin and thrombomodulin results in a shift in the activity of thrombin from a potent procoagulant protease into an anticoagulant protein. The generation of APC by the thrombomodulin-thrombin complex is facilitated by the presence of the endothelial protein C receptor (EPCR). Tissue factor is the predominant initiator of the coagulation cascade, triggered by complex formation with activated factor VII (factor VIIa). The tissue factor-factor VIIa complex is inhibited by TFPI, whereas antithrombin is the foremost inhibitor of thrombin and factor Xa.

Under physiologic conditions, the endothelial cell glycocalyx plays a crucial role in the function of anticoagulant proteins and thereby in preventing unwanted clotting. The glycocalyx is a gel-like structure consisting of membrane-associated proteoglycans, glycoproteins, and glycosaminoglycans (GAGs) that lines the luminal surface of the vascular endothelium[19,20] (**Figs. 4** and **5**). Proteoglycans, including syndecan-1, are anchored to the endothelial cell membrane and bind GAGs. Heparan sulfate comprises more than half of GAGs in the glycocalyx; other components include chondroitin sulfates and dermatan sulfates. Hyaluronic acid can form complexes with GAGs, which stabilizes the glycocalyx. GAGs can bind thrombomodulin, TFPI, and antithrombin, and heparin sulfate increases the anticoagulant actions of TFPI and antithrombin. The involvement of the glycocalyx in maintaining blood flow in the microcirculation further contributes to its role in preventing microvascular thrombosis.

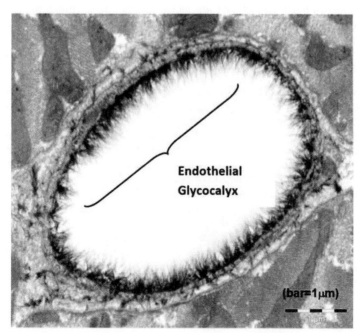

Endothelial
Glycocalyx

(bar=1 μm)

Fig. 4. Electron micrograph of the glycocalyx of vascular endothelial cells.

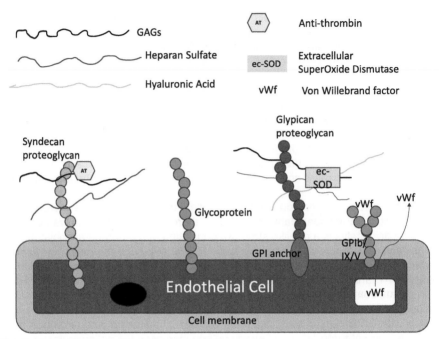

Fig. 5. Various components of the glycocalyx.

Endothelial cells further contribute to hemostasis through the production of vWf, which mediates initial platelet adhesion to areas of vascular injury. Under physiologic conditions, vWf binds to and aggregates platelets under conditions of high shear stress. Ultralarge multimers of vWf are highly thrombogenic; these are cleaved to smaller, less active forms, by ADAMTS13 (A Disintegrin And Metalloproteinase with Thrombospondin type 1 motif, 13).

BARRIER FUNCTION

The endothelium forms a selective and semipermeable barrier between circulating blood and tissues.[17,21] The transport across the endothelium ensues via transcellular and paracellular routes, resulting from passage through endothelial cells by transcytosis and passage in between adjacent cells via opening and closing of intercellular junctions, respectively. During normal homeostasis, the endothelial barrier function is maintained by tight junctions (which seal the intercellular cleft between adjacent cells), adherens junctions (which stabilize tight junctions inside the intercellular space), and the glycocalyx. Tight junctions reduce paracellular permeability and include 3 families: claudins, occludins, and junction adhesion molecules. The integrity of adherens junctions is controlled by the activation status of vascular endothelial (VE)-cadherin. Both adherens and tight junctions are connected to the actin cytoskeleton of endothelial cells, which is closely linked with cell-cell and cell-matrix adhesion complexes, thereby significantly contributing to the stability of endothelial cell junctions and vascular integrity. The small GTPase Rac1 has been implicated as an essential mediator of the preservation of endothelial barrier function.[21] Rac1 increases VE-cadherin abundance at adherens junctions, while, in a reciprocal way, VE-cadherin activates Rac1 on engagement in adherens junctions. Activation of Rac1 under physiologic conditions is regulated by cyclic AMP, as well as by angiopoietin (Ang)1 and sphinosine-1-phosphate (S1P). S1P is a sphingolipid produced by many cell types that regulates barrier function through activation of its receptor S1P1.[22] S1P1 activation contributes to vascular integrity through several mechanisms, including cytoskeletal reorganization and adherens and tight junction assembly.

The Tie receptor family, consisting of Tie1 and Tie2, also play an important role in regulating vascular permeability.[17,23] Tie1 and Tie2 are virtually exclusively expressed by endothelial cells. Tie2 can interact with the Ang family of proteins, which include Ang1, Ang2, and Ang4. In normal homeostasis, mesenchymal cells, such as smooth muscle cells, pericytes, and monocytes, secrete Ang1, which is a strong Tie2 agonist, and the interaction between Ang1 and Tie2 is important for maintaining vascular stability.[24] Tie2 activation by Ang1 enhances Tie2 transassociation at cell-cell junctions and supports the formation of adhesive structures through promoting interaction between Tie2 and extracellular matrix components, such as collagen, fibronectin, and vitronectin. Tie2 activation by Ang1 also results in inhibition of the transcriptional activity of the Forkhead box protein O1 (FOXO1) transcription factor, which further contributes to vessel stability through several mechanisms, including suppression of Ang2 production.[23] As a result, Ang2 is expressed at low levels in quiescent endothelium, where it colocalizes with vWf within Weibel Palade bodies.

PARs comprise another family of receptors involved in endothelial barrier function. PARs, of which 4 types exist in humans (PAR1-4), can either disrupt or protect barrier function, depending on differential activation of intracellular signaling pathways.[17] PARs can be activated by an internal ligand sequestered in their ectodomain that can be removed by the action of serine proteases, such as thrombin.

An intact glycocalyx is vital for maintaining vascular integrity, in part by acting as a negatively charged molecular sieve that limits transvascular movement of negatively charged and/or large molecules.[19,20] In addition, the glycocalyx is important for limiting the interaction between blood leukocytes and the endothelium by "hiding" endothelial cell–associated adhesion molecules such as integrins and immunoglobulin superfamilies. Moreover, the glycocalyx can protect endothelial cells from oxidative stress and is able to sense fluid shear forces, which it transmits to the endothelium, thereby triggering nitric oxide production, which induces vasorelaxation and reduces leukocyte and platelet adherence.

EFFECTS OF INFLAMMATION ON PLATELETS AND HEMOSTASIS

Although the best-known and understood consequence of platelet activation is their role in promoting coagulation and microvascular thrombosis, platelets are now known to play central roles in inflammation, host defenses against pathogens, and in the regulation of vascular tone at the microvascular level (**Table 6**).[15,16,25–28] For the purposes of this review, we focus on the role platelets play in inflammation and host defenses during acute critical illness. Receptor-mediated activation of specific downstream pathways has been found to be an import modulator of host response to critical illness. Activation of Toll-Like Receptor, nuclear factor-κB, ERK/MEK, MAP-kinase, and AKT-associated pathways (among others) has been implicated in this process.[29–32] In addition, platelets have been shown to interact directly and indirectly with immunoeffector cells, including lymphocytes, neutrophils, basophils, and mast cells to modulate host immune responses. This interaction may involve direct binding via cellular adhesion receptors, via platelet expression of secreted cytokines or proteins or via direct transfer of platelet RNA, which may induce new protein synthesis by nucleated cells[6,7](see **Table 4**).

Table 6
Platelet interaction with immune effector cells

Cell Type	Effect	Mechanism

B-lymphocyte	• Germinal center development
	• Antiviral antibody production
		Direct:
		    Platelet CD154/B-Lymphocyte CD40
		    Platelet CD62P/B-Lymphocyte PSGL-1
		Indirect:
		    Platelet sCD154

T-lymphocyte	• Differentiation
	• Cytotoxicity
		Direct:
		    Platelet CD154/T-Lymphocyte CD40
		    Platelet CD62P/T-Lymphocyte PSGL-1

Monocyte	• Survival
	• Differentiation
		Direct:
		    Platelet CD154/Monocyte CD40
		    Platelet CD62P/Monocyte PSGL-1

Neutrophil	• Phagocytosis
	• ROS production
	• Tethering and rolling
	• Activation
		Direct:
		    Platelet CD154/Neutrophil CD40
		    Platelet CD62P/Neutrophil PSGL-1
		Indirect:
		    Complement-mediated NET formation
		        and NETosis
		    Platelet cytokine and chemokine
		        mediated activation of neutrophils

Dendritic cell	• Maturation
	• Antigen presentation
		Direct:
		    Platelet CD154/Dendritic cell CD40
		    Platelet CD62P/Dendritic cell PSGL-1

Abbreviations: CD62P, P-selectin; CD154, CD40 Ligand(CD40L); NET, neutrophil extracellular trap; PSGL-1, P-selectin glycoprotein ligand-1; ROS, reactive oxygen species; sCD154, soluble CD154.

Platelet Role in Neutrophil Extracellular Trap Formation and NETosis

Platelets have been shown to have a role in bacterial killing via synthesis and secretion of platelet-derived bacteriocidal microproteins, and by entrapment in Neutrophil Extracellular Traps (NETs): so-called NETosis (see **Fig.4**). NETs are networks of neutrophil DNA that are extruded from neutrophils when activated by particular mechanisms, one of which is platelet associated. Activation of neutrophils by this mechanism starts a unique neutrophil death process referred to as NETosis. NETosis differs from neutrophil apoptosis or necrosis and is thought to begin with NADPH oxidase activation of protein-arginine deiminase 4 via reactive oxygen species intermediaries, resulting in an increase in intracellular citrulline with consequent increase in citrullinated histones. The neutrophil nuclear chromatin becomes decondensed with rupture of the nucleus and release of nuclear proteins into the cytoplasm. These DNA fibers are ultimately extruded from the cell, creating a "net" that entraps pathogens as well as other blood cells and cellular proteins. Pathogens caught in these NETs are ultimately killed. However, there are data that bacteria also have been shown to use platelets in NETs to evade host immune surveillance. NETs are able to capture and kill various immune cells, including CD4+ and CD8+ T cells, B cells, and monocytes. This effect is seen not only with neutrophils in the blood, but also in various tissues, such as the gut, lung, and liver. When NET development and NETosis occurs within organs, it can result in exacerbation of inflammation-induced organ injury and dysfunction.[33–37] NETs possibly contribute to the hypercoagulable state by trapping platelets, and inducing the expression of tissue factor by trapped leukocytes and monocytes. The linkage of complement activation/inflammation and coagulation has been referred to as "immunothrombosis."[38–40] The formation of NETs in the microvasculature has been shown to contribute to the formation of microthrombi in the microvasculature. In experimental studies, the presence of histidine-rich glycoprotein has been shown to moderate the induction of neutrophil and vascular endothelial cell activation, and induction of thrombosis by a reversible mechanism.[41]

Effect of Critical Illness on Platelet-Mediated Hemostasis

Thrombocytopenia is a common occurrence in critically ill patients, and its presence on intensive care unit admission or subsequent development is associated with increased risk of mortality.[42–45] Thrombocytopenia may reflect decreased production due to marrow failure, infection or drug administration, platelet sequestration, or increased platelet consumption. When due to consumption, it may be an isolated process related to the presence of antibodies directed against platelet epitopes or due to immune complex binding to platelets (eg, immune thrombocytopenia, heparin-induced thrombocytopenia), reflect cell-mediated consumption (eg, hemophagocytosis), represent an early indicator of a global consumptive coagulopathy (eg, DIC) or be secondary to a deficiency of ADAMST13 (eg, thrombotic thrombocytopenic purpura, thrombocytopenia-associated multiorgan failure). Of these etiologic categories, inflammation and complement activation can result in either (or both) a decrease in platelet production and/or the platelet consumption. In addition, thrombocytopenia itself has been shown to produce a dysregulation in immune response.[46]

In vivo studies have demonstrated that the template bleeding time is progressively prolonged once the circulating platelet count falls below 100,000/μL, and this has generally been interpreted as resulting in an increased risk of bleeding. Consequently, in critically ill patients. a platelet count less than this level should warrant evaluation of that patient's risk for bleeding taking into account other aspects of their illness that would affect bleeding risk. Although a platelet count of less than 10,000 to 20,000/μL is often used as a trigger for prophylactic platelet transfusions in the thrombocytopenia that develops following myelosuppressive cancer chemotherapy, transfusion of a higher dose of platelets administered while decreasing donor exposure does not appear to reduce the risk of bleeding.[47–49] Application of this number to trigger platelet transfusion when thrombocytopenia is caused by other mechanisms has not been validated. Indeed, there are data suggesting that common invasive procedures can be safely performed in patients with mild thrombocytopenia without prophylactic platelet transfusion, although to date there are no randomized studies that would enable the determination of the lower limit of a "safe" platelet count for invasive procedures.[49–55] Prophylactic platelet transfusions have also worsened outcome in some patient populations, particularly in neonates.[56–59] Platelets obtained from female donors, even when washed and resuspended in male plasma, still carry a higher risk of inducing transfusion-related acute lung injurey.[60]

Platelet Involvement in Complement Activation and Adaptive Immunity

Platelet activation during thrombotic events is closely associated with complement and contact system activation, and consequently linked with inflammation. Chondroitin sulfate A (CS-A), released from α-granules during platelet activation, is an identified mediator of interactions between platelets and the complement system. This interaction occurs in 3 identifiable processes: platelet interaction with other cellular elements (eg, lymphocytes, monocytes, basophils, mast cells, neutrophils) that require complement (see **Table 5**), complement activation through the classic coagulation cascade (see **Fig. 5**), and complement activation independent of activation of coagulation and the

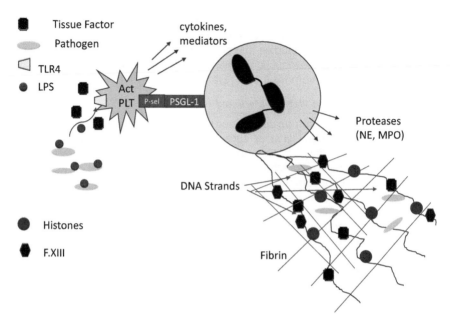

Fig. 6. TLR (Toll-like receptor) or LPS (lipopolysaccharide)-mediated cytokine secretion from activated platelets stimulating neutrophils and the subsequent development of NETs and NETosis. Act PLT, activated platelet; MPO, myeloperoxidase; NE, neutrophil elastase.

complement-mediated clearance of microbial pathogens (**Figs. 6–8**).[61–68] It has been well described that activation of the classic coagulation cascade through the "intrinsic" pathway begins with the "contact phase" complex consisting of clotting factor XII (F.XII) and the complement-related cofactors high molecular weight kininogen and prekallikrein, which cleaves the inactive form of F.XI to the activated F.XIa. In this process, F.XIIa is formed which is able to catalyze the conversion of C1r2 to C1rs beginning the process of complement activation (see **Fig. 5**) Platelet α-granules contain both C1-Inh and polyphosphate, which can inhibit both the conversion of F.XII to XIIa and F.XIIa. Both C1-Inh and polyphosphate interfere with complement activation at other points downstream from initiation. Although complement activation does not occur on the platelet surface, platelets express receptors for both C1q and C3b and the membrane expression of each is increased on platelet activation. As both of these components of complement also bind to several species of bacteria, platelets can participate in response to infection by complement-mediated binding mechanisms (see **Table 4**). This complement-mediated binding of bacterium to platelets has been shown to occur via either the classic or alternative pathways.[66–69] Properidin-dependent Complement activation is affected through the binding of properidin, released from activated neutrophils, to activated platelets.[67] In this model, platelet bound properidin recruits the binding of C3 (or C3H2O) to stimulated platelets with subsequent promotion of C3(H2O)/Bb convertase formation. Complement activation can also be affected through a P-selectin dependent mechanism (see **Fig. 8**).[68] Other investigators have demonstrated alteration in platelet function with inflammation and specifically in the setting of sepsis.[70,71] These studies have shown that how platelets participate in initiation of hemostasis, interact in complement and noncomplement host immune response, and in wound healing may all be affected in sepsis and in clinical situations characterized by a dysregulated inflammatory response.

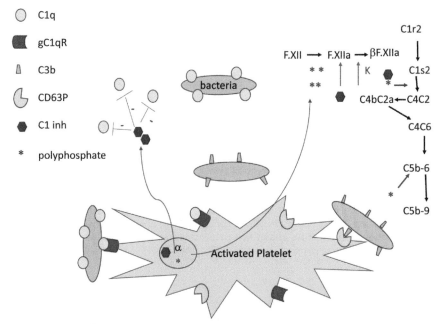

Fig. 7. Complement/platelet interactions in infection, inflammation and coagulation: on activation, platelets overexpress both the C1q receptor (gC1qR) and CD63P, which serves as a receptor for C3b. Bacteria coated with C1q or C3b are subsequently bound by platelets. C1 inhibitor (C1 inh) secreted by platelet alpha (α) granules limit the interactions of C1q with its receptor (gC1qR). In addition, polyphosphate secreted from platelet α-granules inhibits C1q binding to bacterium and also blocks enzymatic activity of clotting factors XIIa and XIa. Platelet-secreted polyphosphate blocks the conversion of F.XII to F.XIIa, and the enzymatic activity of the C5,6 complex. In concert with C1 inh, polyphosphate inhibits C1s2 conversion to C2C4.

DISTURBANCE OF ENDOTHELIAL CELL FUNCTION IN CRITICAL ILLNESS
Hemostasis

Critical illness is virtually always associated with coagulation abnormalities, the extent of which can vary between mild activation of coagulation that can only be recognized by sensitive laboratory measurements, to a subtle fall in platelet count and/or mild prolongation of global clotting assays, to fulminant DIC, manifested by widespread microvascular thrombosis and concurrent hemorrhage.[1,72] A disturbed endothelial function plays an eminent role herein. Proinflammatory stimuli induce tissue factor expression in endothelial cells, a procoagulant receptor molecule also expressed by cells within the vessel wall, monocytes, and extracellular vesicles. Tissue factor is essential for activation of the coagulation system in critical illness. The role of tissue factor has particularly been established in models of sepsis, demonstrating that blocking or inhibiting tissue factor prevents activation of the coagulation system and improves survival.[1,73] In support of these in vitro findings, mice with an almost complete deficiency for tissue factor exhibit reduced coagulation, inflammation, and mortality during endotoxic shock.[74] Tissue factor binds to factor VIIa, resulting in the tissue factor/factor VIIa complex that activates factor X to factor Xa. Factor Xa assembles with factor Va to form the prothrombinase complex on the surface of the endothelium. The prothrombinase complex converts prothrombin to thrombin, which in turn cleaves fibrinogen to fibrin. In addition, proinflammatory

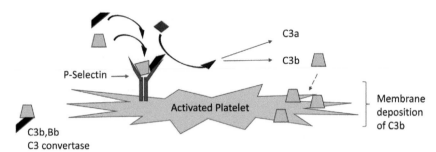

Fig. 8. Platelet-enhanced complement activation. (*A*) P-selectin–dependent complement activation: P-selectin captures and immobilizes labile plasma C3b. Binding of factor B to bound C3b completes formation of C3 convertase (C3b,Bb) on the surface of activated platelet (or endothelial cell). The C3b,Bb C3 convertase complex cleaves C3 and mediates amplification of the complement activation. C3b produced by process deposits on the platelet membrane. MAC, membrane attack complex; PMN, polymorphoneutrophil. (*Adapted from* Del Conde I, Crúz MA, Zhang H, et al. Platelet activation leads to activation and propagation of the complement system. J Exp Med. 2005 Mar 21;201(6):871-9; with permission.)

stimuli trigger the release of vWf from endothelial cells, which in critical illness is accompanied by inactivation of ADAMTS-13. The ensuing relative deficiency in ADAMTS-13 leads to higher concentrations of the prothrombotic ultralarge vWf multimers, which can promote pathologic platelet–vessel wall interactions and microvascular thrombosis.[75] In addition, inflammation causes the release of plasminogen activator inhibitor-1 from endothelial cells, a major inhibitor of fibrinolysis. Adhesion of platelets at sites of vascular injury can further augment endothelial cell and coagulation activation through several mechanisms, including increased adhesion molecule expression and induction of tissue factor.[17] As such, inflammation is associated with a shift in the hemostatic balance of the vascular endothelium toward a prothrombotic state. Conversely, procoagulant and anticoagulant factors modulate inflammation. Thrombin, the tissue factor/factor VIIa complex and factor Xa exert a variety of proinflammatory activities, primarily by activating PARs. Of these, PAR1 has emerged as a major mediator of the link between coagulation and inflammation.[72,76] PAR1 can be activated by several proteases, including thrombin and APC. Proteases involved in the clotting cascade can regulate PAR signaling by either activation or inactivation and can trigger distinct intracellular events. As a consequence, thrombin and APC/EPCR triggering of PAR1 results in different effects (see also the following section "Barrier Function"). Proinflammatory effects of thrombin on endothelial cells include leukocyte adhesion molecule expression and induction of interleukin (IL)-6 and IL-8.

In critical illness, the hemostatic balance is further disturbed by a disruption of the glycocalyx, which is an important injurious event in critically ill patients. Indeed, many studies have reported a decrease in the thickness of the glycocalyx in sepsis. Even a relatively mild stimulus, such as provided by intravenous injection of a low-dose lipopolysaccharide into healthy humans, can result in a 50% reduction in sublingual glycocalyx thickness.[77] Several mediators have been implicated in damaging the glycocalyx in critical illness. For example, hyaluronidase, thrombin, plasmin, cathepsin B, and elastase can degrade hyaluronic acid on the endothelial surface. Matrix metalloproteinases cleave proteoglycans, such as syndecan, and heparanase degrades heparan sulfate. Ang2 can also degrade the glycocalyx. Interestingly, hypervolemia (such as associated with excessive fluid resuscitation) may also cause glycocalyx breakdown, possibly through the release of atrial natriuretic peptide.[78] Loss of the glycocalyx exposes endothelial cell adhesion molecules such as E-selectin and intercellular adhesion molecule-1, and induces recruitment of blood leukocytes and platelets. Aggregation of platelets (and leukocytes) together with loss of endogenous anticoagulant properties results in hypercoagulation and thrombus formation. Although these changes may facilitate pathogen elimination at local sites of infection, in systemic critical illness, destruction of the glycocalyx results in widespread microvascular thrombosis, capillary leakage, reduced vascular responsiveness, and impaired oxygen delivery through the microcirculation. Several biomarkers for impaired glycocalyx function have been reported, including circulating glycocalyx components, such as syndecan-1, endocan, hyaluronic, acid and heparan sulfate, although their correlation with (the extent of) endothelial injury is debated. Nonetheless, a large series of observational studies in patients have documented a correlation between circulating glycocalyx components and severity of disease and/or (adverse) clinical outcomes.[19]

Barrier Function

Disruption of endothelial barrier function not only leads to tissue edema, but also exposes blood to the vessel adventitia with abundant tissue factor (causing coagulation activation) and collagen fibers (causing von Willebrand polymerization and platelet aggregation). As such, endothelial barrier integrity is important for maintaining a balanced hemostasis. Inflammatory mediators can increase paracellular permeability of venules via opening of tight junctions and adherens junctions.[21] The 2 main underlying mechanisms hereof are phosphorylation of adherens junction components and an imbalance of Rac1/RhoA signaling with inactivation of Rac1 together with overactivation of RhoA, which both result in VE-cadherin endocytosis and junction disassembly. In this context, endothelial cyclic AMP is crucial for maintaining barrier integrity, and proinflammatory cytokines, endotoxin, and thrombin can reduce cyclic AMP and inactivate Rac1.

A disturbed function of the Ang/Tie2 axis plays an important role in the disturbed endothelial barrier function.[23] Inflammation is associated with enhanced Ang2 secretion. The net effect of Ang2 on Tie2 signaling is dependent on the extent of inflammation in the surrounding environment. Whereas under quiescent conditions the Tie1/Tie2 heterodimeric complex permits both Ang1 and Ang2 to act as Tie2 agonists, inflammation triggers the release of the Tie1 ectodomain; under these circumstances, Ang2 binding results in Tie2 antagonism.[79] Likewise, Tie1 shedding reduces Ang1 agonistic activity, indicating that Tie1 is necessary for triggering of Tie2. Thus, inflammation, caused by either sterile injury or infection, is accompanied by an increased Ang2/Ang1 balance and blockade of Tie2 activation, resulting in destabilization of the endothelium. Experimental sepsis in animals has documented diminished Tie2 expression and phosphorylation in vivo, further supporting the existence of a disturbed Ang2/Tie2 axis in critical illness.[23] Although endothelial shear stress can reduce Tie2 mRNA expression, diminished Tie2 expression at the surface of the vascular endothelium likely is predominantly caused by enhanced shedding.[80] Elevated circulating levels of soluble Tie2 in critical illness may further inhibit Ang activity by functioning as a decoy receptor. Murine sepsis also is associated with decreased phosphorylation of Tie2, indicating an impaired functional state of this receptor.[81] The plasma levels of (soluble) components of the Ang/Tie2 system are elevated in patients with critical illness and can function as biomarkers of disease severity and outcome.[23,82] Sepsis is characterized by decreased plasma concentrations of Ang1 and increased levels of Ang2 and an increased Ang2/Ang1 ratio is considered to reflect a disturbed endothelial barrier function and bears prognostic significance. The circulating levels of Tie2 signaling components especially associate with lung injury, possibly because Tie2 is strongly expressed in pulmonary vascular endothelium, and Ang2 has been implicated in microvascular leak in the acute respiratory distress syndrome.[83]

The functional importance of the Ang/Tie2 axis has been demonstrated in experimental sepsis models, showing that a rise in Ang1 or decline in Ang2 levels improved survival.[23] Adenoviral overexpression of Ang1 mitigated expression of endothelial adhesion molecules in kidneys and lungs of endotoxemic mice and improved hemodynamic instability and survival.[84] Mice with one functional *Ang2* allele developed less kidney and lung injury, less tissue inflammation, and less vascular leakage compared with normal wild-type mice during abdominal sepsis caused by cecal ligation and puncture, which was associated with a profound survival advantage.[85] Together these animal investigations suggest that increasing circulating Ang1 and reducing Ang2 can improve endothelial function during sepsis.

The effects of thrombi and APC on vascular integrity are complex. Thrombin can activate PAR1 on endothelial cells to induce cytoskeletal derangements and cell contraction and rounding, thereby destabilizing cell-cell contacts.[17] PAR1 activation by high doses of thrombin results in increased permeability of the endothelium, whereas PAR1 activation of APC/EPCR results in protection of the endothelial integrity. Notably, activation of PAR1 by low concentrations of thrombin results in a barrier protective effect[86] and thrombin can transactivate PAR1-PAR2 heterodimers in late sepsis, which also preserves barrier function.[87] APC can inhibit thrombin-induced vascular permeability by a mechanism that includes transactivation of S1P1.

SUMMARY

The interaction between platelets and endothelial cells is critical in the regulation of hemostasis, elements of the immune response, and in the maintenance of vascular intergity. Under conditions of inflammation, the balance of platelet-endothelial interaction shifts from a process that prevents the initiation of thrombus formation to one promoting thrombosis. Additionally, platelets become important players in host defenses against pathogens, and the vascular endothelium exhibits disruption in its barrier function allowing tissue edema to occur. Although these effects on platelets and endothelial cells have the effect of enhancing host response to pathogens, both also serve to increase the likelihood of microvascular thrombosis with resultant organ dysfunction and failure.

REFERENCES

1. Levi M, van der Poll T. Coagulation and sepsis. Thromb Res 2017;149:38–44.
2. Hamilos M, Petousis S, Parthenakis F. Interaction between platelets and endothelium: from pathophysiology to new therapeutic options. Cardiovasc Diagn Ther 2018;8(5):568–80.
3. Jenne CN, Kubes P. Platelets in inflammation and infection. Platelets 2015;26(4): 286–92.
4. Ho-Tin-Noé B, Boulaftali Y, Camerer E. Platelets and vascular integrity: how platelets prevent bleeding in inflammation. Blood 2018 Jan 18;131(3):277–88.
5. Cornelius DC, Baik CH, Travis OK, et al. NLRP3 inflammasome activation in platelets in response to sepsis. Physiol Rep 2019;7(9):e14073.

6. Risitano A, Beaulieu LM, Vitseva O, et al. Platelets and platelet-like particles mediate intercellular RNA transfer. Blood 2012;119:6288–95.

7. Clancy L, Freedman JE. The role of circulating platelet transcripts. J Thromb Haemost 2015;13(Suppl 1):S33–9.

8. Estevez B, Du X. New concepts and mechanisms of platelet activation signaling. Physiology (Bethesda) 2017;32(2):162–77.

9. Yun SH, Sim EH, Goh RY, et al. Platelet activation: the mechanisms and potential biomarkers. Biomed Res Int 2016;2016:9060143.

10. Bye AP, Unsworth AJ, Gibbins JM. Platelet signaling: a complex interplay between inhibitory and activatory networks. J Thromb Haemost 2016;14(5):918–30.

11. Jurk K, Walter U. New insights into platelet signalling pathways by functional and proteomic approaches. Hamostaseologie 2018. https://doi.org/10.1055/s-0038-1675356.

12. Castanon A, Pierre G, Willis R, et al. Performance evaluation and clinical associations of immunoassays that detect antibodies to negatively charged phospholipids other than cardiolipin. Am J Clin Pathol 2018;149(5):401–11.

13. Park HS, Gu JY, Jung HS, et al. Thrombotic risk of non-criteria anti-phospholipid antibodies measured by line immunoassay: superiority of anti-phosphatidylserine and anti-phosphatidic acid antibodies. Clin Lab 2019;65(3). https://doi.org/10.7754/Clin.Lab.2018.171207.

14. Petito E, Amison RT, Piselli E, et al. A dichotomy in platelet activation: evidence of different functional platelet responses to inflammatory versus haemostatic stimuli. Thromb Res 2018;172:110–8.

15. Hubertus K, Mischnik M, Timmer J, et al. Reciprocal regulation of human platelet function by endogenous prostanoids and through multiple prostanoid receptors. Eur J Pharmacol 2014;740:15–27.

16. Rex S, Beaulieu LM, Perlman DH, et al. Immune versus thrombotic stimulation of platelets differentially regulates signaling pathways, intracellular protein–protein interactions, and alpha-granule release. Thromb Haemost 2009;102:97.

17. Opal SM, van der Poll T. Endothelial barrier dysfunction in septic shock. J Intern Med 2015;277(3):277–93.

18. Loghmani H, Conway EM. Exploring traditional and nontraditional roles for thrombomodulin. Blood 2018;132(2):148–58.

19. Uchimido R, Schmidt EP, Shapiro NI. The glycocalyx: a novel diagnostic and therapeutic target in sepsis. Crit Care 2019;23(1):16.

20. Iba T, Levy JH. Derangement of the endothelial glycocalyx in sepsis. J Thromb Haemost 2019;17(2):283–94.

21. Radeva MY, Waschke J. Mind the gap: mechanisms regulating the endothelial barrier. Acta Physiol (Oxf) 2018;222(1).

22. Winkler MS, Nierhaus A, Poppe A, et al. Sphingosine-1-phosphate: a potential biomarker and therapeutic target for endothelial dysfunction and sepsis? Shock 2017;47(6):666–72.

23. Leligdowicz A, Richard-Greenblatt M, Wright J, et al. Endothelial activation: the ang/tie Axis in sepsis. Front Immunol 2018;9:838.

24. Koh GY. Orchestral actions of angiopoietin-1 in vascular regeneration. Trends Mol Med 2013;19(1):31–9.

25. Herter JM, Rossaint J, Zarbock A. Platelets in inflammation and immunity. J Thromb Haemost 2014;12(11):1764–75.

26. Iba T, Levy H. Inflammation and thrombosis: roles of neutrophils, platelets and endothelial cells and their interactions in thrombus formation during sepsis. J Thromb Haemost 2018;16:23–241.

27. Stocker TJ, Ishikawa-Ankerhold H, Massberg S, et al. Small but mighty: platelets as central effectors of host defense. Thromb Haemost 2017;117(4):651–61.

28. Yeaman MR. Platelets in defense against bacterial pathogens. Cell Mol Life Sci 2010;67:525–44.

29. Clark SR, Ma AC, Tavener SA, et al. Platelet TLR4 activates neutrophil extracellular traps to ensnare bacteria in septic blood. Nat Med 2007;13:463–9.

30. Claushuis TAM, Van Der Veen AIP, Horn J, et al. Platelet Toll-like receptor expression and activation induced by lipopolysaccharide and sepsis. Platelets 2019; 30(3):296–304.

31. Scott T, Owens MD. Thrombocytes respond to lipopolysaccharide through Toll-like receptor-4, and MAP kinase and NF-kappaB pathways leading to expression of interleukin-6 and cyclooxygenase-2 with production of prostaglandin E2. Mol Immunol 2008;45(4):1001–8.

32. Mussbacher M, Salzmann M, Brostjan C, et al. Cell type-specific roles of NF-κB linking inflammation and thrombosis. Front Immunol 2019;10:85.

33. Kraemer BF, Campbell RA, Schwertz H, et al. Novel anti-bacterial activities of beta-defensin 1 in human platelets: suppression of pathogen growth and signaling of neutrophil extracellular trap formation. PLoS Pathog 2011;7: e1002355.

34. Wong CH, Jenne CN, Petri B, et al. Nucleation of platelets with blood-borne pathogens on Kupffer cells precedes other innate immunity and contributes to bacterial clearance. Nat Immunol 2013;14:785–92.

35. Youssefian T, Drouin A, Masse JM, et al. Host defense role of platelets: engulfment of HIV and *Staphylococcus aureus* occurs in a specific subcellular compartment and is enhanced by platelet activation. Blood 2002;99:4021–9.

36. Rigg RA, Healy LD, Chu TT, et al. Protease-activated receptor 4 activity promotes platelet granule release and platelet-leukocyte interactions. Platelets 2019;30(1): 126–35.

37. Rossaint J, Margraf A, Zarbock A. Role of platelets in leukocyte recruitment and resolution of inflammation. Front Immunol 2018;9:2712.

38. Gaertner F, Massberg S. Blood coagulation in immunothrombosis—at the frontline of intravascular immunity. Semin Immunol 2016;28(6):561–9.

39. Kimball AS, Obi AT, Diaz JA, et al. The emerging role of NETs in venous thrombosis and immunothrombosis. Front Immunol 2016;7:236.

40. Vazquez-Garza E, Jerjes-Sanchez C, Navarrete A, et al. Venous thromboembolism: thrombosis, inflammation, and immunothrombosis for clinicians. J Thromb Thrombolysis 2017;44(3):377–85.

41. Wake H, Mori S, Liu K, et al. Histidine-rich glycoprotein prevents septic lethality through regulation of immunothrombosis and inflammation. EBioMedicine 2016; 9:180–94.

42. Zarychanski R, Houston DS. Assessing thrombocytopenia in the intensive care unit: the past, present, and future. Hematol Am Soc Hematol Educ Program 2017;2017(1):660–6.

43. Fountain EM, Arepally GM. Etiology and complications of thrombocytopenia in hospitalized medical patients. J Thromb Thrombolysis 2017;43(4):429–36.

44. Menard CE, Kumar A, Houston DS, et al. Evolution and impact of thrombocytopenia in septic shock: a retrospective cohort study. Crit Care Med 2019;47(4): 558–65.

45. Bose S, Wurm E, Popovich MJ, et al. Drug-induced immune-mediated thrombocytopenia in the intensive care unit. J Clin Anesth 2015;27(7):602–5.

46. Claushuis TA, van Vught LA, Scicluna BP, et al. Molecular Diagnosis and Risk Stratification of Sepsis Consortium. Thrombocytopenia is associated with a dys-regulated host response in critically ill sepsis patients. Blood 2016;127(24): 3062–72.

47. Estcourt LJ, Stanworth SJ, Doree C, et al. Comparison of different platelet count thresholds to guide administration of prophylactic platelet transfusion for preventing bleeding in people with haematological disorders after myelosuppressive chemotherapy or stem cell transplantation. Cochrane Database Syst Rev 2015;(11):CD010983.

48. Estcourt LJ, Stanworth S, Doree C, et al. Different doses of prophylactic platelet transfusion for preventing bleeding in people with haematological disorders after myelosuppressive chemotherapy or stem cell transplantation. Cochrane Database Syst Rev 2015;(10):CD010984.

49. Crighton GL, Estcourt LJ, Wood EM, et al. A therapeutic-only versus prophylactic platelet transfusion strategy for preventing bleeding in patients with haematological disorders after myelosuppressive chemotherapy or stem cell transplantation. Cochrane Database Syst Rev 2015;(9):CD010981.

50. Napolitano G, Iacobellis A, Merla A, et al. Bleeding after invasive procedures is rare and unpredicted by platelet counts in cirrhotic patients with thrombocytopenia. Eur J Intern Med 2017;38:79–82.

51. AlRstum ZA, Huynh TT, Huang SY, et al. Risk of bleeding after ultrasound-guided jugular central venous catheter insertion in severely thrombocytopenic oncologic patients. Am J Surg 2019;217(1):133–7.

52. Nandagopal L, Veeraputhiran M, Jain T, et al. Bronchoscopy can be done safely in patients with thrombocytopenia. Transfusion 2016;56(2):344–8.

53. Zeidler K, Arn K, Senn O, et al. Optimal preprocedural platelet transfusion threshold for central venous catheter insertions in patients with thrombocytopenia. Transfusion 2011;51(11):2269–76.

54. Abu-Sbeih H, Ali FS, Coronel E, et al. Safety of endoscopy in cancer patients with thrombocytopenia and neutropenia. Gastrointest Endosc 2019;89(5):937–49.e2.

55. Kumar A, Mhaskar R, Grossman BJ, et al. AABB Platelet Transfusion Guidelines Panel. Platelet transfusion: a systematic review of the clinical evidence. Transfusion 2015;55(5):1116–27 [quiz: 1115].

56. Schmidt AE, Henrichs KF, Kirkley SA, et al. Prophylactic preprocedure platelet transfusion is associated with increased risk of thrombosis and mortality. Am J Clin Pathol 2017;149(1):87–94.

57. Aubron C, Flint AW, Bailey M, et al. Is platelet transfusion associated with hospital-acquired infections in critically ill patients? Crit Care 2017;21(1):2.

58. Estcourt LJ. Platelet transfusion thresholds in premature neonates (PlaNeT-2 trial). Transfus Med 2019;29(1):20–2.

59. Curley A, Stanworth SJ, Willoughby K, et al, PlaNeT2 MATISSE Collaborators. Randomized trial of platelet-transfusion thresholds in neonates. N Engl J Med 2019;380(3):242–51.

60. Vossoughi S, Gorlin J, Kessler DA, et al. Ten years of TRALI mitigation: measuring our progress. Transfusion 2019. https://doi.org/10.1111/trf.15387.

61. Karpman D, Ståhl AL, Arvidsson I, et al. Complement interactions with blood cells, endothelial cells and microvesicles in thrombotic and inflammatory conditions. Adv Exp Med Biol 2015;865:19–42.

62. Ekdahl KN, Teramura Y, Hamad OA, et al. Dangerous liaisons: complement, coagulation, and kallikrein/kinin cross-talk act as a linchpin in the events leading to thromboinflammation. Immunol Rev 2016;274(1):245–69.

63. Verschoor A, Langer HF. Crosstalk between platelets and the complement system in immune protection and disease. Thromb Haemost 2013;110(5):910–9.
64. Nording H, Langer HF. Complement links platelets to innate immunity. Semin Immunol 2018;37:43–52.
65. Hamzeh-Cognasse H, Damien P, Chabert A, et al. Platelets and infections – complex interactions with bacteria. Front Immunol 2015;6:82.
66. Wijeyewickrema LC, Lameignere E, Hor L, et al. Polyphosphate is a novel cofactor for regulation of complement by a serpin, C1 inhibitor. Blood 2016; 128(13):1766–76.
67. Saggu G, Cortes C, Emch HN, et al. Identification of a novel mode of complement activation on stimulated platelets mediated by properdin and C3(H2O). J Immunol 2013;190(12):6457–67.
68. Del Conde I, Crúz MA, Zhang H, et al. Platelet activation leads to activation and propagation of the complement system. J Exp Med 2005;201(6):871–9.
69. Hamad OA, Nilsson PH, Lasaosa M, et al. Contribution of chondroitin sulfate A to the binding of complement proteins to activated platelets. PLoS One 2010;5(9): e12889.
70. Atefi G, Aisiku O, Shapiro N, et al. Complement activation in trauma patients alters platelet function. Shock 2016;46(3 Suppl 1):83–8.
71. Wan P, Tan X, Xiang Y, et al. PI3K/AKT and CD40L signaling regulate platelet activation and endothelial cell damage in sepsis. Inflammation 2018;41(5):1815–24.
72. Gando S, Levi M, Toh CH. Disseminated intravascular coagulation. Nat Rev Dis Primers 2016;2:16037.
73. van der Poll T. Tissue factor as an initiator of coagulation and inflammation in the lung. Crit Care 2008;12(Suppl 6):S3.
74. Pawlinski R, Pedersen B, Schabbauer G, et al. Role of tissue factor and protease-activated receptors in a mouse model of endotoxemia. Blood 2004;103(4): 1342–7.
75. Levi M, Scully M, Singer M. The role of ADAMTS-13 in the coagulopathy of sepsis. J Thromb Haemost 2018;16(4):646–51.
76. Asehnoune K, Moine P. Protease-activated receptor-1: key player in the sepsis coagulation-inflammation crosstalk. Crit Care 2013;17(1):119.
77. Nieuwdorp M, Meuwese MC, Mooij HL, et al. Tumor necrosis factor-alpha inhibition protects against endotoxin-induced endothelial glycocalyx perturbation. Atherosclerosis 2009;202(1):296–303.
78. Bruegger D, Schwartz L, Chappell D, et al. Release of atrial natriuretic peptide precedes shedding of the endothelial glycocalyx equally in patients undergoing on- and off-pump coronary artery bypass surgery. Basic Res Cardiol 2011; 106(6):1111–21.
79. Korhonen EA, Lampinen A, Giri H, et al. Tie1 controls angiopoietin function in vascular remodeling and inflammation. J Clin Invest 2016;126(9):3495–510.
80. Kurniati NF, Jongman RM, vom Hagen F, et al. The flow dependency of Tie2 expression in endotoxemia. Intensive Care Med 2013;39(7):1262–71.
81. Mofarrahi M, Nouh T, Qureshi S, et al. Regulation of angiopoietin expression by bacterial lipopolysaccharide. Am J Physiol Lung Cell Mol Physiol 2008;294(5): L955–63.
82. Parikh SM. Dysregulation of the angiopoietin-Tie-2 axis in sepsis and ARDS. Virulence 2013;4(6):517–24.
83. Terpstra ML, Aman J, van Nieuw Amerongen GP, et al. Plasma biomarkers for acute respiratory distress syndrome: a systematic review and meta-analysis*. Crit Care Med 2014;42(3):691–700.

84. Witzenbichler B, Westermann D, Knueppel S, et al. Protective role of angiopoietin-1 in endotoxic shock. Circulation 2005;111(1):97–105.
85. David S, Mukherjee A, Ghosh CC, et al. Angiopoietin-2 may contribute to multiple organ dysfunction and death in sepsis*. Crit Care Med 2012;40(11):3034–41.
86. Bae JS, Kim YU, Park MK, et al. Concentration dependent dual effect of thrombin in endothelial cells via Par-1 and Pi3 Kinase. J Cell Physiol 2009;219(3):744–51.
87. Kaneider NC, Leger AJ, Agarwal A, et al. Role reversal' for the receptor PAR1 in sepsis- induced vascular damage. Nat Immunol 2007;8(12):1303–12.

Role of Antithrombin III and Tissue Factor Pathway in the Pathogenesis of Sepsis

Sarah Sungurlu, DO, Jessica Kuppy, MD, Robert A. Balk, MD*

KEYWORDS

- Antithrombin • Tissue factor • Sepsis • Coagulopathy • Multiple organ failure

KEY POINTS

- The pathobiology of sepsis reflects a complex interrelationship of inflammation and disorders of the coagulation system resulting in a dysregulated host response and organ dysfunction.
- Sepsis-associated coagulation system effects include both procoagulation (from tissue factor release, decreased levels of protein S, protein C, thrombomodulin, and antithrombin) and impaired fibrinolysis (related to PAI-1 and TAFI) combined with anticoagulation from factor and platelet consumption.
- Attempts to modify the sepsis outcome by administering supratherapeutic doses of antithrombin did not improve survival or reduce the development of organ dysfunction.
- Attempts to modify the septic process and improve mortality by administering tissue factor pathway inhibitor to impact the coagulation cascade did not improve survival.
- At this time, there is no mortality benefit associated with strategies to modify the coagulation system as part of the management strategy for sepsis or septic shock.

INTRODUCTION

Sepsis and septic shock are common in critically ill patients and are among the leading causes of morbidity and mortality despite efforts to improve early diagnosis and to streamline care with the aid of bundles and guidelines for optimum management.[1,2] The new definition of sepsis moves the focus away from an overwhelming proinflammatory response to infection to one that highlights the complexity of the sepsis pathobiology.[1,3] This complex relationship to pathogenesis takes into account contributions of the pathogen and host factors along with the pathobiologic sepsis process that results in an aberrant or dysregulated host response to infection and ultimately leads to organ dysfunction.[1,3,4] To date, there is no specific treatment that has been shown to

Division of Pulmonary, Critical Care, and Sleep Medicine, Rush Medical College and Rush University Medical Center, 1725 West Harrison Street, Suite 054, Chicago, IL 606012, USA
* Corresponding author.
E-mail address: Robert_Balk@rush.edu

Crit Care Clin 36 (2020) 255–265
https://doi.org/10.1016/j.ccc.2019.12.002
0749-0704/20/© 2019 Elsevier Inc. All rights reserved.
criticalcare.theclinics.com

improve the outcome of septic patients by either blocking or interrupting the systemic inflammatory response or the activation of the clotting system.[5] As many may remember, in 2001 it appeared that drotrecogin alfa (activated) (activated protein C [APC] marked as Xigris by Eli Lilly and Company) would be the first approved drug specifically for the treatment of severe sepsis and septic shock; however, the drug was taken off the market after subsequent clinical trials failed to demonstrate the needed survival benefit and side-effect profile.[6,7]

The present understanding of the sepsis pathobiologic pathways includes an appreciation of the complex interrelationship between the inflammatory response and perturbation of the coagulation system that may result in inappropriate microvascular coagulation, bleeding, or both.[5] The sepsis process appears to include activation of proinflammatory cytokines and other inflammatory molecules and the resultant damage to the endothelial cells of the microvasculature, which can lead to activation of the coagulation pathways by tissue factor (TF), production of coagulation abnormalities related to changes in concentration of protein C, protein S, thrombomodulin, and Antithrombin (AT) III, and the inhibition of the normal fibrinolytic pathways can result in microvascular thrombosis, organ ischemia/dysfunction/failure, and potentially, death.[1,5] It is not surprising that many of these components have been the target of innovative treatment strategies, which have attempted to improve the outcome of patients with sepsis and septic shock.[1,5] This article specifically highlights the role and impact of ATIII and TF in both the production and the possible treatment of sepsis and septic shock.

NORMAL PATHOPHYSIOLOGY AND ALTERATIONS IN SEPSIS

In the normal physiologic state, blood circulates through the vasculature in a relatively anticoagulated state as a consequence of the interaction of thrombomodulin coupling with thrombin with subsequent activation of protein C. APC is responsible for inhibiting factors Va and VIIIa (cofactors of the extrinsic and intrinsic procoagulant pathway, respectively) as shown in **Fig. 1**. In addition, plasminogen activator initiates fibrinolysis to reduce clot formation.[8] In the setting of sepsis, infectious agents and proinflammatory cytokines (tumor necrosis factor alpha [TNF-α], interleukin-1 [IL-1], IL-6) can activate the coagulation system by stimulating the release of TF from monocytes and the vascular endothelial cells.[9] Proinflammatory cytokines also inhibit the production of protein C and protein S, thrombomodulin, and ATIII. All the major physiologic anticoagulation mechanisms are thus impaired. In addition, tissue factor pathway inhibitor (TFPI) is also reduced as a result of the endothelial dysfunction.[10] Plasminogen activator inhibitor type 1 (PAI-1) and thrombin-activatable fibrinolysis inhibitor (TAFI) shut down the fibrinolytic system. The inflammatory mediators cause reduced thrombomodulin expression, making APC anticoagulation inefficient. Increased TF thus drives generation of thrombin, which subsequently converts fibrinogen to fibrin and activates platelets leading to clot formation and potentially disseminated intravascular coagulation (DIC), as demonstrated in **Fig. 2**.[8,11]

DISSEMINATED INTRAVASCULAR COAGULATION IN SEPSIS

Inflammation-induced activation of the clotting system, deposition of fibrin, and inhibition of fibrinolysis can be part of the host's defense system for containing inflammatory activity to sites of infection. However, increased generation of thrombin and coagulation pathway proteases may act as proinflammatory stimuli releasing excess cytokines and chemokines, thus amplifying the process.[4] This overly exuberant response may result in DIC as depicted in **Fig. 3**.[4] DIC is characterized by impaired

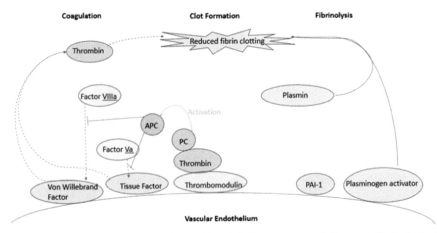

Fig. 1. Normal physiology in circulating blood: balancing coagulation and fibrinolysis. In normal physiology, anticoagulation is necessary in order to preserve blood flow. The thrombin-thrombomodulin complex interacts with protein C (PC) to form APC. APC prevents factor Va from interacting with TF (extrinsic pathway) and factor VIIIa from interacting with von Willebrand factor (intrinsic pathway), thereby inhibiting further thrombin formation. Plasminogen activator and plasmin also add to fibrinolysis to reduce any formed clots. (*Adapted from* Toussaint S, Gerlach H. Activated protein C for sepsis. *The New England journal of medicine.* Dec 31 2009;361(27):2646-2652.)

fibrinolysis and enhanced intravascular thrombin generation, leading clinically to a combination of excessive clot generation and bleeding tendency that can culminate in organ failure and death.[10] The excessive thrombin generation owing to overexpression of TF results in consumption of natural coagulation inhibitors (AT and protein C) and enhances platelet activation. Activated platelets form phospholipid surfaces, which complex with activated coagulation factors, thereby accelerating the clotting cascade.[10] The accelerated clotting cascade is the mechanism for the

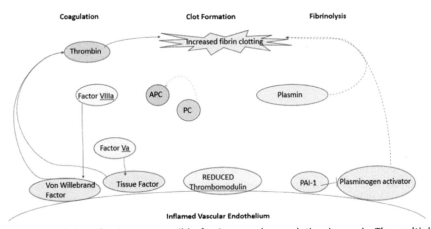

Fig. 2. Potential mechanisms responsible for increased coagulation in sepsis. The multiple potential mechanisms responsible for the production of increased coagulation in the setting of sepsis. (*Adapted from* Toussaint S, Gerlach H. Activated protein C for sepsis. *The New England journal of medicine.* Dec 31 2009;361(27):2646-2652.)

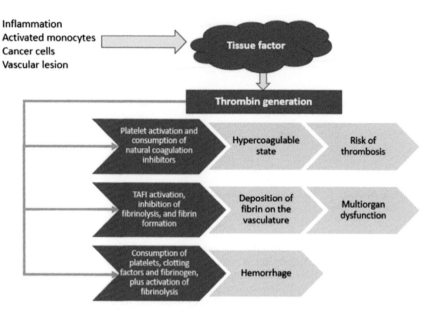

Fig. 3. Pathogenesis of DIC. The mechanism associated with the production of a hypercoagulable state, leading to the development of thrombosis, multiple organ dysfunction, and hemorrhage in the setting of DIC. (*Adapted from* Papageorgiou C, Jourdi G, Adjambri E, et al. Disseminated Intravascular Coagulation: An Update on Pathogenesis, Diagnosis, and Therapeutic Strategies. *Clinical and applied thrombosis/hemostasis : official journal of the International Academy of Clinical and Applied Thrombosis/Hemostasis.* Oct 8 2018:1076029618806424.)

hypercoagulable state of DIC. In addition, sustained thrombin generation leads to ongoing consumption of the clotting factors, fibrinogen, and platelets, resulting in the hemorrhagic state of DIC. The insufficient fibrinolysis secondary to PAI-1 and TAFI increases fibrin formation and deposition leading to thrombosis of the microvasculature, which can impair organ perfusion/function and result in the production of organ system dysfunction/failure. In addition, macrovascular thrombi may result in venous or arterial emboli.[12] A detailed discussion of the causes and ramifications of DIC is beyond the scope of this article and is covered in greater detail (See Ram Kalpatthi and Joseph E. Kiss's article, "Thrombotic Thrombocytopenic Purpura, Heparin Induced Thrombocytopenia and Disseminated Intravascular Coagulation," in this issue).

MULTIORGAN DYSFUNCTION/FAILURE

Critically ill patients are at increased risk for the development of organ system dysfunction/failure, and DIC is one of the potential mechanisms for the development of this significant complication in the critically ill septic patient.[4] As mentioned, insufficient fibrinolysis and resultant fibrin deposition can result in microvasculature thrombosis contributing to impaired organ perfusion and/or function and result in dysfunction/failure.[4] Studies have found no significant correlation between the plasma thrombin-AT complex (TAT) levels and the subsequent degree of multiorgan failure (MOF), although increased levels of circulating TAT are suspected to contribute to the development of this process. In addition, the inhibition of the fibrinolytic system by markedly elevated PAI-1 and TAFI levels plays a significant role in the development of MOF in septic patients who develop DIC. Extremely high levels of PAI and low levels of plasmin inhibitor complex have been correlated with the development of MOF in patients with DIC.[13]

ROLE OF ANTITHROMBIN IN THE COAGULOPATHY OF SEPSIS

ATIII, now commonly referred to as AT, is a single-chain glycoprotein produced by the liver. AT is a member of the serine protease inhibitor superfamily, which inhibits the intrinsic (factor XIa), extrinsic (factor VIIa), and common coagulation pathways (factor Xa, thrombin).[14] In its natural state, AT works to slowly neutralize serine enzymes. Glycosaminoglycans within vessel walls further increase AT activity.[15] AT is potentiated by heparin administration, which increases its activity by a factor of 1000, by competitively binding AT and preventing its interaction with heparan sulfate on endothelial cells.[16]

AT has been postulated to have anti-inflammatory properties, some of which are attributed to its inhibition of the clotting cascade and antithrombin effect. Thrombin activates platelets and endothelial cells, resulting in increased local inflammation. Platelets respond to local inflammation and secrete additional inflammatory mediators, recruiting neutrophils and other inflammatory cells, thus propagating the inflammatory process. In addition, AT induces prostacyclin release, which inhibits platelet aggregation and activation, and works further downstream by blocking neutrophil activity. AT binds to leukocyte and lymphocyte receptors, blocking their interaction with endothelial cells, thereby decreasing local inflammation. AT levels have been reported to be decreased in sepsis and septic shock patients, likely as a result of decreased synthesis, increased degradation by neutrophil elastase, and increased consumption related to increased thrombin generation as seen in DIC.[11] Various proinflammatory cytokines have been shown to further reduce synthesis of endogenous glycosaminoglycans, thereby indirectly decreasing AT activity.

ANTITHROMBIN TREATMENT OF SEPSIS

Recognizing that both inflammation and abnormal coagulation are important contributors to the septic response, it is not surprising that AT replacement therapy was proposed as a possible therapeutic strategy for patients with sepsis and DIC since the 1980s.[17] The observation that serum levels of AT, protein C, and protein S are all severely deficient in patients with sepsis provided additional support for this therapeutic strategy. Fourrier and colleagues[18] found that initial ATIII levels less than 50% predicted short-term mortality with a sensitivity of 96% and specificity of 76%. In a small clinical trial, Fourrier and coworkers[19] discovered that AT replacement in patients with sepsis and DIC reduced mortality by 44%, although this reduction was not statistically significant because of the small sample size. Harper and colleagues[20] administered AT replacement to patients with ATIII levels less than 70% of normal, and despite not finding a mortality benefit, they did discover that supplementation led to reduced renal impairment. Another small randomized clinical trial comparing AT versus placebo treatment in 42 patients with severe sepsis found a 39% reduction in mortality associated with AT treatment (25% mortality [5 of 20 patients] vs 41% mortality [9 of 22 patients]).[21] AT replacement therapy was found to be safe and well tolerated with minimal side effects. Although these initial clinical trials were too small to demonstrate a statistical survival benefit, the results were encouraging enough to lead to larger, multicenter clinical trials designed to evaluate the potential treatment benefit of AT replacement in sepsis.

In 2001, Warren and colleagues[22] conducted the largest prospective, randomized, multicenter, placebo-controlled, double-blind clinical trial evaluating the therapeutic effect of AT administration in 2314 patients with severe sepsis in the KyberSept trial. Patients were randomized to either receive high-dose AT or placebo, and the primary outcome was 28-day all-cause mortality. Secondary endpoints included mortality at 56 and 90 days, length of intensive care unit (ICU) stay, and occurrence of new organ dysfunction. Baseline AT levels were less than 60% of normal in more than 50% of patients in both treatment groups. No difference was observed in any of the designated primary or secondary outcomes of interest, including mortality at 28, 56, or 90 days. There was no difference in ICU length of stay between the groups. Furthermore, there was no difference in new-onset organ dysfunction. Again, this study confirmed that AT was safe and well tolerated (when administered without concomitant heparin). Finally, patients treated with AT did demonstrate an average of 115% increase in ATIII serum levels, whereas placebo-treated patients showed no significant increase.

In their discussion of the trial, the investigators postulated several theories to explain the observed lack of significant benefit. One of the theories was that less than 60% of patients enrolled in either group had reduced levels of circulating ATIII. Therefore, additional ATIII supplementation would not be expected to be beneficial. Furthermore, some suggest that a serum of level of 200% to 250% of normal would be required to achieve maximum benefit of AT administration, and that level was not achieved even with the high-dose supplementation used in this study. Finally, the subgroup of patients receiving concomitant heparin may have adversely impacted the outcome of the study because other trials have suggested that heparin can inhibit the natural anti-inflammatory properties of AT by blocking the binding to the glycosaminoglycans on the endothelial surface.[23,24] A subgroup analysis of ATIII administration with concomitant low-dose heparin for routine venous thromboembolism prophylaxis found that patients who received both did not respond as favorably to AT administration. Although there was no statistically significant difference in mortalities, they did find that there were more significant bleeding events with heparin coadministration.[23]

At present, there is little interest in further investigations of the role of AT treatment of sepsis and the coagulopathy of sepsis in the United States and Europe, but there remains an interest in Japan because of some encouraging findings in the early 2010s. A small study by Gando and coworkers[25] demonstrated that AT supplementation improved recovery from DIC. Another observational study of more than 1000 patients found a significant mortality benefit with AT supplementation in those patients with very low AT levels ($\leq$43% of normal).[26]

There has also been interest in the combination of AT and thrombomodulin, in sepsis with coagulation abnormalities. Thrombomodulin is an endothelial cell surface protein that activates protein C, producing APC, which works to inhibit thrombin formation.[27] As with AT, levels are greatly decreased in sepsis. In 2007, a small Japanese trial enrolled 234 patients with DIC randomized patients to receive either recombinant human soluble thrombomodulin or low-dose heparin and found that thrombomodulin supplementation improved DIC.[28] Thrombomodulin supplementation has been a treatment strategy in Japan since 2008, although no large prospective controlled trials have yet confirmed a survival benefit.

The recently published SCARLET trial was a randomized, double-blind, placebo-controlled, multinational, multicenter phase 3 clinical study conducted at 159 sites in 26 countries.[29] Eight hundred sixteen patients with sepsis-associated coagulopathy (defined as sepsis with an international normalized ratio [INR] >1.4 without other known cause and a platelet count of 30–150 $\times$ 10^9/L or a >30% decrease in platelet count in 24 hours) were randomized to receive either thrombomodulin supplementation or placebo for a period of 6 days. Unfortunately, there was no statistically significant mortality benefit at 28 days (26.8% mortality vs 29.4% mortality) for thrombomodulin versus placebo, respectively. The risk of serious bleeding complications was higher in the thrombomodulin group (5.8%) as compared with the placebo-treated group (4.0%).[29] There are some data to suggest that there may be a mortality benefit in highly selected patients with a severe coagulopathy who are treated with thrombomodulin, but more research is clearly needed regarding this claim.[30]

To date, there have not been any head-to-head trials comparing thrombomodulin and ATIII supplementation. A small trial of 129 patients with sepsis-induced DIC compared treatment with recombinant thrombomodulin and AT versus AT alone and found that combination therapy improved platelet counts and decreased D-dimer levels more quickly than AT monotherapy.[31] In addition, the 28-day mortality was significantly lower in the combination group than the monotherapy group. These data are encouraging, but larger, prospective, placebo-controlled, double-blind, multicenter clinical trials are needed to help establish the potential benefit of combination therapy in sepsis-associated coagulopathy.

In summary, at the present time, neither AT nor thrombomodulin supplementation is an approved therapy for the treatment of sepsis-induced coagulopathy in the United States. Although initial phase 2 research was encouraging, phase 3 trials have not found a significant mortality benefit associated with the use of replacement therapy for natural anticoagulants. There is some research to suggest that supplementation in highly selected patients with more severe coagulopathies may have some benefit, but this remains unconfirmed.

ROLE OF TISSUE FACTOR IN THE COAGULOPATHY OF SEPSIS

TF (thromboplastin) is a 47-kDa glycoprotein expressed as a transmembrane cell surface receptor in various cells in the vasculature.[32] Because the potent activating properties of TF make it highly thrombogenic, only minimal amounts are exposed in the circulating blood under normal physiology. However, in sepsis, TF is induced, secondary to bacterial endotoxins producing proinflammatory cytokines, including TNF-α, IL-1, IL-6, and IL-8 resulting in to the expression of TF on the surface of circulating monocytes and endothelial cells.[9] On exposure to blood, TF complexes with factor VII (in zymogen or activated form), creating the TF–factor VIIa complex (**Fig. 4**). This complex catalyzes the conversion of factors IX and X to their activated forms. Factor IXa and Xa then enhance the activation of factor X and prothrombin, respectively, effectively activating the common coagulation pathway and leading to the formation of thrombin.[10,33] Thus, TF initiates extrinsic clotting pathway leading to coagulation through activation of factor X and supports amplification through factor IX.[9]

The activation of TF and the extrinsic clotting system is inhibited by the natural anticoagulant TFPI. TFPI is a 276-amino-acid glycoprotein that has only 10% to 25% circulation in blood and normally is bound to the vessel wall through low-affinity binding to glycosaminoglycans. Circulating TFPI is bound to lipoproteins, and the levels vary in sepsis. The functional properties of circulating TFPI are not fully understood.[32] It acts as a Kunitz-type protease inhibitor, directly inhibiting the TF/factor VIIa complex when factor Xa is present by forming a quaternary complex.[11,34] This quaternary complex then blocks the generation of thrombin from prothrombin. DIC develops when there is an imbalance between TF and TFPI.

TISSUE FACTOR TREATMENT STRATEGIES IN SEPSIS

As previously discussed, endothelial damage occurs in sepsis and precipitates coagulation abnormalities. Endothelial cells respond and release cytokines and express adhesion molecules and growth factors, which affect the coagulation response.[10]

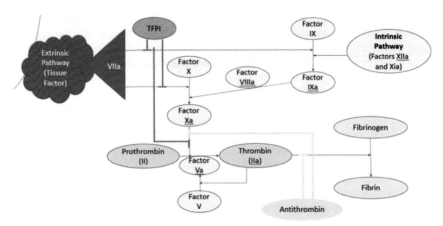

Fig. 4. Coagulation cascade: intrinsic, extrinsic, and common coagulation pathways. The activation of both the intrinsic and the extrinsic clotting pathways and their relationship to the common coagulation pathway. In addition, the action of the inhibitory molecules TFPI and AT is also shown as potential regulators of the coagulation cascade. (*Adapted from* reference Doshi SN, Marmur JD. Evolving role of tissue factor and its pathway inhibitor. *Critical care medicine*. May 2002;30(5 Suppl):S241-250.)

TFPI has been hypothesized to protect the microvasculature endothelium from excess coagulation during severe sepsis.[32,34] The relevance of TFPI has been illustrated in various experimental animal models.[34] For example, TFPI depletion sensitized rabbits to DIC, and recombinant TFPI infusion protected primates from DIC and improved hemodynamics when exposed to *Escherichia coli*. Recombinant protein tissue factor pathway inhibitor (rTFPI [tifacogin]) has an additional alanine residue on the aminoterminus, which resists glycosylation when expressed in bacteria.[34] In intraperitoneal infection rabbit models of sepsis, rTFPI was able to improve hematologic parameters of DIC and also reduce circulating levels of proinflammatory cytokines.[34]

In a clinical trial conducted in healthy human volunteers, exogenous recombinant TFPI blocked inflammation-induced thrombin generation, thereby raising hope that high concentrations of TFPI may modulate TF-mediated DIC.[10] A small phase 1 and 2 study enrolled 14 patients to receive rTFPI (at either 0.33 mg/kg/h or 0.66 mg/kg/h) versus placebo in patients with sepsis.[34] Three subjects in the treatment group had greater than expected anticoagulation (prolonged prothrombin time), and there was an apparent increase in serious adverse events involving bleeding. Lower dosages of rTFPI were subsequently studied using doses between 0.025 and 0.1 mg/kg/h without evidence of increased bleeding events.[34] Another phase 2 study was performed on 16 healthy patients who received intravenous bacterial lipopolysaccharide or endotoxin as an experimental simulator of gram-negative sepsis.[35] The infusion of rTFPI induced inhibition of thrombin generation without influencing the fibrinolytic or cytokine response.[12,35] There was a trend toward reduction in all-cause mortality in the rTFPI-treated group, which led Abraham[34] to evaluate the clinical value of rTFPI in the OPTIMIST phase 3 study.[12]

The primary objective of the OPTIMIST trial was to evaluate safety and efficacy of rTFPI (tifacogin) infused for 96 hours in patients with severe sepsis and a coagulopathy as manifested by an elevated INR ($\geq$1.2).[32] Unfortunately, the primary study population demonstrated no survival benefit with the administration of tifacogin.[32] There was an interesting time-dependent change in the outcome of the trial. The first 722 patients demonstrated a large difference in mortality, which favored patients receiving the rTFPI (38.9% vs 29.1%). However, the survival difference was not large enough to stop the study, and the subsequent 28-day mortality declined to the point of the final analysis, leading to no evidence of a survival advantage in patients receiving rTFPI versus placebo (34.2% vs 33.9%). Post hoc analysis could not find any bias or error (clerical, systematic, manufacturing) to explain this change.[36] The OPTIMIST trial also suggested that concomitant low-dose heparin may have influenced survival. Mortality was similar in TFPI recipients whether or not they received heparin (34.6% vs 34.0%, respectively), but in the placebo group, those who received heparin had a much lower mortality (29.8% vs 42.7%). A parallel cohort of patients who had low INR (<1.2) was also recruited, and it was found that in this subgroup the trend suggested that patients who received rTFPI were less likely to die (12% vs 23%); however, the sample size of this subgroup analysis was low, and this observation did not reach statistical significance.[32]

SUMMARY

The high rate of morbidity and mortality associated with sepsis and septic shock generated great interest if identifying a specific treatment. The first identified specific treatment to achieve Food and Drug Administration (FDA) approval was APC (drotrecogin alfa [activated], brand name Xigris).[6] This discovery centered a great deal of attention on targeting activation of the clotting system, an important component of sepsis pathobiology.[5] Among the additional strategies identified were administration of AT, TFPI, and thrombomodulin.[5,29] Observational studies and clinical trials then followed with some semblance of hope for additional therapies, but the additional trials of APC mandated by the FDA after the initial PROWESS study were terminated early for a significant improvement and failed to substantiate such improvement, and there were even concerns for potential harm in selected patients.[7] The FDA approval of APC was subsequently removed, and Xigris was taken off the market.

Unfortunately, subsequent large prospective, randomized, double-blind, placebo-controlled, multicenter clinical trials of AT, thrombomodulin, and TFPI have failed to demonstrate a significant survival benefit. With the withdrawal of the APC approval, the enthusiasm of the clinical and pharmaceutical community to continue costly investigations with clinical trials targeting the coagulation cascade faded rapidly. Japanese investigators and clinicians are still pursuing the investigation and participating in clinical use of some of these agents; however, before they rekindle the enthusiasm anticoagulation strategies had in the early 2000s, some substantial beneficial data from well-conducted large prospective, randomized clinical trials are needed. In the United States, this therapeutic strategy to treat sepsis and septic shock remains unsupported, and the potential bleeding risks outweigh the potential therapeutic benefits.

DISCLOSURE

The authors have no significant relationships to disclose related to this article.

REFERENCES

1. Prucha M, Zazula R, Russwurm S. Immunotherapy of sepsis: blind alley or call for personalized assessment? Arch Immunol Ther Exp (Warsz) 2017;65(1):37–49.
2. Rhodes A, Evans LE, Alhazzani W, et al. Surviving sepsis campaign: international guidelines for management of sepsis and septic shock: 2016. Intensive Care Med 2017;43(3):304–77.

3. Singer M, Deutschman CS, Seymour CW, et al. The third international consensus definitions for sepsis and septic shock (SEPSIS-3). JAMA 2016;315(8):801–10.

4. Abraham E, Singer M. Mechanisms of sepsis-induced organ dysfunction. Crit Care Med 2007;35(10):2408–16.

5. van der Poll T, van de Veerdonk FL, Scicluna BP, et al. The immunopathology of sepsis and potential therapeutic targets. Nat Rev Immunol 2017;17(7):407–20.

6. Bernard GR, Vincent JL, Laterre PF, et al. Efficacy and safety of recombinant human activated protein C for severe sepsis. N Engl J Med 2001;344(10):699–709.

7. Ranieri VM, Thompson BT, Barie PS, et al. Drotrecogin alfa (activated) in adults with septic shock. N Engl J Med 2012;366(22):2055–64.

8. Toussaint S, Gerlach H. Activated protein C for sepsis. N Engl J Med 2009; 361(27):2646–52.

9. Doshi SN, Marmur JD. Evolving role of tissue factor and its pathway inhibitor. Crit Care Med 2002;30(5 Suppl):S241–50.

10. Levi M, de Jonge E, van der Poll T. New treatment strategies for disseminated intravascular coagulation based on current understanding of the pathophysiology. Ann Med 2004;36(1):41–9.

11. Levi M, de Jonge E, van der Poll T. Rationale for restoration of physiological anticoagulant pathways in patients with sepsis and disseminated intravascular coagulation. Crit Care Med 2001;29(7 Suppl):S90–4.

12. Papageorgiou C, Jourdi G, Adjambri E, et al. Disseminated intravascular coagulation: an update on pathogenesis, diagnosis, and therapeutic strategies. Clin Appl Thromb Hemost 2018. https://doi.org/10.1177/1076029618806424.

13. Asakura H, Ontachi Y, Mizutani T, et al. An enhanced fibrinolysis prevents the development of multiple organ failure in disseminated intravascular coagulation in spite of much activation of blood coagulation. Crit Care Med 2001;29(6): 1164–8.

14. Ilias W, List W, Decruyenaere J, et al. Antithrombin III in patients with severe sepsis: a pharmacokinetic study. Intensive Care Med 2000;26(6):704–15.

15. Levi M, van der Poll T. Inflammation and coagulation. Crit Care Med 2010;38(2 Suppl):S26–34.

16. Opal SM, Kessler CM, Roemisch J, et al. Antithrombin, heparin, and heparan sulfate. Crit Care Med 2002;30(5 Suppl):S325–31.

17. Levi M. Antithrombin in sepsis revisited. Crit Care 2005;9(6):624–5.

18. Fourrier F, Chopin C, Goudemand J, et al. Septic shock, multiple organ failure, and disseminated intravascular coagulation. Compared patterns of antithrombin III, protein C, and protein S deficiencies. Chest 1992;101(3):816–23.

19. Fourrier F, Chopin C, Huart JJ, et al. Double-blind, placebo-controlled trial of antithrombin III concentrates in septic shock with disseminated intravascular coagulation. Chest 1993;104(3):882–8.

20. Harper PL, Williamson L, Park G, et al. A pilot study of antithrombin replacement in intensive care management: the effects on mortality, coagulation and renal function. Transfus Med 1991;1(2):121–8.

21. Eisele B, Lamy M, Thijs LG, et al. Antithrombin III in patients with severe sepsis. A randomized, placebo-controlled, double-blind multicenter trial plus a meta-analysis on all randomized, placebo-controlled, double-blind trials with antithrombin III in severe sepsis. Intensive Care Med 1998;24(7):663–72.

22. Warren BL, Eid A, Singer P, et al. Caring for the critically ill patient. High-dose antithrombin III in severe sepsis: a randomized controlled trial. JAMA 2001;286(15): 1869–78.

23. Opal SM. Therapeutic rationale for antithrombin III in sepsis. Crit Care Med 2000; 28(9 Suppl):S34–7.

24. Okajima K, Uchiba M. The anti-inflammatory properties of antithrombin III: new therapeutic implications. Semin Thromb Hemost 1998;24(1):27–32.

25. Gando S, Saitoh D, Ishikura H, et al. A randomized, controlled, multicenter trial of the effects of antithrombin on disseminated intravascular coagulation in patients with sepsis. Crit Care 2013;17(6):R297.

26. Hayakawa M, Kudo D, Saito S, et al. Antithrombin supplementation and mortality in sepsis-induced disseminated intravascular coagulation: a multicenter retrospective observational study. Shock 2016;46(6):623–31.

27. Iba T, Yamada A, Hashiguchi N, et al. New therapeutic options for patients with sepsis and disseminated intravascular coagulation. Pol Arch Med Wewn 2014; 124(6):321–8.

28. Saito H, Maruyama I, Shimazaki S, et al. Efficacy and safety of recombinant human soluble thrombomodulin (ART-123) in disseminated intravascular coagulation: results of a phase III, randomized, double-blind clinical trial. J Thromb Haemost 2007;5(1):31–41.

29. Vincent JL, Francois B, Zabolotskikh I, et al. Effect of a recombinant human soluble thrombomodulin on mortality in patients with sepsis-associated coagulopathy: the SCARLET randomized clinical trial. JAMA 2019;321(20):1993–2002.

30. Kato T, Matsuura K. Recombinant human soluble thrombomodulin improves mortality in patients with sepsis especially for severe coagulopathy: a retrospective study. Thromb J 2018;16:19.

31. Yasuda N, Goto K, Ohchi Y, et al. The efficacy and safety of antithrombin and recombinant human thrombomodulin combination therapy in patients with severe sepsis and disseminated intravascular coagulation. J Crit Care 2016;36:29–34.

32. Abraham E, Reinhart K, Opal S, et al. Efficacy and safety of tifacogin (recombinant tissue factor pathway inhibitor) in severe sepsis: a randomized controlled trial. JAMA 2003;290(2):238–47.

33. Ten Cate H. Pathophysiology of disseminated intravascular coagulation in sepsis. Crit Care Med 2000;28(9 Suppl):S9–11.

34. Abraham E. Tissue factor inhibition and clinical trial results of tissue factor pathway inhibitor in sepsis. Crit Care Med 2000;28(9 Suppl):S31–3.

35. de Jonge E, Dekkers PE, Creasey AA, et al. Tissue factor pathway inhibitor dose-dependently inhibits coagulation activation without influencing the fibrinolytic and cytokine response during human endotoxemia. Blood 2000;95(4):1124–9.

36. Angus DC, Linde-Zwirble WT, Clermont G, et al. Cost-effectiveness of drotrecogin alfa (activated) in the treatment of severe sepsis. Crit Care Med 2003; 31(1):1–11.

Red Blood Cell Dysfunction in Critical Illness

Stephen Rogers, PhD, Allan Doctor, MD*

KEYWORDS

- Erythrocyte • Red blood cell • O_2 delivery • Vasoregulation • Blood flow

KEY POINTS

- Together, all red blood cells (RBCs) at each stage of development may be considered an organ (termed the erythron), now appreciated to participate in active regulation of regional blood flow distribution as well as oxygen (O_2) and carbon dioxide (CO_2) transport.
- RBCs are subject to intense biochemical, biomechanical, and physiologic stress during repeated circulatory transit and, as such, possess unique properties and robust energetic and antioxidant systems to maintain functionality for a 3-month to 4-month lifetime.
- RBCs actively regulate blood flow volume and distribution to maintain coupling between O_2 delivery and demand. The trapping, processing, and delivery of nitric oxide (NO) by RBCs has emerged as a conserved mechanism through which regional blood flow is linked to biochemical cues of perfusion sufficiency.
- A new paradigm for O_2 delivery homeostasis has emerged, based on coordinated gas transport and vascular signaling by RBCs. By coordinating vascular signaling in a fashion that links O_2 and NO flux, RBCs couple vessel caliber (and thus blood flow) to O_2 need in tissue. Malfunction of this signaling system is implicated in a wide array of pathophysiologies and may in part explain the dysoxia frequently encountered in the critical care setting.

INTRODUCTION: THE ERYTHRON

Recently, the red blood cell (RBC) series, from progenitor cells to mature erythrocytes, has, collectively, been termed the erythron. The erythron comprises RBCs at all stages of development and is the organ (primarily composed of anucleated cells in suspension) responsible for oxygen (O_2) transport from lungs to tissue.[1] This role is newly appreciated to include active (by RBCs) vasoregulation that links regional blood flow to O_2 availability in the lung and to consumption in the periphery.[2] A considerable portion of the human

Funding: NIH R01GM113838, R42HL135965, U01AI126610 and Department of Defense W81XWH-17-1-0668.
Department of Pediatrics, Center for Blood Oxygen Transport and Hemostasis, University of Maryland School of Medicine, HSF III, 8th Floor, 670 West Baltimore Street, Baltimore, MD 21204, USA
* Corresponding author.
E-mail address: adoctor@som.umaryland.edu

nutritional and energy budget is devoted to maintaining a robust RBC population (20–30 trillion cells circulate in the average adult; approximately 85% of the cells in the body are RBCs); 1.4 million RBCs are released into the circulation per second, replacing ~1% of the circulating mass per day. Mature RBCs have a life span of ~4 months, most of which is spent traversing the microcirculation. It is estimated that RBCs travel approximately 400 km during this interval, having made 170,000 circuits through the vascular tree. Circulating RBCs show unique physiology and are adapted to withstand significant biomechanical and biochemical stress. As RBCs age, energy and antioxidant systems fail; key proteins (including hemoglobin [Hb] and lipids) suffer oxidative injury, negatively affecting performance (rheology, adhesion, gas transport, vascular signaling). Such cells acquire marks of senescence and are cleared by the spleen or undergo eryptosis (a process unique to RBCs, similar to apoptosis). Of importance, this process may be accelerated in the course of critical illness and thereby, by limiting O_2 delivery, influence organ failure progression and outcome.

Moreover, it is essential to note that, in the setting of insufficient O_2 delivery, blood flow (rather than content) is the focus of O_2 delivery regulation: O_2 content is relatively fixed, whereas flow is modulated by several orders of magnitude. Thus, blood flow volume and distribution are the physiologic parameters most actively regulated to maintain coupling between O_2 delivery and demand. Specifically, the trapping, processing, and delivery of nitric oxide (NO) by RBCs has emerged as a conserved mechanism through which regional blood flow is linked to biochemical cues of perfusion sufficiency. By coordinating vascular signaling in a fashion that links O_2 and NO flux, RBCs couple vessel caliber (and thus blood flow) to O_2 need in tissue. Malfunction of this signaling system is implicated in a wide array of pathophysiologies and may be explanatory in part for the dysoxia frequently encountered in the critical care setting.

CAPTURE AND RELEASE OF OXYGEN BY RED BLOOD CELLS

Hb is formed of 2 α and 2 β polypeptide chains, each carrying a heme prosthetic group, composed of a porphyrin ring bearing a ferrous atom that can reversibly bind an O_2 molecule. In the deoxygenated state, the Hb tetramer is electrostatically held in a tense (T) conformation. Binding of the first O_2 molecule leads to mechanical disruption of these bonds, an increase in free energy, and transition to the relaxed (R) conformation. Each successive O_2 captured by T-state Hb shifts the Hb tetramer closer to the R state, which has an estimated 500-fold increase in O_2 affinity.[3] This concept of thermodynamically coupled cooperativity in O_2 binding was first described by Bohr[4] and explains the sigmoidal appearance of the O_2-Hb binding curve, also known as the oxy-Hb dissociation curve (ODC) (**Fig. 1**). Moreover, understanding allosteric influence of protein function by heterotropic effectors (eg, for Hb, O_2, which binds to the active site [heme] is the homotropic ligand and all other molecules influencing the Hb-O_2 binding relationship are termed heterotropic effectors) was first achieved following description of Hb-O_2 affinity variation.[5] In addition to the homotropic effects of ligand binding on quaternary conformational changes (eg, cooperativity), primary ligand binding affinity (O_2) is also affected by multiple heterotropic effectors of significant physiologic relevance. The major heterotropic effectors that influence Hb O_2 affinity are hydrogen ion (H^+), chloride ion (Cl^-), carbon dioxide (CO_2), and 2,3-diphosphoglycerate (DPG).[3]

P_{50}, the oxygen tension at which 50% of Hb binding sites are saturated, is used as a standard means to quantify change in Hb-O_2 affinity and is inversely related to the binding affinity of Hb for O_2.[6] Increased levels of H^+, Cl^-, and CO_2 reduce O_2 binding affinity (eg, increase P_{50}). This allosteric shift in O_2 affinity, called the Bohr effect,[7]

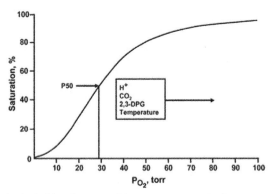

Fig. 1. The normal whole-blood O2 equilibrium curve. P_{50} is the P_{O_2} at which Hb is half-saturated with O_2. The principal effectors that alter the position and shape of the curve under physiologic conditions are indicated. DPG, 2,3-diphosphoglycerate. (*From* Winslow RM. The role of hemoglobin oxygen affinity in oxygen transport at high altitude. Respir Physiol Neurobiol 2007; 158:121-127; with permission.)

arises from the interactions among the heterotropic effectors listed earlier bound to different sites on Hb, all of which serve to stabilize the low-energy, low-affinity, T-state Hb conformation.[8] This effect is achieved by complex interactions among carbonic anhydrase (CA) and the band 3 (B3) membrane protein (also known as anion exchange protein 1 [AE1]). Specifically, CA generates H^+ and HCO_3^- from CO_2 encountered in the microcirculation; HCO_3^- then exchanges for Cl^- across the RBC membrane through AE1. As a consequence, extraerythrocytic CO_2 is converted into intraerythrocytic HCl by the CA-AE1 complex, thus acidifying RBC cytoplasm and increasing p50 (reducing affinity, also termed right-shifting the ODC). In addition, through the Haldane effect, CO_2 more directly decreases O_2 affinity (by binding to the N terminus of the globin chains to form a carbamino, further stabilizing T-state Hb); carbamino formation also releases another hydrogen ion (further reinforcing the right shift in ODC)[3] (**Fig. 2**). This set of reactions is reversed in the alkaline (and low-CO_2) milieu in the pulmonary circulation, leading to increased Hb-O_2 binding affinity (lower P_{50}). In sum, this physiology vastly improves O_2 transport efficiency by enhancing gas capture in the lung and release to tissue, and does so in proportion to perfusion sufficiency (in the setting of perfusion lack, acidosis and hypercapnia improve O_2 release). Of note, this tightly regulated modulation of O_2 affinity may become impaired in the setting of critical illness[9–12] and may, in part explain the dysoxia commonly observed in this setting.

Less acute modulation of P_{50} is achieved by DPG, a glycolytic intermediate that binds in an electrically charged pocket between the β chains of Hb, which stabilizes the T conformation, decreasing O_2 affinity and increasing P_{50}. DPG binding also releases protons, decreasing intracellular pH and further reinforcing the Bohr effect. DPG in RBCs increases whenever O_2 availability is diminished (as in hypoxia or anemia) or when glycolytic flux is stimulated.[13] In addition, temperature significantly influences Hb-O_2 affinity. As body temperature increases, affinity lessens (P_{50} increases, ODC shifts right); the reverse happens in hypothermia. This feature is of physiologic importance during heavy exercise, fever, or induced hypothermia. Note that clinical co-oximetry results and blood gas values are reported at 37°C, not at true in vivo temperature, and can lead to either underestimation or overestimation of true Hb O_2 saturation percentage (HbSo_2%) values and blood O_2 tension.[14]

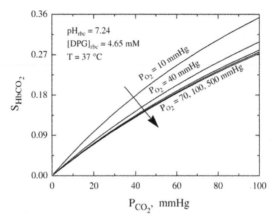

Fig. 2. The quantitative behavior of the carbaminohemoglobin (HbCO₂) dissociation curves at various oxygen tension levels. (*From* Dash RK, Bassingthwaighte JB. Erratum to: Blood HbO2 and HbCO2 dissociation curves at varied O2, CO2, pH, 2,3-DPG and temperature levels. Annals of biomedical engineering 2010; 38:1683-1701; with permission.)

RED BLOOD CELL BIOPHYSICAL FACTORS INFLUENCING TISSUE PERFUSION
Blood Rheology

Disease-based variation in blood fluidity has been recognized since the early twentieth century[15] and there is substantive evidence that this property strongly influences tissue perfusion.[16] Plasma is a newtonian fluid (viscosity is independent of shear rate); its viscosity is closely related to protein content, and, in critical illness, physiologically significant changes in viscosity may vary with concentration of acute phase reactants. However, whole blood is considered a non-newtonian suspension (fluidity cannot be described by a single viscosity value); whole-blood fluidity is determined by combined rheological properties of plasma and the cellular components.

The cellular components of blood, particularly RBCs, influence blood viscosity as a function of both number and deformability. RBC concentration in plasma (hematocrit) has an exponential relationship with viscosity and meaningfully diminishing tissue perfusion when hematocrit exceeds ~60 to 65%. RBC deformability, or behavior under shear stress, also strongly influences blood fluidity. Normal RBCs behave like fluid drops under most conditions, are highly deformable under shear, and orient with flow streamlines. However, during inflammatory stress, RBCs tend to aggregate into linear arrays like a stack of coins (rouleaux); fibrinogen and other acute phase reactants in plasma stabilize such aggregates, significantly increasing blood viscosity. Such a change in viscosity most affects O_2 delivery during low-flow (eg, low-shear) states (such as in critical illness) in the microcirculation.[17] RBC biomechanics and aggregation affect blood viscosity, strongly influencing the volume and distribution of O_2 delivery (again, more so in the low-shear microcirculation, or when vessel tone is abnormal).[18] This hemorheological physiology is perturbed by oxidative stress (common in critical illness)[19] and in sepsis,[20] which has been attributed to increased intracellular 2,3-DPG concentration,[21] intracellular free Ca^{2+},[22] and decreased intraerythrocytic ATP with subsequent decreased sialic acid content in RBC membranes.[23] Both increased direct contact between RBCs and white blood cells (WBCs) and reactive oxygen species released during sepsis have also been shown to alter RBC membrane properties.[24]

Red Blood Cell Aggregation and Adhesion

As noted earlier, in the absence of shear, RBCs suspended in autologous plasma stack in large aggregates, known as rouleaux. Acute phase reactants, especially fibrinogen, C-reactive protein, serum amyloid A, haptoglobin, and ceruloplasmin, have been shown to increase RBC aggregation.[25] Pathophysiologic conditions such as sepsis and ischemia-reperfusion injury have been shown to alter RBC surface proteins and increase RBC aggregability.[19] Activated WBCs are also thought to cause structural changes in the RBC glycocalyx and increase RBC aggregability.[26]

Under normal conditions, RBC adherence to endothelial cells (ECs) is insignificant and RBC deformability permits efficient passage through the microcirculation. Again, under normal conditions, enhanced EC adherence plays a role in the removal of senescent RBCs in the spleen. However, during critical illness, RBC-endothelial interactions are altered by RBC injuries associated with sepsis[27,28] and/or oxidative stress.[19] This finding is more prominent, with activated endothelium, as frequently occurs in critical illness.[29,30] Such RBC-endothelial aggregates create a physiologically significant increase in apparent blood viscosity.[18] Moreover, RBC adhesion directly damages the endothelium[31,32] and augments leukocyte adhesion,[33–35] further impairing apparent viscosity and microcirculatory flow. This phenomenon is commonly appreciated in the pathophysiology of vaso-occlusive crises in patients with sickle cell disease, malaria, diabetic vasculopathy, polycythemia vera, and central retinal vein thrombosis, but it may be more widespread than was originally appreciated.

Red Blood Cell Deformability

Tissue deformation can be defined as the relative displacement of specific points within a cell or structure. Mature RBCs are biconcave disks ranging from 2 to 8 μm in thickness, which act like droplets that deform reversibly under the shear encountered during circulatory transit.[18] Unique RBC geometry and deformability arise from (1) cytoplasmic viscosity and (2) specific interactions between the plasma membrane and underlying protein skeleton[23] (**Fig. 3**). Cytoplasmic viscosity is mainly determined by Hb concentration, which varies with intraerythrocytic hydration, which is actively regulated by ATP-dependent cation pumps.[36] The integral transmembrane membrane proteins AE-1 (also called B3) and glycophorins are reversibly anchored to a submembrane filamentous protein mesh composed of spectrin, actin, and protein 4.1. Linear extensibility of this mesh defines the limits of RBC deformability.[37] Maintenance of membrane-mesh interactions and robust RBC mechanical behavior depend on ATP-dependent ion pumps as well as support from NADPH (nicotinamide adenine dinucleotide phosphate, reduced form)-dependent antioxidant systems.[36] The sole energy source in RBCs is anaerobic glycolysis, which is discussed in detail later. RBC geometric and mechanical alterations secondary to impaired metabolism (leading to RBC dehydration, increased intraerythrocytic calcium level, and ATP/NADPH depletion) is a well-described consequence in blood stored for prolonged periods[38] and in RBCs subjected to significant metabolic stress during critical illness.[39,40]

REGULATION OF BLOOD FLOW DISTRIBUTION BY RED BLOOD CELLS

Microcirculatory blood flow is physiologically regulated to instantaneously match O_2 delivery to metabolic demand. This extraordinarily sensitive programmed response to tissue hypoperfusion is termed hypoxic vasodilation (HVD).[41] This process involves the detection of point-to-point variations in arteriolar O_2 content[42] with the subsequent initiation of signaling mechanisms capable of immediate modulation of vascular tone (**Fig. 4**).

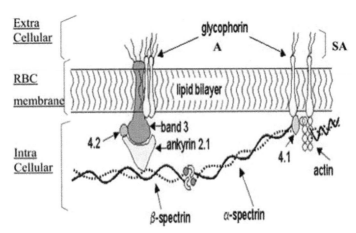

Fig. 3. The RBC membrane is composed of a phospholipid membrane bilayer and transmembrane proteins, including glycophorin A and B, and 3 proteins. Glycophorin A is the major sialoglycoprotein of the RBC. Sialic acid (SA) bound to glycophorin A is responsible for the negative charge of the RBC membrane. The intracellular compartment is constituted by spectrin (α and β subunits), actin, protein 4.1, and ankyrin. (*From*: Piagnerelli M, et al. Red blood cell rheology in sepsis. Intensive Care Med. 2003; 29(7):1052-1061; with permission.)

More than 30 years ago, intracellular RBC Hb was identified as a potential circulating O_2 sensor, following identification that, in severe hypoxia, O_2 content was more important than partial pressure of O_2 (Po_2) in the maintenance of regional O_2 supply.[43] It was later shown in vivo that $HbSo_2$ was independent of plasma or tissue Po_2 but was directly correlated with blood flow.[44] These findings implicated a role for RBCs in the regulation of O_2 supply, given the following evidence: (1) the Hb molecule within the RBC is the only component in the O_2 transport pathway directly influenced by O_2 content, and (2) the level of O_2 content of the RBC at a particular point in the circulation is linked to the level of O_2 use.[45]

With the vascular O_2 sensor identified, the mechanism involved in mediating the vasoactive response has remained in debate. To date, 3 $HbSo_2$-dependent RBC-derived signaling mechanisms have been proposed, the first 2 linked to the vasoactive effector NO, and the third to RBC ATP: (1) formation and export of S-nitrosothiols, "catalyzed" by Hb (SNO-Hb hypothesis),[46–48] (2) reduction of nitrite (NO_2^-) to NO by deoxygenated Hb (nitrite hypothesis),[49] and (3) hypoxia-responsive release of ATP (ATP hypothesis).[45,50] Each of these hypotheses is addressed further later.

Role of Red Blood Cell–Nitric Oxide Interactions in Vasoregulation

Interest in the free radical NO began with the identification of EDRF (endothelium-derived relaxing factor), first reported in 1980,[51] which resolved the apparent paradox as to why acetylcholine, an agent known to be a vasodilator in vivo, often caused vasoconstriction in vitro. Experiments performed with dissected segments of rabbit thoracic aorta mounted on a force transducer showed that handling of the tissue in a fashion that preserved endothelium always resulted in acetylcholine having relaxant properties. However, removal of the endothelium eradicated this action.[51,52] Identification of EDRF consequently led to a race to discover its chemical identity. It was not until 7 years later that 2 groups simultaneously published definitive studies

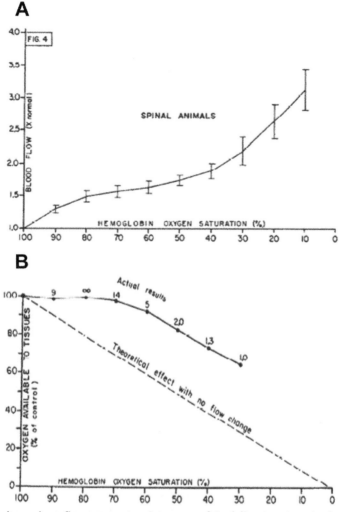

Fig. 4. Local vascular reflexes support maintenance of O_2 delivery to tissue in the setting of progressive hypoxia. In a classic article, Guyton[41] showed regional autoregulation of systemic blood flow in normal dogs (following spinal anesthesia) by observing variation in blood flow during constant-pressure blood perfusion of the femoral artery, while reducing the Hb O_2saturation percentage ($HbSo_2\%$) from 100% to 0% in the perfusing blood. (*A*) Stepwise reduction in $HbSo_2\%$ caused a progressive increase in blood flow through the leg. (*B*) These data show that autoregulation of blood flow occurs at a local level and this regulation serves to improve O_2supply when blood O_2content decreases. In addition, effects on blood flow were replicated by injecting partially deoxygenated versus oxygenated red blood cells into the artery, showing that effects could be elicited during arteriovenous transit (<1 second). (*From* Ross JM, Fairchild HM, Weldy J, Guyton AC. Autoregulation of blood flow by oxygen lack. *Am J Physiol.* 1962;202:21-24; with permission.)

characterizing and identifying EDRF as NO.[53,54] However, the means by which NO exerted its physiologic effects remained unknown, and effort focused on identifying the NO receptors. This effort characterized the classic signaling pathway for NO via soluble guanylate cyclase (sGC) and cyclic guanosine 3',5'-monophosphate (cGMP), which seemed to clarify the means by which NO achieves its myriad effects.[55] However, it is now appreciated that this pathway has little to do with the vasoregulation that governs regional blood flow distribution.

In terms of the HVD response (which underlies blood flow regulation), it is essential to appreciate that endothelium-derived NO plays no direct role in this reflex.[44,56] Because of O_2 substrate limitation, NO production by endothelial NO synthase (eNOS) is most likely attenuated by hypoxia.[57,58] NO derived from eNOS[46] (and perhaps other NOS isoforms[59] and/or nitrite[60]) is taken up by RBCs, transported, and subsequently dispensed in proportion to regional O_2 gradients to effect HVD at a time and place remote from the original site of NO synthesis. This key process enables RBCs to instantaneously modulate vascular tone in concert with cues of perfusion insufficiency, including hypoxia, hypercarbia, and acidosis.[46,47]

Metabolism of Endothelium-Derived Nitric Oxide by Red Blood Cells: Historical View

In the original NO paradigm, NO derived from (eNOS) was thought to play a purely paracrine role in the circulation, acting within the vicinity of its release.[61] Its metabolic fate was explained by the diffusion of the gas in solution and its terminal reactions (1) in vascular smooth muscle cells with the ferrous heme iron (Fe^{2+}) of sGC[62]; and (2) in the vessel lumen, with the heme group (Fe^{2+}) of oxy-Hb (the resultant oxidation reaction forming MetHb and nitrate), or deoxy-Hb (the resultant addition reaction forming iron nitrosyl Hb [HbNO]), or in plasma with dissolved O_2 (the resultant autoxidation reaction),[63] and/or O_2-derived free radicals including superoxide (O_2^-), hydrogen peroxide (H_2O_2), or hydroxyl radicals (OH^-). Several barriers were presumed to retard NO diffusing into the blood vessel lumen to react avidly with the abundance of Hb, including the RBC membrane, the submembrane protein matrix, and an unstirred layer around the RBC,[64,65] in addition to laminar blood flow.[66] These barriers were thought to limit these luminal reactions, thus allowing the local concentration of NO adjacent to ECs to increase sufficiently to provide a diffusional gradient for NO to activate the underlying vascular smooth muscle sGC. Reactions of NO in the bloodstream were assumed only to scavenge/inactivate NO via the formation of metabolites unable to activate sGC.[62]

Metabolism of Endothelium-Derived Nitic Oxide by Red Blood Cells: Modern View

A much broader biological chemistry of endothelial NO has been elucidated.[67–69] Most notable is the covalent binding of NO^+ to cysteine thiols, forming S-nitrosothiols (SNOs). This paradigm developed following the discovery that endogenously produced NO circulated in human plasma primarily complexed to the protein albumin (S-nitrosoalbumin[70]), which transformed the understanding of blood-borne NO signaling. SNO proteins thus offered a means to conserve NO bioactivity, allowing the storage, transport, and potential release of NO remote from its location of synthesis.[71] The SNO hypothesis was extended to include a reactive thiol of Hb (Cysβ93) that was shown to undergo S-nitrosylation and sustain bioactivity under oxygenated conditions and NO release under low-O_2 conditions (the SNO-Hb hypothesis).[46]

In this SNO paradigm, the NO radical must be oxidized to an NO^+ (nitrosonium) equivalent, which can then be passed between thiols in peptides and proteins preserving NO bioactivity.[67,68] S-nitrosylation then is akin to protein phosphorylation in terms of regulating protein function. SNO biochemistry offers NO a far broader signaling repertoire and has enabled awareness that the heme in sGC is not the sole, or even the principal, target of NO generated by endothelium. A wide array of alternative sGC (cyclic guanosine monophosphate)-independent reactions following eNOS activation have been identified.[69,72]

Processing and Export of S-nitrosothiols by Red Blood Cells

Hb S-nitrosylation (HbSNO), which has been characterized by both mass spectrometry[73] and X-ray crystallography,[74] provides an explanation as to how NO circumvents terminal reactions with Hb, enabling RBCs to conserve NO bioactivity and transport it throughout the circulation[46,47] (**Fig. 5**). The formation and export of NO groups by Hb is governed by the transition in Hb conformation that occurs in the course of O_2 loading/unloading during arteriovenous (AV) transit. This transition is caused by conformational-dependent change in reactivity of the $Cys\beta93$ residue toward NO, which is higher in the R (oxygenated) Hb state and lower in the T (deoxygenated) Hb state.[46,47]

In a tightly regulated fashion, Hb captures and binds NO at its β hemes and then passes the NO group from the heme to a thiol ($Cys-\beta93-SNO$).[60,75] Transfer of NO between heme and thiol requires heme-redox–coupled activation of the NO group, which is controlled by its allosteric transition across the lung.[76] Once in R state, the $Cys-\beta93$-SNO is protected through confinement to a hydrophobic pocket.[74] NO group export from $Cys-\beta93$-SNO occurs when steep O_2 gradients are encountered in the periphery (HVD). The R-state to T-state conformational transition that occurs on $Cys-\beta93$-SNO deoxygenation (or oxidation) results in a shift in the location of the β chain from its hydrophobic niche toward the aqueous cytoplasmic solvent.[74] This allows the $Cys-\beta93$-SNO to be chemically available for transfer to target thiol-containing proteins, including those associated with the RBC membrane protein AE-1 (band 3)[77] and extra-erythrocytic thiols.[78,79] Resultant plasma or other cellular SNOs, then become vasoactive at low-nanomolar concentrations.[46,47] Importantly, all NO transfers in this process involve NO^+,[46,48] which protects bioactivity from Fe^{2+} heme recapture and/or inactivation. SNOs are the only known endogenous NO compounds that retain bioactivity in the presence of Hb.[46,79,80]

Extensive evidence supports SNO-Hb biology, whereby RBCs exert graded vasodilator and vasoconstrictor responses across the physiologic microcirculatory O_2 gradient. RBCs dilate preconstricted aortic rings at low Po_2 (1% O_2), whereas they constrict at high Po_2 (95% O_2).[47,80–82] The vasodilatory response at low O_2 is enhanced following the addition of NO (or SNO) to RBCs, commensurate with SNO-Hb formation.[46,77,80,83] In addition, the vasodilatory response is enhanced in the presence of extracellular free thiol,[80] occurs in the absence of endothelium[48,80] (which is consistent with in vivo observation that HVD is endothelium independent[84]), and transpires in the time frame of circulatory transit, as confirmed by measurements of AV gradients in SNO-Hb.[46,78,81,82] In addition to these ex vivo experiments, numerous groups have also shown bioactivity of inhaled NO, commensurate with SNO-Hb formation.[85–89]

Metabolism of Nitrite by Red Blood Cells

Nitrite (NO_2^-), formed mainly via hydration reactions involving NOs, was long viewed as an inactive oxidation product of NO metabolism. More recently it has been proposed as circulating pool of bioactive NO.[90] Some investigators have suggested that the reduction of nitrite by deoxy-Hb may serve as the RBC-derived signaling mechanism regulating HVD.[91] However, this hypothesis has 2 major shortcomings in terms of known NO chemistry/biochemistry and HVD physiology. First, to influence vascular tone, the NO radical produced from NO_2^- must escape RBCs at low O_2 tension in order to elicit a vasodilatory response. However, experimental evidence

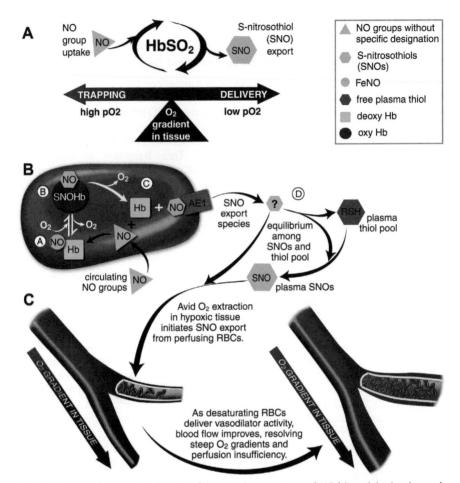

Fig. 5. RBCs transduce regional O_2 gradients in tissue to control NO bioactivity in plasma by trapping or delivering NO groups as a function of HbSo$_2$ saturation. (*A*) In this fashion, circulating NO groups are processed by Hb into the highly vasoactive (thiol-based) NO congener, S-nitrosothiol (SNO). By exporting SNOs as a function of Hb deoxygenation, RBCs precisely dispense vasodilator bioactivity in direct proportion to regional blood flow lack. (*B*) O_2 delivery homeostasis requires biochemical coupling of vessel tone to environmental cues that match perfusion sufficiency to metabolic demand. Because oxy-Hb and deoxy-Hb process NO differently (see text), allosteric transitions in Hb conformation afford context-responsive (O_2-coupled) control of NO bioavailability, thereby linking the sensor and effector arms of this system. Specifically, Hb conformation governs the equilibria among deoxy-HbFeNO (A; NO sink), SNO-oxy-Hb (B; NO store), and acceptor thiols including the membrane protein SNO-AE-1 (C; bioactive NO source). Direct SNO export from RBCs or S-transnitrosylation from RBCs to plasma thiols (D) or to endothelial cells directly (not shown) yields vasoactive SNOs, which influence resistance vessel caliber and close this signaling loop. Thus, RBCs either trap (A) or export (D) NO groups to optimize blood flow. (*C*) NO processing in RBCs (*A, B*) couples vessel tone to tissue Po$_2$; this system subserves hypoxic vasodilation in the arterial periphery and thereby calibrates blood flow to regional tissue hypoxia. (*From* Doctor A, Stamler JS. NO Transport in Blood: A third gas in the respiratory cycle. In: Comprehensive Physiology: Respiratory Physiology. Wagner P and Hlastala M, Ed's. American Physiological Society. Compr Physiol 1:541-568, 2011; with permission.)

unambiguously refutes the possibility of NO escaping RBCs as an authentic radical, especially given the proximity, high concentration, and diffusion limited reaction kinetics of authentic NO with deoxy-Hb. The only plausible reconciliation of this is that bioactivity from this reaction may derive from heme-captured NO ($HbFe^{2+}NO$) being further converted into SNO-Hb,[60,75] because $HbFe^{2+}NO$ itself acts as a vasoconstrictor rather than vasodilator.[92] The second shortcoming relates to the NO_2^- reductase activity of deoxy-Hb purportedly being symmetric across the physiologic O_2 gradient,[93,94] with maximal activity occurring at the P_{50} of Hb (~ 27 mm Hg).[93,95] This reaction profile does not match the HVD response, which increases in a steadily graded fashion as Po_2 decreases in the physiologic range from 100 mm Hg down to approximately 5 mm Hg ($HbSo_2 \sim 1\%-2\%$).[41,44] If RBC-based vasoactivity were maximal at Hb's P_{50}, then blood flow would be diverted away from regions with Po_2 less than 27 mm Hg, where it would be needed most. In addition, based on the symmetry of Hb nitrite reductase activity at the P_{50}, RBCs traversing vascular beds with Po_2 at 25 or 75 mm Hg would generate equal NO-based activity,[91] where different blood flow demands are required.

Vasoregulation by Red Blood Cell–Derived ATP

ATP has long been known to act as an endothelium-dependent vasodilator in humans,[45] binding to P_2Y purinergic receptors to induce local and conducted vasodilation via stimulation of vasoactive signals, including endothelial NO, prostaglandins, and endothelial-derived hyperpolarization factors. More recently, RBCs have been identified as sources of vascular ATP,[45,96] with release stimulated by conditions associated with diminished O_2 supply relative to demand, hypoxia, hypercapnia, and low pH.[45,97] O_2 offloading from membrane-associated Hb is thought to initiate RBC ATP release,[96] stimulating heterotrimeric G protein,[98] as a result of membrane deformation. This process leads to activation of adenylyl cyclase and an increase in cAMP,[99] which activates protein kinase A (PKA).[99] PKA stimulates cystic fibrosis transmembrane conductance regulator (CFTR),[100] which activates release of ATP from the RBC via pannexin 1.[101] Release of ATP via this pathway requires an increase in intracellular cyclic AMP (cAMP), which is controlled by the relative activities of adenylyl cyclase and phosphodiesterase 3 (PDE3B).[50]

Despite potential as an HVD mediator, RBC-derived ATP falls short on 2 fronts. First, HVD is unaltered by both endothelial denudation and eNOS deletion,[48] but ATP vasoactivity is endothelial dependent. Second, blood levels of ATP increase and decrease over a period of minutes, which is not commensurate with the HVD response that occurs in the course of AV transit over a couple of seconds. Despite its shortcomings in terms of acting as a primary mediator of HVD, it is likely that Hb and ATP serve complementary vasoactive roles, in acute local and prolonged systemic hypoxia respectively.[48]

RED BLOOD CELL ENERGETICS AND CONSEQUENCES OF ANTIOXIDANT SYSTEM FAILURE

RBCs produce ATP by glycolysis only, with 2 branches:[102] the Embden-Meyerhof pathway (EMP) and the hexose monophosphate pathway (HMP).[103] Importantly, the HMP is the sole means for recycling NADPH,[104] which powers the thiol-based antioxidant system.[104] HMP flux is gated by protein complex assembly on the cytoplasmic domain of the band 3 membrane protein (cdB3 metabolon).[105–112] HMP flux oscillates with Po_2, as a function of Hb conformation and cdB3 phosphorylation (**Fig. 6** A, B).[107,108,113–117] Of note, RBC antioxidant systems fail when HMP flux is blunted by

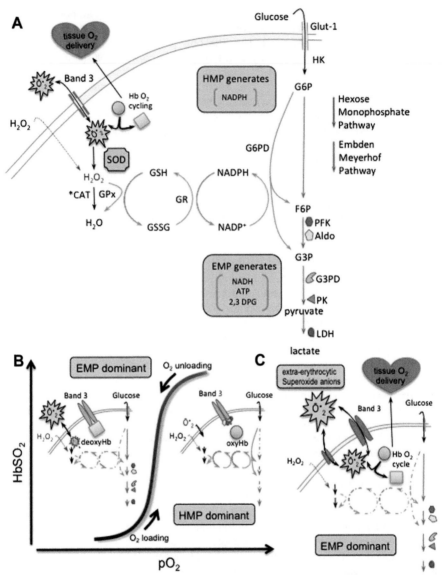

Fig. 6. Simplified scheme of cdB3-based control of RBC metabolism and proposed causal path for sepsis-induced red cell dysfunction. (*A*) Energy metabolism in RBCs proceeds through either the EMP (*orange arrows*), or the HMP (*blue arrows*, also called the pentose shunt). Both share glucose-6 phosphate (G6P) as initial substrate. The HMP is the sole source of NADPH in RBCs and generates fructose-6-phosphate (F6P) or glyceraldehyde-3-phosphate (G3P), which rejoin the EMP before G3P dehydrogenase (G3PD/GAPDH), a key regulatory point. The EMP generates NADH (nicotinamide adenine dinucleotide plus hydrogen; used by methemoglobin reductase), as well as ATP (to drive ion pumps) and 2,3-DPG (to modulate Hb P_{50}). H_2O_2 and O_2^- are the principal endogenous reactive O_2 species (ROS) that are generated/encountered by RBCs. Both ROS are generated internally in the course of HbO_2 cycling.[220–222] Notably, only H_2O_2 can cross the membrane directly. O_2^- enters/departs RBCs via the band 3 channel (anion exchange protein 1, or AE-1). O_2^- and H_2O_2 are ultimately reduced to water by catalase (CAT) or glutathione peroxidase (GPx). (*B*) O_2 content

altered cdB3 protein assembly/phosphorylation caused by aberrant Hbs or hypoxia.[102,118] Strikingly similar perturbations to cdB3 are reported in sepsis,[119,120] possibly arising from caspase 3 activation[121-123] and/or direct endotoxin or complement membrane binding[124-131] (altering metabolon assembly, glycolysis, and ROS clearance).[110,132,133] As such, it seems that that sepsis (particularly, in the setting of hypoxic and/or uremic/oxidative[134-141] environments) disturbs cdB3-based metabolic control (**Fig. 6**C), leading to (1) EMP activation, (2) limited glucose-6-phosphate availability, (3) HMP flux constraint, (4) depowered NADPH/glutathione (GSH) recycling, (4) antioxidant system failure, and (5) injury to proteins/lipids that are key to O_2 delivery homeostasis (sepsis-induced red cell dysfunction [SiRD]). This full pattern has been reported in other settings affecting protein assembly at cdB3[102,118]; further, such an HMP constraint has functional similarity to glucose-6 phosphate dehydrogenase (G6PD) deficiency,[102] which amplifies vulnerability to sepsis.[142-144] Moreover, hypoxia critically limits RBC energetics and depowers RBC antioxidant systems.[102,118] In health, $O_2\bullet$ abundance is tightly regulated by the superoxide dismutase (SOD) family[145]; however, overwhelming $O_2\bullet$ genesis[146] is implicated in sepsis-associated injury cascades.[147,148] Of note, sepsis-associated $O_2\bullet$ excess injures RBCs, impairing O_2 delivery by altering control of O_2 affinity,[9-12] NO processing,[78,149,150] rheology,[20,23,127,128,151-153] and adhesion.[154,155] $O_2\bullet$ excess also disrupts vasoregulation via NO consumption and catecholamine inactivation in plasma.[156-162] Specifically, ROS sourced directly to RBCs[163-166] injure vessels.[167,168] Such reciprocal injuries mutually escalate and, as such, the dysoxia characteristic of septic shock (ischemia despite adequate blood O_2 content and cardiac output)[169-172] may arise from SiRD-vascular interactions.[27,28] Notably, ROS excess is also a common consequence of uremia/kidney injury,[134-141] particularly during sepsis.[173-179] As such, the combination of lung injury (hypoxia) and kidney injury (uremia) simultaneously constrains RBC energetics and antioxidant systems and presents substantive oxidant loading conditions, meaningfully increasing RBC injury risk.

ACQUIRED RED BLOOD CELL INJURY, ERYPTOSIS, AND CLEARANCE

After maturation to an anucleated cell furnished with the metabolic systems described earlier, the estimated normal life span of a mature RBC is 110 to 120 days.[180] To date, clearance of normal senescent RBCs has not been clearly understood. Two mechanisms have been proposed: clustering of the B3 membrane protein[181-184] and externalization of membrane phosphatidyl serine (PS),[185-188] and both of these processes may be accelerated in the setting of critical illness, impairing O_2 transport capacity.

---

modulates EMP/HMP balance via reciprocal binding for cdB3 between deoxy-Hb and key EMP enzymes (phosphofructokinase, aldolase, G3PD, pyruvate kinase, and lactate dehydrogenase;). In oxygenated RBCs (right half of stylized O_2 dissociation plot), EMP enzyme sequestration to cdB3 inactivates this pathway, resulting in HMP dominance and maximal NADPH (and thus GSH) recycling capacity. In deoxygenated RBCs (left half of O_2 dissociation plot), deoxy-Hb binding to cdB3 disperses bound EMP enzymes, activating the EMP, creating G6P substrate competition, constraining HMP flux, limiting NADPH and GSH recycling capacity, and weakening resilience to ROS such as O_2^-. (C) In sepsis, data suggest cdB3-complex assembly may be prevented (particularly with coincident hypoxia; see text). As in settings similarly affecting the cdB3 complex, it seems that this disturbs normal EMP/HMP balance (disfavoring HMP), depowering antioxidant systems and rendering RBCs vulnerable to oxidant attack. GR, glutathione reductase; GSH, glutathione.

Oxidatively modified Hb forms hemichrome aggregates, which associate with the cytoplasmic domain of the abundant membrane protein B3. Subsequent clustering of B3 exofascial domains increases affinity of naturally occurring anti-B3 autoantibodies, which activate the complement system leading to RBC uptake and destruction by macrophages.[189] Normally, PS is asymmetrically distributed in the plasma membrane (a process regulated by flippases). Disruption of this pattern is a well-documented mark of RBC senescence,[185–188] signaling RBC removal by the reticuloendothelial system.[188] Alternatively, RBCs may proceed through a form of stimulated suicide similar to apoptosis (termed eryptosis), which is characterized by cell shrinkage and cell membrane scrambling and is stimulated by Ca^{2+} entry through Ca^{2+}-permeable, prostaglandin E2 –activated cation channels, by ceramide, caspases, calpain, complement, hyperosmotic shock, energy depletion, oxidative stress, and deranged activity of several common kinases. Eryptosis has been described in the setting of ethanol intoxication, malignancy, hepatic failure, diabetes, chronic renal insufficiency, hemolytic uremic syndrome, dehydration, phosphate depletion, fever, sepsis, mycoplasma infection, malaria, iron deficiency, sickle cell anemia, thalassemia, G6PD deficiency, and Wilson disease.[144,188,190]

INFLUENCE OF RED BLOOD CELLS ON HEMOSTASIS

The principal impact of RBCs in clot formation in vivo is rheological, because RBC laminar shearing promotes platelet margination,[191] as well as RBC aggregation and deformability of RBCs, which also support clot assembly/retraction.[192] In addition, RBCs interact directly and indirectly with ECs and platelets during thrombosis.[193] Both the stiffness of RBCs and the extent to which they form a procoagulant surface to generate thrombin through exposure of phosphatidylserine seem to play important roles, both in clot initiation and completion.[194,195] Moreover, RBC-derived microparticles (MPs) transfused with stored RBCs or formed in various pathologic conditions associated with hemolysis have strong procoagulant potential along with prothrombotic effects of the extracellular Hb and heme.[196] In addition, RBCs directly interact with fibrin(ogen) and affect the structure, mechanical properties, and lytic resistance of clots and thrombi.[197] In addition, tessellated polyhedral RBCs (polyhedrocytes) are recognized to be a significant structural component of contracted clots, enabling the impermeable barrier important for hemostasis and wound healing.[198]

SUMMARY: RED BLOOD CELL DYSFUNCTION DISRUPTS OF OXYGEN DELIVERY DURING CRITICAL ILLNESS

Evidence is mounting in support of a causal relationship between acquired RBC dysfunction and a host of perfusion-related morbidities that complicate critical illness.[82,163,164,199–212] Recently, it has been observed that levels of SNO-Hb are altered in several disease states characterized by disordered tissue oxygenation.[82,83,89,149,150,213–217] In addition, where examined, RBCs from such patients show impaired vasodilatory capacity.[78,82,83,214,216–218] These data suggest that altered RBC-derived NO bioactivity may contribute to human pathophysiology. Specifically, alterations in thiol-based RBC NO metabolism have been reported in congestive heart failure,[82] diabetes,[83,213] pulmonary hypertension,[81,89] and sickle cell disease,[214,219] all of which are conditions characterized by inflammation, oxidative stress, and dysfunctional vascular control. Moreover, known crosstalk between SNO signaling and cellular communication via carbon monoxide, serotonin, prostanoids, catecholamines, and endothelin may permit broad dispersal of signals generated by dysfunctional RBCs. Precise understanding of the roles of dysregulated RBC-based

NO transport in the spread of vasomotor dysfunction from stressed vascular beds may open novel therapeutic approaches to a range of disorders.

CONFLICTS OF INTEREST

A. Doctor has received research funding and/or consulting fees from Viasys Inc, Entegrion Inc, Terumo BCT, Fresenius Kabi, Galleon Pharmaceuticals, Nitrox LLD, Nitric BioTherapeutics, Galera Inc, and Novartis. A. Doctor holds intellectual property related to biosynthetic artificial RBCs and holds equity in and is CSO of KaloCyte, Inc, which is developing this technology. S. Rogers has no conflicts to declare.

REFERENCES

1. Kaushansky K. Williams hematology. 8th edition. New York: McGraw-Hill; 2010.
2. Doctor A, Stamler JS. Nitric oxide transport in blood: a third gas in the respiratory cycle. Compr Physiol 2011;1(1):541–68.
3. Hsia CC. Respiratory function of hemoglobin. N Engl J Med 1998;338(4): 239–47.
4. Edsall JT. Understanding blood and hemoglobin: an example of international relations in science. Perspect Biol Med 1986;29(3 Pt 2):S107–23.
5. Edsall JT. Hemoglobin and the origins of the concept of allosterism. Fed Proc 1980;39(2):226–35.
6. Winslow RM. The role of hemoglobin oxygen affinity in oxygen transport at high altitude. Respir Physiol Neurobiol 2007;158(2–3):121–7.
7. Bohr C, Hasselbalch K, Krogh A. Ueber einen in biologischer Beziehung wichtigen Einfluss, den die Kohlensäurespannung des Blutes auf dessen Sauerstoffbindung übt. Skand Arch Physiol 1904;16:402–12.
8. Margaria R, Green AA. The first dissociation constant, pK 1, of carbonic acid in hemoglobin solutions and its relation to the existence of a combination of hemoglobin with carbon dioxide. J Biol Chem 1933;102:611–34.
9. Leon K, Pichavant-Rafini K, Quemener E, et al. Oxygen blood transport during experimental sepsis: effect of hypothermia*. Crit Care Med 2012;40(3):912–8.
10. Ibrahim Eel D, McLellan SA, Walsh TS. Red blood cell 2,3-diphosphoglycerate concentration and in vivo P50 during early critical illness. Crit Care Med 2005; 33(10):2247–52.
11. Tuynman HA, Thijs LG, Straub JP, et al. Effects of glucose-insulin-potassium (GIK) on the position of the oxyhemoglobin dissociation curve, 2.3-diphosphoglycerate, and oxygen consumption in canine endotoxin shock. J Surg Res 1983;34(3):246–53.
12. Johnson G Jr, McDevitt NB, Proctor HJ. Erythrocyte 2,3-diphosphoglycerate in endotoxic shock in the subhuman primate: response to fluid and-or methylprednisolone succinate. Ann Surg 1974;180(5):783–6.
13. Bunn HF, Jandl JH. Control of hemoglobin function within the red cell. N Engl J Med 1970;282(25):1414–21.
14. Severinghaus JW. Oxyhemoglobin dissociation curve correction for temperature and pH variation in human blood. J Appl Physiol 1958;12(3):485–6.
15. Robin Fahraeus TL. The viscosity of the blood in narrow capillary tubes. Am J Physiol 1931;96:562–8.
16. Copley AL. Fluid mechanics and biorheology. Thromb Res 1990;57(3):315–31.
17. McHedlishvili G, Varazashvili M, Gobejishvili L. Local RBC aggregation disturbing blood fluidity and causing stasis in microvessels. Clin Hemorheol Microcirc 2002;26(2):99–106.

18. Baskurt OK, Meiselman HJ. Blood rheology and hemodynamics. Semin Thromb Hemost 2003;29(5):435–50.
19. Baskurt OK, Temiz A, Meiselman HJ. Effect of superoxide anions on red blood cell rheologic properties. Free Radic Biol Med 1998;24(1):102–10.
20. Piagnerelli M, Boudjeltia KZ, Vanhaeverbeek M, et al. Red blood cell rheology in sepsis. Intensive Care Med 2003;29(7):1052–61.
21. Suzuki Y, Nakajima T, Shiga T, et al. Influence of 2,3-diphosphoglycerate on the deformability of human erythrocytes. Biochim Biophys Acta 1990;1029(1): 85–90.
22. Todd JC 3rd, Mollitt DL. Effect of sepsis on erythrocyte intracellular calcium homeostasis. Crit Care Med 1995;23(3):459–65.
23. Piagnerelli M, Boudjeltia KZ, Brohee D, et al. Alterations of red blood cell shape and sialic acid membrane content in septic patients. Crit Care Med 2003;31(8): 2156–62.
24. Machiedo GW, Powell RJ, Rush BF Jr, et al. The incidence of decreased red blood cell deformability in sepsis and the association with oxygen free radical damage and multiple-system organ failure. Arch Surg 1989;124(12):1386–9.
25. Somer T, Meiselman HJ. Disorders of blood viscosity. Ann Med 1993;25(1):31–9.
26. Baskurt OK, Meiselman HJ. Activated polymorphonuclear leukocytes affect red blood cell aggregability. J Leukoc Biol 1998;63(1):89–93.
27. Aird WC. The hematologic system as a marker of organ dysfunction in sepsis. Mayo Clin Proc 2003;78(7):869–81.
28. Goyette RE, Key NS, Ely EW. Hematologic changes in sepsis and their therapeutic implications. Semin Respir Crit Care Med 2004;25(6):645–59.
29. Anniss AM, Sparrow RL. Variable adhesion of different red blood cell products to activated vascular endothelium under flow conditions. Am J Hematol 2007; 82(6):439–45.
30. Tissot Van Patot MC, MacKenzie S, Tucker A, et al. Endotoxin-induced adhesion of red blood cells to pulmonary artery endothelial cells. Am J Physiol 1996;270(1 Pt 1):L28–36.
31. Zoukourian C, Wautier MP, Chappey O, et al. Endothelial cell dysfunction secondary to the adhesion of diabetic erythrocytes. Modulation by iloprost. Int Angiol 1996;15(3):195–200.
32. Sirois E, Charara J, Ruel J, et al. Endothelial cells exposed to erythrocytes under shear stress: an in vitro study. Biomaterials 1998;19(21):1925–34.
33. Munn LL, Melder RJ, Jain RK. Role of erythrocytes in leukocyte-endothelial interactions: mathematical model and experimental validation. Biophys J 1996;71(1): 466–78.
34. Migliorini C, Qian Y, Chen H, et al. Red blood cells augment leukocyte rolling in a virtual blood vessel. Biophys J 2002;83(4):1834–41.
35. Zennadi R, Chien A, Xu K, et al. Sickle red cells induce adhesion of lymphocytes and monocytes to endothelium. Blood 2008;112(8):3474–83.
36. Mohandas N, Shohet SB. The role of membrane-associated enzymes in regulation of erythrocyte shape and deformability. Clin Haematol 1981;10(1):223–37.
37. Mohandas N. The red blood cell membrane. In: Hoffman RBE, Shattil SJ, Furie B, et al, editors. Hematology: basis, principles and practice. New York: Churchill-Livingstone; 1991. p. 264–9.
38. Rendell M, Luu T, Quinlan E, et al. Red cell filterability determined using the cell transit time analyzer (CTTA): effects of ATP depletion and changes in calcium concentration. Biochim Biophys Acta 1992;1133(3):293–300.

39. Kayar E, Mat F, Meiselman HJ, et al. Red blood cell rheological alterations in a rat model of ischemia-reperfusion injury. Biorheology 2001;38(5–6):405–14.
40. Baskurt O. Activated granulocyte induced alterations in red blood cells and protection by antioxidant enzymes. Clin Hemorheol Microcirc 1996;16:49–56.
41. Ross JM, Fairchild HM, Weldy J, et al. Autoregulation of blood flow by oxygen lack. Am J Physiol 1962;202:21–4.
42. Roy CS, Brown JG. The blood-pressure and its variations in the arterioles, capillaries and smaller veins. J Physiol 1880;2(5–6):323–446.
43. Stein JC, Ellsworth ML. Capillary oxygen transport during severe hypoxia: role of hemoglobin oxygen affinity. J Appl Physiol 1985;75(4):1601–7.
44. Gonzalez-Alonso J, Richardson RS, Saltin B. Exercising skeletal muscle blood flow in humans responds to reduction in arterial oxyhaemoglobin, but not to altered free oxygen. J Physiol 2001;530(Pt 2):331–41.
45. Ellsworth ML, Forrester T, Ellis CG, et al. The erythrocyte as a regulator of vascular tone. Am J Physiol 1995;269(6 Pt 2):H2155–61.
46. Jia L, Bonaventura C, Bonaventura J, et al. A dynamic activity of blood involved in vascular control. Nature 1996;380(6571):221–6.
47. Stamler JS, Jia L, Eu JP, et al. Blood flow regulation by S-nitrosohemoglobin in the physiological oxygen gradient. Science 1997;276(5321):2034–7.
48. Singel DJ, Stamler JS. Chemical physiology of blood flow regulation by red blood cells: the role of nitric oxide and S-nitrosohemoglobin. Annu Rev Physiol 2005;67:99–145.
49. Gladwin MT, Shelhamer JH, Schechter AN, et al. Role of circulating nitrite and S-nitrosohemoglobin in the regulation of regional blood flow in humans. Proc Natl Acad Sci U S A 2000;97(21):11482–7.
50. Ellsworth ML, Ellis CG, Goldman D, et al. Erythrocytes: oxygen sensors and modulators of vascular tone. Physiology (Bethesda) 2009;24:107–16.
51. Furchgott RF, Zawadzki JV. The obligatory role of endothelial cells in the relaxation of arterial smooth muscle by acetylcholine. Nature 1980;288(5789):373–6.
52. Furchgott RF. Endothelium-derived relaxing factor: discovery, early studies, and identification as nitric oxide. Biosci Rep 1999;19(4):235–51.
53. Ignarro LJ, Buga GM, Wood KS, et al. Endothelium-derived relaxing factor produced and released from artery and vein is nitric oxide. Proc Natl Acad Sci U S A 1987;84(24):9265–9.
54. Palmer RM, Ferrige AG, Moncada S. Nitric oxide release accounts for the biological activity of endothelium-derived relaxing factor. Nature 1987;327(6122):524–6.
55. Arnold WP, Mittal CK, Katsuki S, et al. Nitric oxide activates guanylate cyclase and increases guanosine 3':5'-cyclic monophosphate levels in various tissue preparations. Proc Natl Acad Sci U S A 1977;74(8):3203–7.
56. Gonzalez-Alonso J, Mortensen SP, Dawson EA, et al. Erythrocytes and the regulation of human skeletal muscle blood flow and oxygen delivery: role of erythrocyte count and oxygenation state of haemoglobin. J Physiol 2006;572(Pt 1):295–305.
57. Kantrow SP, Huang YC, Whorton AR, et al. Hypoxia inhibits nitric oxide synthesis in isolated rabbit lung. Am J Physiol 1997;272(6 Pt 1):L1167–73.
58. Rengasamy A, Johns RA. Determination of Km for oxygen of nitric oxide synthase isoforms. J Pharmacol Exp Ther 1996;276(1):30–3.
59. Mamone G, Sannolo N, Malorni A, et al. In vitro formation of S-nitrosohemoglobin in red cells by inducible nitric oxide synthase. FEBS Lett 1999;462(3):241–5.

60. Angelo M, Singel DJ, Stamler JS. An S-nitrosothiol (SNO) synthase function of hemoglobin that utilizes nitrite as a substrate. Proc Natl Acad Sci U S A 2006; 103(22):8366–71.

61. Schechter AN, Gladwin MT. Hemoglobin and the paracrine and endocrine functions of nitric oxide. N Engl J Med 2003;348(15):1483–5.

62. Hobbs AJ. Soluble guanylate cyclase: the forgotten sibling. Trends Pharmacol Sci 1997;18(12):484–91.

63. Gow AJ, Ischiropoulos H. Nitric oxide chemistry and cellular signaling. J Cell Physiol 2001;187(3):277–82.

64. Liu X, Miller MJ, Joshi MS, et al. Diffusion-limited reaction of free nitric oxide with erythrocytes. J Biol Chem 1998;273(30):18709–13.

65. Huang KT, Han TH, Hyduke DR, et al. Modulation of nitric oxide bioavailability by erythrocytes. Proc Natl Acad Sci U S A 2001;98(20):11771–6.

66. Liao JC, Hein TW, Vaughn MW, et al. Intravascular flow decreases erythrocyte consumption of nitric oxide. Proc Natl Acad Sci U S A 1999;96(15):8757–61.

67. Gow AJ, Farkouh CR, Munson DA, et al. Biological significance of nitric oxide-mediated protein modifications. Am J Physiol Lung Cell Mol Physiol 2004; 287(2):L262–8.

68. Hess DT, Matsumoto A, Kim SO, et al. Protein S-nitrosylation: purview and parameters. Nat Rev Mol Cell Biol 2005;6(2):150–66.

69. Stamler JS, Singel DJ, Loscalzo J. Biochemistry of nitric oxide and its redox-activated forms. Science 1992;258(5090):1898–902.

70. Stamler JS, Jaraki O, Osborne J, et al. Nitric oxide circulates in mammalian plasma primarily as an S-nitroso adduct of serum albumin. Proc Natl Acad Sci U S A 1992;89(16):7674–7.

71. Stamler JS, Simon DI, Osborne JA, et al. S-nitrosylation of proteins with nitric oxide: synthesis and characterization of biologically active compounds. Proc Natl Acad Sci U S A 1992;89(1):444–8.

72. Arnelle DR, Stamler JS. NO+, NO, and NO- donation by S-nitrosothiols: implications for regulation of physiological functions by S-nitrosylation and acceleration of disulfide formation. Arch Biochem Biophys 1995;318(2):279–85.

73. Ferranti P, Malorni A, Mamone G, et al. Characterisation of S-nitrosohaemoglobin by mass spectrometry. FEBS Lett 1997;400(1):19–24.

74. Chan NL, Rogers PH, Arnone A. Crystal structure of the S-nitroso form of liganded human hemoglobin. Biochemistry 1998;37(47):16459–64.

75. Luchsinger BP, Rich EN, Gow AJ, et al. Routes to S-nitroso-hemoglobin formation with heme redox and preferential reactivity in the beta subunits. Proc Natl Acad Sci U S A 2003;100(2):461–6.

76. Gow AJ, Stamler JS. Reactions between nitric oxide and haemoglobin under physiological conditions. Nature 1998;391(6663):169–73.

77. Pawloski JR, Hess DT, Stamler JS. Export by red blood cells of nitric oxide bioactivity. Nature 2001;409(6820):622–6.

78. Doctor A, Platt R, Sheram ML, et al. Hemoglobin conformation couples erythrocyte S-nitrosothiol content to O2 gradients. Proc Natl Acad Sci U S A 2005; 102(16):5709–14.

79. Palmer LA, Doctor A, Chhabra P, et al. S-nitrosothiols signal hypoxia-mimetic vascular pathology. J Clin Invest 2007;117(9):2592–601.

80. Diesen DL, Hess DT, Stamler JS. Hypoxic vasodilation by red blood cells: evidence for an s-nitrosothiol-based signal. Circ Res 2008;103(5):545–53.

81. McMahon TJ, Moon RE, Luschinger BP, et al. Nitric oxide in the human respiratory cycle. Nat Med 2002;8(7):711–7.

82. Datta B, Tufnell-Barrett T, Bleasdale RA, et al. Red blood cell nitric oxide as an endocrine vasoregulator: a potential role in congestive heart failure. Circulation 2004;109(11):1339–42.
83. James PE, Lang D, Tufnell-Barret T, et al. Vasorelaxation by red blood cells and impairment in diabetes: reduced nitric oxide and oxygen delivery by glycated hemoglobin. Circ Res 2004;94(7):976–83.
84. Saltin B, Radegran G, Koskolou MD, et al. Skeletal muscle blood flow in humans and its regulation during exercise. Acta Physiol Scand 1998;162(3):421–36.
85. Fox-Robichaud A, Payne D, Kubes P. Inhaled NO reaches distal vasculatures to inhibit endothelium- but not leukocyte-dependent cell adhesion. Am J Physiol 1999;277(6 Pt 1):L1224–31.
86. Fox-Robichaud A, Payne D, Hasan SU, et al. Inhaled NO as a viable antiadhesive therapy for ischemia/reperfusion injury of distal microvascular beds. J Clin Invest 1998;101(11):2497–505.
87. Kubes P, Payne D, Grisham MB, et al. Inhaled NO impacts vascular but not extravascular compartments in postischemic peripheral organs. Am J Physiol 1999;277(2 Pt 2):H676–82.
88. Cannon RO 3rd, Schechter AN, Panza JA, et al. Effects of inhaled nitric oxide on regional blood flow are consistent with intravascular nitric oxide delivery. J Clin Invest 2001;108(2):279–87.
89. McMahon TJ, Ahearn GS, Moya MP, et al. A nitric oxide processing defect of red blood cells created by hypoxia: deficiency of S-nitrosohemoglobin in pulmonary hypertension. Proc Natl Acad Sci U S A 2005;102(41):14801–6.
90. Reutov VP, Sorokina EG. NO-synthase and nitrite-reductase components of nitric oxide cycle. Biochemistry (Mosc) 1998;63(7):874–84.
91. Gladwin MT. Evidence mounts that nitrite contributes to hypoxic vasodilation in the human circulation. Circulation 2008;117(5):594–7.
92. Luchsinger BP, Rich EN, Yan Y, et al. Assessments of the chemistry and vasodilatory activity of nitrite with hemoglobin under physiologically relevant conditions. J Inorg Biochem 2005;99(4):912–21.
93. Huang Z, Shiva S, Kim-Shapiro DB, et al. Enzymatic function of hemoglobin as a nitrite reductase that produces NO under allosteric control. J Clin Invest 2005; 115(8):2099–107.
94. Rifkind JM, Ramasamy S, Manoharan PT, et al. Redox reactions of hemoglobin. Antioxid Redox Signal 2004;6(3):657–66.
95. Crawford JH, Isbell TS, Huang Z, et al. Hypoxia, red blood cells, and nitrite regulate NO-dependent hypoxic vasodilation. Blood 2006;107(2):566–74.
96. Jagger JE, Bateman RM, Ellsworth ML, et al. Role of erythrocyte in regulating local O2 delivery mediated by hemoglobin oxygenation. Am J Physiol Heart Circ Physiol 2001;280(6):H2833–9.
97. Bergfeld GR, Forrester T. Release of ATP from human erythrocytes in response to a brief period of hypoxia and hypercapnia. Cardiovasc Res 1992;26(1):40–7.
98. Sprague RS, Bowles EA, Olearczyk JJ, et al. The role of G protein beta subunits in the release of ATP from human erythrocytes. J Physiol Pharmacol 2002;53(4 Pt 1):667–74.
99. Sprague RS, Ellsworth ML, Stephenson AH, et al. Participation of cAMP in a signal-transduction pathway relating erythrocyte deformation to ATP release. Am J Physiol Cell Physiol 2001;281(4):C1158–64.
100. Sprague RS, Ellsworth ML, Stephenson AH, et al. Deformation-induced ATP release from red blood cells requires CFTR activity. Am J Physiol 1998;275(5 Pt 2):H1726–32.

101. Sridharan M, Adderley SP, Bowles EA, et al. Pannexin 1 is the conduit for low oxygen tension-induced ATP release from human erythrocytes. Am J Physiol Heart Circ Physiol 2010;299(4):H1146–52.
102. Rogers SC, Said A, Corcuera D, et al. Hypoxia limits antioxidant capacity in red blood cells by altering glycolytic pathway dominance. FASEB J 2009;23(9): 3159–70.
103. Bossi D, Giardina B. Red cell physiology. Mol Aspects Med 1996;17(2):117–28.
104. Siems WG, Sommerburg O, Grune T. Erythrocyte free radical and energy metabolism. Clin Nephrol 2000;53(1 Suppl):S9–17.
105. Sterling D, Reithmeier RAF, Casey JR. A transport metabolon. J Biol Chem 2001; 276(51):47886–94.
106. Bruce LJ, Beckmann R, Ribeiro ML, et al. A band 3-based macrocomplex of integral and peripheral proteins in the RBC membrane. Blood 2003;101(10): 4180–8.
107. Messana I, Orlando M, Cassiano L, et al. Human erythrocyte metabolism is modulated by the O2-linked transition of hemoglobin. FEBS Lett 1996; 390(1):25–8.
108. Barvitenko NN, Adragna NC, Weber RE. Erythrocyte signal transduction pathways, their oxygenation dependence and functional significance. Cell Physiol Biochem 2005;15(1–4):1–18.
109. Campanella ME, Chu H, Low PS. Assembly and regulation of a glycolytic enzyme complex on the human erythrocyte membrane. Proc Natl Acad Sci U S A 2005;102(7):2402–7.
110. Low PS, Rathinavelu P, Harrison ML. Regulation of glycolysis via reversible enzyme binding to the membrane protein, band 3. J Biol Chem 1993;268(20): 14627–31.
111. Chu H, Low PS. Mapping of glycolytic enzyme-binding sites on human erythrocyte band 3. Biochem J 2006;400(1):143–51.
112. Chu H, Breite A, Ciraolo P, et al. Characterization of the deoxyhemoglobin binding site on human erythrocyte band 3: implications for O2 regulation of erythrocyte properties. Blood 2008;111(2):932–8.
113. Hald B, Madsen MF, Dano S, et al. Quantitative evaluation of respiration induced metabolic oscillations in erythrocytes. Biophys Chem 2009;141(1):41–8.
114. Kinoshita A, Tsukada K, Soga T, et al. Roles of hemoglobin allostery in hypoxia-induced metabolic alterations in erythrocytes: simulation and its verification by metabolome analysis. J Biol Chem 2007;282(14):10731–41.
115. Barbul A, Zipser Y, Nachles A, et al. Deoxygenation and elevation of intracellular magnesium induce tyrosine phosphorylation of band 3 in human erythrocytes. FEBS Lett 1999;455(1–2):87–91.
116. Bordin L, Ion-Popa F, Brunati AM, et al. Effector-induced Syk-mediated phosphorylation in human erythrocytes. Biochim Biophys Acta 2005;1745(1):20–8.
117. Harrison ML, Rathinavelu P, Arese P, et al. Role of band 3 tyrosine phosphorylation in the regulation of erythrocyte glycolysis. J Biol Chem 1991;266(7): 4106–11.
118. Rogers SC, Ross JG, d'Avignon A, et al. Sickle hemoglobin disturbs normal coupling among erythrocyte O2 content, glycolysis and antioxidant capacity. Blood 2013;121(9):1651–62.
119. Condon MR, Feketova E, Machiedo GW, et al. Augmented erythrocyte band-3 phosphorylation in septic mice. Biochim Biophys Acta 2007;1772(5):580–6.
120. Serroukh Y, Djebara S, Lelubre C, et al. Alterations of the erythrocyte membrane during sepsis. Crit Care Res Pract 2012;2012:702956.

121. Suzuki Y, Ohkubo N, Aoto M, et al. Participation of caspase-3-like protease in oxidation-induced impairment of erythrocyte membrane properties. Biorheology 2007;44(3):179–90.

122. Foller M, Huber SM, Lang F. Erythrocyte programmed cell death. IUBMB Life 2008;60(10):661–8.

123. Mandal D, Baudin-Creuza V, Bhattacharyya A, et al. Caspase 3-mediated proteolysis of the N-terminal cytoplasmic domain of the human erythroid anion exchanger 1 (band 3). J Biol Chem 2003;278(52):52551–8.

124. Birmingham DJ. Erythrocyte complement receptors. Crit Rev Immunol 1995; 15(2):133–54.

125. Pascual M, Schifferli JA. The binding of immune complexes by the erythrocyte complement receptor 1 (CR1). Immunopharmacology 1992;24(2):101–6.

126. Pascual M, Schifferli JA. Another function of erythrocytes: transport of circulating immune complexes. Infusionsther Transfusionsmed 1995;22(5):310–5.

127. Poschl JM, Leray C, Ruef P, et al. Endotoxin binding to erythrocyte membrane and erythrocyte deformability in human sepsis and in vitro. Crit Care Med 2003;31(3):924–8.

128. Todd JC 3rd, Poulos ND, Mollitt DL. The effect of endotoxin on the neonatal erythrocyte. J Pediatr Surg 1993;28(3):334–6 [discussion: 336–7].

129. Todd JC 3rd, Poulos ND, Davidson LW, et al. Role of the leukocyte in endotoxin-induced alterations of the red cell membrane. Second place winner of the Conrad Jobst Award in the Gold Medal paper competition. Am Surg 1993; 59(1):9–12.

130. Todd JC 3rd, Poulos ND, Mollitt DL. The effect of endotoxin on neonatal erythrocyte intracellular calcium concentration. J Pediatr Surg 1994;29(6):805–7.

131. Godin DV, Tuchek JM, Garnett ME. Studies on the interaction of Escherichia coli endotoxin with erythrocyte membranes. Can J Physiol Pharmacol 1982;60(7): 977–85.

132. Lewis IA, Campanella ME, Markley JL, et al. Role of band 3 in regulating metabolic flux of red blood cells. Proc Natl Acad Sci U S A 2009;106(44):18515–20.

133. Low PS. Structure and function of the cytoplasmic domain of band 3: center of erythrocyte membrane–peripheral protein interactions. Biochim Biophys Acta 1986;864(2):145–67.

134. Buranakarl C, Trisiriroj M, Pondeenana S, et al. Relationships between oxidative stress markers and red blood cell characteristics in renal azotemic dogs. Res Vet Sci 2009;86(2):309–13.

135. Vaziri ND. Oxidative stress in uremia: nature, mechanisms, and potential consequences. Semin Nephrol 2004;24(5):469–73.

136. Zingraff J, Kamoun P, Lebreton P, et al. Plasma inhibitors of the erythrocyte hexose monophosphate shunt in uraemia. Proc Eur Dial Transplant Assoc 1979;16: 475–80.

137. Yawata Y, Jacob HS. Abnormal red cell metabolism in patients with chronic uremia: nature of the defect and its persistence despite adequate hemodialysis. Blood 1975;45(2):231–9.

138. Poulianiti KP, Kaltsatou A, Mitrou GI, et al. Systemic redox imbalance in chronic kidney disease: a systematic review. Oxid Med Cell Longev 2016;2016: 8598253.

139. Eggert W, Scigalla P, Noack C, et al. Effect of uremic plasma fractions of different molecular sizes on the filterability of red blood cells. Z Urol Nephrol 1981;74(5):391–9 [in German].

140. Eggert W, Schmidt G, Devaux S. Uremic plasma as cause of metabolic changes in red blood cells. Z Urol Nephrol 1981;74(2):141–7 [in German].

141. Lucchi L, Bergamini S, Iannone A, et al. Erythrocyte susceptibility to oxidative stress in chronic renal failure patients under different substitutive treatments. Artif Organs 2005;29(1):67–72.

142. Spolarics Z, Condon MR, Siddiqi M, et al. Red blood cell dysfunction in septic glucose-6-phosphate dehydrogenase-deficient mice. Am J Physiol Heart Circ Physiol 2004;286(6):H2118–26.

143. van Wijk R, van Solinge WW. The energy-less red blood cell is lost: erythrocyte enzyme abnormalities of glycolysis. Blood 2005;106(13):4034–42.

144. Lang F, Abed M, Lang E, et al. Oxidative stress and suicidal erythrocyte death. Antioxid Redox Signal 2014;21(1):138–53.

145. Droge W. Free radicals in the physiological control of cell function. Physiol Rev 2001;82:47–95.

146. Fantone JC, Ward PA. Role of oxygen-derived free radicals and metabolites in leukocyte-dependent inflammatory reactions. Am J Pathol 1982;107(3): 395–418.

147. Andrades ME, Morina A, Spasic S, et al. Bench-to-bedside review: sepsis - from the redox point of view. Crit Care 2011;15(5):230.

148. Salvemini D, Cuzzocrea S. Oxidative stress in septic shock and disseminated intravascular coagulation. Free Radic Biol Med 2002;33(9):1173–85.

149. Crawford JH, Chacko BK, Pruitt HM, et al. Transduction of NO-bioactivity by the red blood cell in sepsis: novel mechanisms of vasodilation during acute inflammatory disease. Blood 2004;104(5):1375–82.

150. Liu L, Yan Y, Zeng M, et al. Essential roles of S-nitrosothiols in vascular homeostasis and endotoxic shock. Cell 2004;116(4):617–28.

151. Bellary SS, Anderson KW, Arden WA, et al. Effect of lipopolysaccharide on the physical conformation of the erythrocyte cytoskeletal proteins. Life Sci 1995; 56(2):91–8.

152. Piagnerelli M, Cotton F, Van Nuffelen M, et al. Modifications in erythrocyte membrane protein content are not responsible for the alterations in rheology seen in sepsis. Shock 2012;37(1):17–21.

153. Condon MR, Kim JE, Deitch EA, et al. Appearance of an erythrocyte population with decreased deformability and hemoglobin content following sepsis. Am J Physiol Heart Circ Physiol 2003;284(6):H2177–84.

154. Eichelbronner O, Sielenkamper A, Cepinskas G, et al. Endotoxin promotes adhesion of human erythrocytes to human vascular endothelial cells under conditions of flow. Crit Care Med 2000;28(6):1865–70.

155. Eichelbronner O, Sibbald WJ, Chin-Yee IH. Intermittent flow increases endotoxin-induced adhesion of human erythrocytes to vascular endothelial cells. Intensive Care Med 2003;29(5):709–14.

156. Behonick GS, Novak MJ, Nealley EW, et al. Toxicology update: the cardiotoxicity of the oxidative stress metabolites of catecholamines (aminochromes). J Appl Toxicol 2001;21(Suppl 1):S15–22.

157. Gryglewski RJ, Palmer RM, Moncada S. Superoxide anion is involved in the breakdown of endothelium-derived vascular relaxing factor. Nature 1986; 320(6061):454–6.

158. Jonsson LM, Rees DD, Edlund T, et al. Nitric oxide and blood pressure in mice lacking extracellular-superoxide dismutase. Free Radic Res 2002;36(7):755–8.

159. Macarthur H, Westfall TC, Riley DP, et al. Inactivation of catecholamines by superoxide gives new insights on the pathogenesis of septic shock. Proc Natl Acad Sci U S A 2000;97(17):9753–8.

160. Misra HP, Fridovich I. The role of superoxide anion in the autoxidation of epinephrine and a simple assay for superoxide dismutase. J Biol Chem 1972; 247(10):3170–5.

161. Thomas DD, Ridnour LA, Espey MG, et al. Superoxide fluxes limit nitric oxide-induced signaling. J Biol Chem 2006;281(36):25984–93.

162. Wink DA, Cook JA, Kim SY, et al. Superoxide modulates the oxidation and nitro-sation of thiols by nitric oxide-derived reactive intermediates. J Biol Chem 1997; 272:11147–51.

163. Kiefmann R, Rifkind JM, Nagababu E, et al. Red blood cells induce hypoxic lung inflammation. Blood 2008;111(10):5205–14.

164. Huertas A, Das SR, Emin M, et al. Erythrocytes induce proinflammatory endothelial activation in hypoxia. Am J Respir Cell Mol Biol 2013;48(1):78–86.

165. Rattan V, Shen Y, Sultana C, et al. Diabetic RBC-induced oxidant stress leads to transendothelial migration of monocyte-like HL-60 cells. Am J Physiol 1997; 273(2 Pt 1):E369–75.

166. Sultana C, Shen Y, Rattan V, et al. Interaction of sickle erythrocytes with endothelial cells in the presence of endothelial cell conditioned medium induces oxidant stress leading to transendothelial migration of monocytes. Blood 1998;92(10): 3924–35.

167. Darley-Usmar V, Halliwell B. Blood radicals: reactive nitrogen species, reactive oxygen species, transition metal ions, and the vascular system. Pharm Res 1996;13(5):649–62.

168. Li JM, Shah AM. Endothelial cell superoxide generation: regulation and relevance for cardiovascular pathophysiology. Am J Physiol Regul Integr Comp Physiol 2004;287(5):R1014–30.

169. Abraham E, Singer M. Mechanisms of sepsis-induced organ dysfunction. Crit Care Med 2007;35(10):2408–16.

170. Sibbald WJ, Messmer K, Fink MP. Roundtable conference on tissue oxygenation in acute medicine, Brussels, Belgium, 14-16 March 1998. Intensive Care Med 2000;26(6):780–91.

171. Elbers PW, Ince C. Mechanisms of critical illness–classifying microcirculatory flow abnormalities in distributive shock. Crit Care 2006;10(4):221.

172. Ince C. Mechanism of impaired oxygen extraction in sepsis. Shunt and the pO2 gap. Minerva Anestesiol 1999;65(6):337–9.

173. Martensson J, Bellomo R. Sepsis-induced acute kidney injury. Crit Care Clin 2015;31(4):649–60.

174. McCullough PA, Shaw AD, Haase M, et al. Diagnosis of acute kidney injury using functional and injury biomarkers: workgroup statements from the tenth acute dialysis quality initiative consensus conference. Contrib Nephrol 2013;182: 13–29.

175. Nguyen MT, Devarajan P. Biomarkers for the early detection of acute kidney injury. Pediatr Nephrol 2008;23(12):2151–7.

176. O'Neal JB, Shaw AD, Billings FTT. Acute kidney injury following cardiac surgery: current understanding and future directions. Crit Care 2016;20(1):187.

177. Okusa MD, Jaber BL, Doran P, et al. Physiological biomarkers of acute kidney injury: a conceptual approach to improving outcomes. Contrib Nephrol 2013; 182:65–81.

178. Prowle JR, Bellomo R. Sepsis-associated acute kidney injury: macrohemody-namic and microhemodynamic alterations in the renal circulation. Semin Nephrol 2015;35(1):64–74.

179. Zuk A, Bonventre JV. Acute kidney injury. Annu Rev Med 2016;67:293--307.

180. Landaw SA. Factors that accelerate or retard red blood cell senescence. Blood Cells 1988;14(1):47–67.

181. Kay MM. Localization of senescent cell antigen on band 3. Proc Natl Acad Sci U S A 1984;81(18):5753–7.

182. Kay MM, Bosman GJ, Johnson GJ, et al. Band-3 polymers and aggregates, and hemoglobin precipitates in red cell aging. Blood cells 1988;14(1):275–95.

183. Low PS, Waugh SM, Zinke K, et al. The role of hemoglobin denaturation and band 3 clustering in red blood cell aging. Science 1985;227(4686):531–3.

184. Lutz HU, Bussolino F, Flepp R, et al. Naturally occurring anti-band-3 antibodies and complement together mediate phagocytosis of oxidatively stressed human erythrocytes. Proc Natl Acad Sci U S A 1987;84(21):7368–72.

185. Boas FE, Forman L, Beutler E. Phosphatidylserine exposure and red cell viability in red cell aging and in hemolytic anemia. Proc Natl Acad Sci U S A 1998;95(6):3077–81.

186. Bratosin D, Mazurier J, Tissier JP, et al. Cellular and molecular mechanisms of senescent erythrocyte phagocytosis by macrophages. A review. Biochimie 1998;80(2):173–95.

187. Kiefer CR, Snyder LM. Oxidation and erythrocyte senescence. Curr Opin Hematol 2000;7(2):113–6.

188. Kuypers FA, de Jong K. The role of phosphatidylserine in recognition and removal of erythrocytes. Cell Mol Biol 2004;50(2):147–58.

189. Lutz HU. Naturally occurring anti-band 3 antibodies in clearance of senescent and oxidatively stressed human red blood cells. Transfus Med Hemother 2012;39(5):321–7.

190. Lang KS, Lang PA, Bauer C, et al. Mechanisms of suicidal erythrocyte death. Cell Physiol Biochem 2005;15(5):195–202.

191. Aarts PA, van den Broek SA, Prins GW, et al. Blood platelets are concentrated near the wall and red blood cells, in the center in flowing blood. Arteriosclerosis 1988;8(6):819–24.

192. Hellem AJ, Borchgrevink CF, Ames SB. The role of red cells in haemostasis: the relation between haematocrit, bleeding time and platelet adhesiveness. Br J Haematol 1961;7:42–50.

193. Andrews DA, Low PS. Role of red blood cells in thrombosis. Curr Opin Hematol 1999;6(2):76–82.

194. Turitto VT, Weiss HJ. Red blood cells: their dual role in thrombus formation. Science 1980;207(4430):541–3.

195. Whelihan MF, Zachary V, Orfeo T, et al. Prothrombin activation in blood coagulation: the erythrocyte contribution to thrombin generation. Blood 2012;120(18):3837–45.

196. Du VX, Huskens D, Maas C, et al. New insights into the role of erythrocytes in thrombus formation. Semin Thromb Hemost 2014;40(1):72–80.

197. van Gelder JM, Nair CH, Dhall DP. Erythrocyte aggregation and erythrocyte de-formability modify the permeability of erythrocyte enriched fibrin network. Thromb Res 1996;82(1):33–42.

198. Gersh KC, Nagaswami C, Weisel JW. Fibrin network structure and clot mechanical properties are altered by incorporation of erythrocytes. Thromb Haemost 2009;102(6):1169–75.

199. Besarab A, Bolton WK, Browne JK, et al. The effects of normal as compared with low hematocrit values in patients with cardiac disease who are receiving hemodialysis and epoetin. N Engl J Med 1998;339(9):584–90.
200. Wu WC, Rathore SS, Wang Y, et al. Blood transfusion in elderly patients with acute myocardial infarction. N Engl J Med 2001;345(17):1230–6.
201. Hart RG, Kanter MC. Hematologic disorders and ischemic stroke. A selective review. Stroke 1990;21(8):1111–21.
202. Cirillo M, Laurenzi M, Trevisan M, et al. Hematocrit, blood pressure, and hypertension. The gubbio population study. Hypertension 1992;20(3):319–26.
203. Stephansson O, Dickman PW, Johansson A, et al. Maternal hemoglobin concentration during pregnancy and risk of stillbirth. JAMA 2000;284:2611–7.
204. Hebert PC, Wells G, Blajchman MA, et al. A multicenter, randomized, controlled clinical trial of transfusion requirements in critical care. Transfusion requirements in critical care investigators, canadian critical care trials group. N Engl J Med 1999;340(6):409–17.
205. Vincent JL, Baron JF, Reinhart K, et al. Anemia and blood transfusion in critically ill patients. JAMA 2002;288(12):1499–507.
206. Crawford JH, Chacko BK, Kevil CG, et al. The red blood cell and vascular function in health and disease. Antioxid Redox Signal 2004;6(6):992–9.
207. Rao SV, Jollis JG, Harrington RA, et al. Relationship of blood transfusion and clinical outcomes in patients with acute coronary syndromes. JAMA 2004; 292(13):1555–62.
208. Qing DY, Conegliano D, Shashaty MG, et al. Red blood cells induce necroptosis of lung endothelial cells and increase susceptibility to lung inflammation. Am J Respir Crit Care Med 2014;190(11):1243–54.
209. Mohanty JG, Nagababu E, Rifkind JM. Red blood cell oxidative stress impairs oxygen delivery and induces red blood cell aging. Front Physiol 2014;5:84.
210. Purtle SW, Moromizato T, McKane CK, et al. The association of red cell distribution width at hospital discharge and out-of-hospital mortality following critical illness. Crit Care Med 2014;42(4):918–29.
211. Bazick HS, Chang D, Mahadevappa K, et al. Red cell distribution width and all-cause mortality in critically ill patients. Crit Care Med 2011;39(8):1913–21.
212. Reggiori G, Occhipinti G, De Gasperi A, et al. Early alterations of red blood cell rheology in critically ill patients. Crit Care Med 2009;37(12):3041–6.
213. Milsom AB, Jones CJ, Goodfellow J, et al. Abnormal metabolic fate of nitric oxide in Type I diabetes mellitus. Diabetologia 2002;45(11):1515–22.
214. Pawloski JR, Hess DT, Stamler JS. Impaired vasodilation by red blood cells in sickle cell disease. Proc Natl Acad Sci U S A 2005;102(7):2531–6.
215. Sonveaux P, Kaz AM, Snyder SA, et al. Oxygen regulation of tumor perfusion by S-nitrosohemoglobin reveals a pressor activity of nitric oxide. Circ Res 2005; 96(10):1119–26.
216. Reynolds JD, Ahearn GS, Angelo M, et al. S-nitrosohemoglobin deficiency: a mechanism for loss of physiological activity in banked blood. Proc Natl Acad Sci U S A 2007;104(43):17058–62.
217. Bennett-Guerrero E, Veldman TH, Doctor A, et al. Evolution of adverse changes in stored RBCs. Proc Natl Acad Sci U S A 2007;104(43):17063–8.
218. James PE, Tufnell-Barret T, Milsom AB, et al. Red blood cell-mediated hypoxic vasodilatation: a balanced physiological viewpoint. Circ Res 2004;95(2):e8–9.
219. Hammerman SI, Klings ES, Hendra KP, et al. Endothelial cell nitric oxide production in acute chest syndrome. Am J Physiol Heart Circ Physiol 1999;277(4): H1579–92.

220. Balagopalakrishna C, Manoharan PT, Abugo OO, et al. Production of superoxide from hemoglobin-bound oxygen under hypoxic conditions. Biochemistry 1996;35(20):6393–8.

221. Misra HP, Fridovich I. The generation of superoxide radical during the autoxidation of hemoglobin. J Biol Chem 1972;247(21):6960–2.

222. Cimen MYB. Free radical metabolism in human erythrocytes. Clin Chim Acta 2008;390(1–2):1–11.

A Review on Microvascular Hemodynamics

The Control of Blood Flow Distribution and Tissue Oxygenation

Carlos J. Munoz, MS, Alfredo Lucas, MS,
Alexander T. Williams, BS, Pedro Cabrales, PhD*

KEYWORDS

- Microcirculation • Microvascular hemodynamics • Microvascular measurements
- Microvascular regulation

KEY POINTS

- Mechanotransduction produces nitric oxide to regulate the flow in the microcirculation.
- Unlike previously thought tissue oxygenation occurs in the arteriole end, whereas capillary perfusion correlates to metabolite washout.
- Microvascular hemodynamics vary with the type of vessel; flow in the arterial and venous differs from the high shear stress environment of the capillaries.
- Microvascular measurements quantify the flow inside the microvasculature using a cross-correlating algorithm, and oxygen tension is quantified using phosphorescence quenching microscopy.

INTRODUCTION—MICROCIRCULATION AT A GLANCE

The microcirculation is a functionally independent entity that encompasses of arterioles, venules, and capillaries, with diameters ranging from 5 μm to 100 μm. The primary goal of the microcirculation is to adjust blood flow to *match* the changing nutritional needs of parenchymal cells and to remove byproducts of metabolism. Although the primary purpose of the microcirculation is to facilitate the delivery of oxygen and nutrients to the tissues, its endogenous vasomotor activity also influences control of blood perfusion at all levels.

Living organisms have localized organs, such as the brain, lungs, heart, skin, etc. or complex, distributed systems, such as the circulation, nervous system, and immune

Department of Bioengineering, University of California, 9500 Gilman Drive, La Jolla, CA 92093-0412, USA
* Corresponding author. Department of Bioengineering, University of California, San Diego, 0412, 9500 Gilman Drive, La Jolla, CA 92093-0412.
E-mail address: pcabrales@ucsd.edu

system. The microcirculation belongs to the latter. The angiogenesis of the microvasculature seems to branch at random and ultimately becomes a network whose smallest components, the capillaries, have a minimal internal diameter that allows passage of one blood cell. The circulation has a fixed design and structure, whereas the microcirculation's growth and changes are driven by local tissue factors.[1,2]

One of the principal determinants of microvascular structure is the rate of oxygen consumption. The configuration of blood vessels is optimized to achieve the most efficient blood flow distribution.[3] This optimization manipulates vessel diameter and length to minimize cardiac energy expenditure in order to ensure maximal oxygen .delivery and removal of metabolic waste from the tissue.[4] The process of angiogenesis is controlled by chemical signals, such as vascular endothelial growth factor, which bind to receptors on the surface of normal endothelial cells.[5]

MICROCIRCULATION—ARTERIOLES AND VENULES

The structural integrity of the arteriole and venular vessels are composed of several layers. An inner layer of endothelial cells creates the lumen for the passage of fluids, cells, and proteins. A thin sheet of smooth muscle composes the central part of the wall and connective tissue outer layer that provides an inelastic outer boundary to the blood vessel.[6] The general structure is depicted in **Fig. 1**.

The microcirculation diverges into smaller branching points until it reaches the capillary network. The capillary network then converges back into progressively larger diameter vessels, through a network of venules, which are the starting point of the system of veins that returns blood to the heart. Arterioles are configured in 2 basic branching patterns, a dichotomous tree or arcading tree.[7] In the dichotomous tree, the main branch gives rise to two daughter branches that branch progressively until the capillary level is reached. In the arcading network, branch points can connect with other segments of the same tree, producing a polygonal network. Arcading networks are found in the intestinal mesenteric circulation, skeletal muscle, and the thermoregulatory cutaneous vasculature. Arcading structures are typical of organs that are subjected to significant deformation frequently, which may result in the occlusion of arterioles, in which case the arcading network provides alternative flow pathways for maintaining tissue nutritive flow, regulating temperature, and equalizing blood pressure at specific arteriolar vessel size.[8]

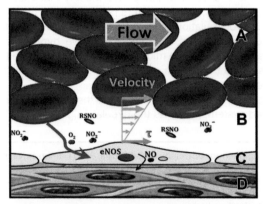

Fig. 1. Blood flow through arterioles or venules. (A) RBC flow. (B) Cell-free layer generated by the Segre-Silberberg effect with various biochemical proteins. (C) Endothelial cell lining generating eNOS from mechanotransduction. (D) Smooth muscle layer encapsulating the entire vessel. eNOS, endothelium-derived nitric oxide synthase; RBC, red blood cell.

The position, size, and configuration of blood vessels in the microcirculation are associated with regulatory functions beyond the simple distribution of flow. The process is centered on oxygen delivery by red blood cells (RBCs), where oxygen release to the tissues is determined by the O_2 affinity of hemoglobin (Hb) within RBCs, and the local O_2 concentration gradient between RBCs and tissues.[9] *As oxygen diffuses through the microvessels, it can diffuse radially to a distance ranging 100 to 200 μm.*[10] The first level of local regulation is governed by the arterioles, where the predominant cellular component is smooth muscle, which maintains vascular tone via a latch-bridge mechanism, which is a mechanism analogous to a ratchet-like apparatus.[11] The latch-bridge mechanism occurs as a result of myosin light chain adenosine triphosphatase inhibition by phosphatases, thus preventing the hydrolysis of adenosine triphosphate.[12] Arterioles and venules maintain a dynamic state of partial constriction (ie, vascular tone), regulated by smooth muscle cells (SMCs) that constitute much of the vascular wall. SMCs are arranged in multiple layers embedded in a tough and elastic matrix of connective tissue, wrapping around the vessel in a low-pitch spiral, so that, when they shorten, the diameter of the vascular lumen decreases.

The layers of SMCs are separated from the blood by a monolayer of flat, polygonal endothelial cells. *As blood flows over the endothelial cell lining, the shear stress applied to the endothelial cells by the flowing blood causes a release of nitric oxide (NO).* NO has myogenic properties resulting in vasodilation. NO reacts with guanylyl cyclase in SMCs, increasing the concentration of guanosine monophosphate (cGMP) and causing a decrease in intracellular calcium resulting in smooth muscle relaxation.[13]

MECHANOTRANSDUCTION AND NITRIC OXIDE REGULATION

A major source of NO production occurs as a result of endothelial mechanotransduction. *The mechanical stimulus on the endothelial cells from the flowing blood is a potent signal to activate the endothelium-derived nitric oxide synthase (eNOS), which is depicted in* **Fig. 1**. Activation of eNOS results in the production of NO, L-citrulline from L-arginine, and O_2.[14,15] Mechanotransduction is sensitive to blood flow through local vessels, as well as blood viscosity. *The greater the shear stress on the endothelial cells the greater the eNOS production.* NO in the vasculature, whether it be in the microcirculation or the macrocirculation, is concentration dependent. As NO stimulates the receptors of this G-protein–coupled cascade, the SMCs become desensitized; NO receptors are endocytosed as the initialization step of the cascade, so the number of NO receptors diminishes and the rate of endocytosis exceeds the rate of receptor reappearance on the cell surface with increasing concentration.[16] As these receptors become saturated, the NO concentration increases in the lumen of the vessel. Because of rapid and irreversible scavenging of NO by Hb, cell-free Hb can effectively block NO bioactivity, resulting in vasoconstriction.[17–19] Hb is also known for its involvement in NO deoxygenation converting NO to nitrate (NO_3) and met (ferric) heme when reacted with oxygenated heme.[20–22] Therefore, the NO reactions with Hb depend on the redox and ligation state of the heme iron modulated by O_2 levels. However, these reactions are slowed 1000x when the Hb is contained within the protective RBC membrane.[23,24] If not regulated, NO at high concentrations is toxic as it begins to target aconitase and cytochrome oxidase, enzymes used in cellular respiration, thus making this process a natural defense against high concentrations of NO, but at low concentration a whole host of other side effects become apparent.[25,26]

OXYGEN EXCHANGE IN THE MICROCIRCULATION

Around 60% to 70% of the oxygen supply in the tissues occurs as oxygen diffuses through the microcirculation.[27–29] Oxygen is a major driving force for several biochemical processes. A significant amount of the oxygen transport occurs in the larger arterioles[27–29]; this is evident as studies have previously shown Hb oxygen saturation decreased from 69.9% to 56.7% between large and small arterioles and the periarteriolar Po_2 decreased from 35 to 20 mm Hg in the same vessels.[29] The continuous branching of the arterioles reduces the arteriole size and reduces the arteriolar blood oxygen content proportional to the change in cross-sectional area.[30] *An approach to understand oxygen delivery and consumption of the tissue, microvascular Po_2 and Hb saturation must be coupled with the microvascular blood flow.*[31] Traditional measurements of Po_2 are done using invasive methods such as oxygen-sensitive polarographic microcathodes or phosphorescence quenching microscopy; another method that is not as invasive to determine Hb saturation (SO_2) is spectrophotometry of Hb.[32] Regardless of the measurement, SO_2 and Po_2 are related via the hill equation so long as the hill coefficient of your oxygen carrier is known.

MICROCIRCULATION—CAPILLARIES

As the microvasculature diverges from arterioles to capillaries, vessel diameter continues to decrease ultimately limiting transit to single RBCs. The capillary's inner diameter can be significantly smaller than the RBC diameter ($\sim 8\ \mu m$), particularly in tissues such as the spleen and the liver where capillary diameters are as small as 4 to 5 μm, pushing RBC deformability to the extreme. The precise hydraulic radius of capillaries is not well defined due to the presence of the vascular endothelial glycocalyx, a glycoprotein layer that covers the luminal membrane of vascular endothelial cells and occupies a significant cross-sectional area within the capillaries.[33] The outer structure of capillary is composed by a single layer of vascular endothelial cells supported on their basement membrane.[34]

The compliance of the capillary system is heterogeneous throughout the body and is determined primarily by the organ or tissue the capillary network supplies. Capillaries in connective and muscle tissue are relatively rigid,[35] whereas pulmonary capillaries tend to be more compliant, varying as a function of lung volume. The differences in the elasticity of the capillaries are thought to be associated with varying amounts of tissue surrounding the capillary bed.[36] *For example, pulmonary capillaries are often represented as a tight 3-dimensional mesh of capillaries. The capillary bed around the alveoli is described as a parking garage with floors, ceilings, and intervening collagen enriched posts that provides elastic support.*[37,38] The idea of the sheet model is illustrated in **Fig. 2**. In contrast, muscle tissue capillaries are embedded in dense muscle fibers or connective tissue, which need significantly lower compliance to remain patent. The patency of the capillary is important, as the metabolic needs of the tissue can be matched only if blood is actively flowing through the tissue. Thus, capillary beds (networks) experience changes in perfusion according to the metabolic activity of the tissue. The adaptive behavior of the capillary bed preserves their ability to remain perfused regardless of the compression stress of the surrounding tissues.[39] *However, the sensitivity of the arteriole vascular smooth muscle should not be overlooked to be sensitive to the change of Po_2.*[38] *The regulation of blood flow to the tissues depend on the idea of precapillary sphincters to limit local blood flow and prevent over oxygenation of tissue.*[40]

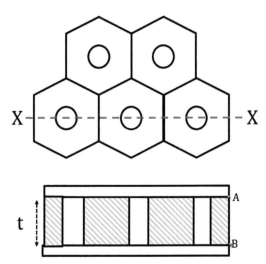

Fig. 2. Sheet fold model. (*Top*) Plain view. (*Bottom*) Cross section view from X to X. The clear rectangular spaces are the nonvascular posts. The striped areas indicate the flow channels. Sheet thickness = t. A and B are contact of posts with endothelial surface.

MICROCIRCULATION—HEMODYNAMICS

The flow through the circulation, whether it be the arterial or venous end, experiences similar phenomena. In the microcirculation blood and plasma flow is influenced by shear stress forces developed at the vessel walls, which result in partially blunted velocity blood profiles.[41,42] *Unlike a normal parabolic profile with a peak indicating the maximum flow, this flow profile is blunted, thus lacking a peak of max flow as a result of a core of fast-moving RBCs.* **Fig. 3** *portrays a comparative view between a parabolic profile and a blunted profile. The degree of blunting depends on the ratio of tube diameter (D) and particle thickness (d), D/d. With increasing flow rates, the flow profile*

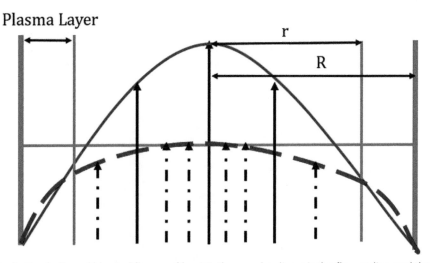

Fig. 3. Parabolic and blunted flow profiles. R is the vessel radius, r is the flow radius, and the plasma layer illustrates the CFL. CFL, cell-free layer.

continues to become more parabolic as the shear rate on the particles increases. This is likely due to a shear-dependent particle-particle interaction, which results in an increase of particle size at higher shears by formation of rouleaux or other aggregates.[42] With the same train of thought these blunted profiles tend to move closer to a normal parabolic profile as the diameter of the vessel decreases.[42,43] The flow inside these vessels have another interesting characteristic, the presence of thin zone between the column of blood and the endothelial membrane, the cell-free layer (CFL). *The CFL is occasionally randomly intruded by RBCs and leukocytes and contains a gel like surface made of different sugars attached to the endothelial membrane known as the glycocalyx. The CFL is similar to a mechanical system that is generated due to dynamic conditions as cells and other formed elements draft away from the vessel wall due to the velocity gradient. The CFL works similar to a lubricating layer of moving mechanical parts as a viscous medium between blood and the vessel wall.* Thus, the presence of the CFL significantly reduces the resistance to blood flow. The CFL is possible because of the Segre-Silberberg effect, which describes that the radial forces act on the neutrally buoyant particles creating an equilibrium at approximately 60% of the tube's radii from the central axis.[44] *The RBCs near the wall experience drag forces that drive cells along in the direction of the velocity vectors and inertial forces that create lateral movement perpendicular to the velocity vectors.* This lateral movement forces RBCs away from the vessel wall, leaving an annulus of plasma with very low concentration of cells near the wall.[45,46]

MICROCIRCULATION—CAPILLARY HEMODYNAMICS

To better understand the capillary hemodynamics, the authors separate the analysis of how plasma flows from that of how RBC flow. *An example of blood flow in a capillary is seen in* **Fig. 4**. The flow of the incompressible Newtonian plasma, *where the shear stress is proportionally related to shear velocity*, is governed by Stokes flow, because plasma is mostly water.[47] As the plasma enters the capillary from a diverging arteriole branch it has a characteristic non-Poiseuille profile, the pressure drop cannot be described across the capillary tube due to the viscosity of the fluid. Considering the radial velocities inside the capillary, the radial velocities can reach as much as 30% of the mean axial velocity.[47] As the plasma flows downstream, the flow reverts back to a parabolic profile that can be characterized as Poiseuille flow *whose pressure drop can be characterized by the viscosity of the fluid* (see **Fig. 2**). This occurs at a distance 0.65 times the diameter of the capillary tube from the entry section.[48]

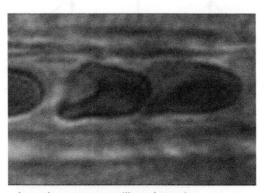

Fig. 4. RBCs flowing through a narrow capillary channel.

Adding a layer of complexity, consider the deformable RBC entering the capillary. If 2 RBCs have a distance apart greater than 1.3x the capillary diameter, the plasma's velocity profile between the cells remains nearly parabolic.[48] This type of flow is named bolus flow.[49] As long as the distance between 2 consecutive RBCs is greater than the capillary diameter, the cells have very little interaction and the flow is essentially a superposition of 2 independent entry flows. There is a benefit in terms of reducing the resistance the RBCs experience in the capillaries by decreasing their distance apart. As the distance between RBCs in the capillary decreases, the interaction between the RBCs reduces the total resistance experienced by each RBC. Therefore, close packing of RBC results in a lower hydrodynamic resistance than when RBCs flow separately.[50]

Similar to the arterioles and venules, capillaries have a CFL and a gel-like glycocalyx. The thin plasma layer between the endothelial lining of the capillary blood vessel and the RBCs experiences extremely high shear stress from the *flowing RBCs in contact with it, as the diameter of the vessel is less than that of the RBC diameter. This CFL between the vessel wall and the RBC as previously mentioned can be thought of as the lubrication zone created by the CFL.* Performing the proper analysis on this CFL can better characterize the flow of the RBC through the capillary. The thickness of the CFL or lubrication layer is related to RBCs velocity by the square root of the velocity, and the resistance is related to the velocity by the inverse square of the RBC's velocity.[51,52] As the thickness of the CFL decreases, the RBC's velocity decreases and can potentially "seize up" due to lubrication failure.

Assessing the flow of RBCs at bifurcations was extensively studied by Fung in 1972.[53] RBCs at bifurcations tend to move into the branch with higher velocity. The channel of a bifurcation with higher flow has a higher axial pressure gradient. The pressure gradient in both bifurcations drives plasma to skim past the RBC, resulting in uneven shear stress across the cell, which ultimately drives the RBC down the path with greater flow. As additional RBCs reach the same junction, they experience similar pressure and shear forces, resulting in all RBCs following in the same path at the bifurcation, assuming all RBCs were uniform. However, there is actual deviation in RBC flow due to randomness in the RBC shape and size, nonuniformity in vessel geometry, asymmetric flow, rotation of the RBC, and other factors. As most things in nature, nature seeks balance, and capillary flow is no different. Although, capillaries will favor one side of the bifurcation over another; the continuous flow of red cells down a particular path increases its resistance forcing a change in direction at the bifurcation.[53]

MICROCIRCULATION DYSFUNCTION

The pathophysiology of the microcirculation can illuminate the intricacies involved with tissue perfusion. These hemodynamic alterations are known as circulatory shock, which includes variations in systemic hemodynamics or endothelial dysfunction. Alterations in microcirculatory blood flow have been identified, and the severity of these differences is associated with a poor outcome. For example, during hemorrhagic or *septic shock*, a dramatic drop in oxygen delivery to the tissues is seen.[54] Thus, the microvascular pressure decreases, reducing the density of functional capillaries (the number of capillaries perfused with RBCs), limiting the washout of metabolic by-products that can lead to mitochondrial disfunction.[55] In the event of severe shock, some of the most apparent changes to the microcirculation are a reduction in oxygen-carrying capacity; a decrease in blood viscosity; a decrease in vessel wall shear stress; and shedding of the protective glycocalyx barrier,[56] pathologic hyperfibrinolysis, and diffuse coagulopathy.[57,58] In the first few moments of shock, reduction in blood pressure and an increase in the heart rate are observed. The decrease in blood pressure corresponds to a drastic reduction in hydrostatic pressure at the arteriolar end of the capillaries. The reduced hydrostatic pressure promotes interstitial fluid reabsorption in the capillaries.[59] The primary goal of resuscitation from shock is to restore balance via blood volume and microvascular pressure. Restoring microcirculatory function is a must to ensure a positive outcome following shock. The longer shock proceeds the longer an oxygen debt accumulates in the tissues, a debt that can only be repaid in the microcirculation.

EXPERIMENTAL MICROVASCULAR MEASUREMENTS

To further understand the complexities of the microcirculation and its tendencies, a variety of techniques were developed to properly measure microcirculatory oxygen tension and hemodynamics. Better understanding of the intricacies of this complex network aids in engineering new techniques that promote more positive outcomes.

Intravital Microscopy

Observation of the microcirculation in humans is normally completed using laser Doppler techniques or orthogonal polarization spectral imaging on the skin, nail flap, or lip.[60] However, a common model to observe the microcirculation and oxygen delivery to the tissues uses hamsters and their dorsal skin flap. The skin is lifted from the animal, creating a skin fold, which is supported by 2 titanium frames with 12 mm circular openings. One frame is sutured on one side of the skin fold. The opposite skin layer is removed following the outline of the window, leaving only a thin layer of retractor muscle, connective tissue, and intact skin. The exposed tissue is sealed with a glass cover held by the other frame creating an environment that allows for clear optical measurements of the microcirculation in vivo (**Fig. 5**).[61] Furthermore, 2 blood vessels are typically cannulated: the carotid artery for monitoring blood pressure and the femoral or jugular vein for the infusion of fluids and contrast agents. *Hamsters are mammals that adapt to a fossorial environment and in normal conditions have low central Pao$_2$ (57 mm Hg corresponding to an Hb saturation of 84%) and a similar arteriolar Po$_2$ (57 mm Hg corresponding to a Hb saturation of 81%). This suggests that hamsters are effective animals in delivering oxygen to the tissue in the microcirculation with minimal oxygen before reaching the microcirculation.*[31]

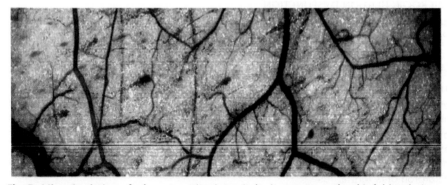

Fig. 5. Microcirculation of a hamster using intravital microscopy on the skinfold technique.

Velocity Measurements

Velocity measurements in microvessels can be obtained via frame-by-frame analysis of short videos filmed through the high-magnification microscopy. Neither laser Doppler methods, nor ultrasound Doppler methods, have been refined to achieve reliable analytical results from vessels less than 100 μm in diameter.

The flow of blood in microvessels gives the appearance of the passage of a granular surface. This is quantified by placing a photo sensor over the microvessel videos and displaying the voltage of the photo sensor. This gives a time-varying signal, which depends on the local light intensity in a small area of the microvessel image. The frequency and amplitude characteristics of this signal are directly related to the size of the objects that pass through the observed area and their velocity.

Previous iterations of this method used a single photometric sensor; however, a single sensor resulted in frequency ambiguity and made determination of velocity difficult. As such, the method evolved to incorporate a second photometric sensor aligned along the axis of flow, allowing velocity to be determined by measuring the time delay between upstream and downstream signals. This is readily accomplished by measuring the time delay between the signals that maximizes their cross-correlation, a process that can be done online and in real time. Wayland and Johnson in 1967 refined the 2-slit photometric method into a convenient quantitative tool, capable of online presentation of velocity data for capillaries.[62–64]

Measurement of Oxygen Tension

High-resolution microvascular Po_2 measurements can be made using phosphorescence quenching microscopy (PQM). PQM is based on the relationship between the phosphorescent decay of palladium-meso-tetra-(4-carboxyphenyl)-porphyrin bound to albumin and the partial pressure of oxygen, according to the Stern-Volmer equation. A 10-mg/mL intravenous injection of the porphyrin dye is given approximately10 minutes before Po_2 measurements. A series of flashes causes phosphorescence of the dye, and the oxygen concentration is measured in an adjustable optical window.[65]

Phosphorescence is the emission of photons as the molecules of an excited phosphorescent material, such as Pd-porphyrin, falls from the excited triplet state back to the singlet ground state. The energy required to excite the electrons of molecular oxygen is approximately the same as the energy released by phosphorescent decay of Pd-porphyrin. O_2 can absorb this energy before a photon is released, and a much faster rate than a photon can be released, thus "quenching" the phosphorescence. Naturally, this is a concentration-dependent effect, as the O_2 must be in close contact with the phosphorescent molecule. As such, a decrease in the rate of phosphorescent emission (a faster time constant) can be correlated with a higher local concentration of Po_2 via the Stern-Volmer equation.

SUMMARY

The microcirculation is an incredibly complex and vital network of vessels that are specifically designed to maintain the surrounding tissues. As this field of research continues to grow and new techniques are developed, questions revolving around oxygen transport will begin to be answered with clarity. As these questions are answered, engineers can adapt these fundamental understandings of oxygen transport to create nonspecific blood substitutes. Furthermore, microcirculatory research also promotes further research on blood pathologies such as sickle cell and thalassemia. All in all, the microcirculation is a corner stone of the human body.

DISCLOSURE

The authors have nothing to disclose.

REFERENCES

1. Fukumura D, Jain RK. Role of nitric oxide in angiogenesis and microcirculation in tumors. Cancer Metastasis Rev 1998;17(1):77–89.
2. Drevs J, Müller-Driver R, Wittig C, et al. PTK787/ZK 222584, a specific vascular endothelial growth factor-receptor tyrosine kinase inhibitor, affects the anatomy of the tumor vascular bed and the functional vascular properties as detected by dynamic enhanced magnetic resonance imaging. Cancer Res 2002;62(14): 4015–22.
3. Wei HS, Kang H, Rasheed I-YD, et al. Erythrocytes are oxygen-sensing regulators of the cerebral microcirculation. Neuron 2016;91(4):851–62.
4. Khanin MA, Bukharov IB. Optimal structure of the microcirculatory bed. J Theor Biol 1994;169(3):267–73.
5. Ferrara N, Gerber H-P, LeCouter J. The biology of VEGF and its receptors. Nat Med 2003;9(6):669–76.
6. Martinez-Lemus LA. The dynamic structure of arterioles. Basic Clin Pharmacol Toxicol 2012;110(1):5–11.
7. Less JR, Skalak TC, Sevick EM, et al. Microvascular architecture in a mammary carcinoma: branching patterns and vessel dimensions. Cancer Res 1991;51(1): 265–73.
8. le Noble F, Fleury V, Pries A, et al. Control of arterial branching morphogenesis in embryogenesis: go with the flow. Cardiovasc Res 2005;65(3):619–28.
9. Pittman RN. Regulation of tissue oxygenation. San Rafael (CA): Morgan & Claypool Life Sciences; 2011. Chapter 4, Oxygen Transport.
10. Dewhirst MW. Concepts of oxygen transport at the microcirculatory level. Semin Radiat Oncol 1998;8(3):143–50.
11. Hai CM, Murphy RA. Cross-bridge phosphorylation and regulation of latch state in smooth muscle. Am J Physiol Cell Physiol 1988;254(1):C99–106.
12. Dillon PF, Aksoy MO, Driska SP, et al. Myosin phosphorylation and the cross-bridge cycle in arterial smooth muscle. Science 1981;211(4481):495–7.
13. Schlossmann J, Feil R, Hofmann F. Signaling through NO and cGMP-dependent protein kinases. Ann Med 2003;35(1):21–7.
14. Hill MA, Meininger GA. Arteriolar vascular smooth muscle cells: mechanotransducers in a complex environment. Int J Biochem Cell Biol 2012;44(9):1505–10.
15. Moncada S, Higgs A. The L-arginine-nitric oxide pathway. N Engl J Med 1993; 329(27):2002–12.
16. Bellamy TC, Wood J, Goodwin DA, et al. Rapid desensitization of the nitric oxide receptor, soluble guanylyl cyclase, underlies diversity of cellular cGMP responses. Proc Natl Acad Sci U S A 2000;97(6):2928–33.
17. Sakai H, Hara H, Yuasa M, et al. Molecular dimensions of Hb-based O2 carriers determine constriction of resistance arteries and hypertension. Am J Physiol Heart Circ Physiol 2000;279(3):H908–15.
18. Olson JS, Foley EW, Rogge C, et al. No scavenging and the hypertensive effect of hemoglobin-based blood substitutes. Free Radic Biol Med 2004;36(6):685–97.
19. Buehler PW, Alayash AI. All hemoglobin-based oxygen carriers are not created equally. Biochim Biophys Acta 2008;1784(10):1378–81.
20. Sharma VS, Traylor TG, Gardiner R, et al. Reaction of nitric oxide with heme proteins and model compounds of hemoglobin. Biochemistry 1987;26(13):3837–43.

21. Olson JS, Mathews AJ, Rohlfs RJ, et al. The role of the distal histidine in myoglobin and haemoglobin. Nature 1988;336(6196):265.
22. Eich RF, Li T, Lemon DD, et al. Mechanism of NO-induced oxidation of myoglobin and hemoglobin. Biochemistry 1996;35(22):6976–83.
23. Azarov I, Liu C, Reynolds H, et al. Mechanisms of slower nitric oxide uptake by red blood cells and other hemoglobin-containing vesicles. J Biol Chem 2011; 286:33567–79.
24. Han TH, Hyduke DR, Vaughn MW, et al. Nitric oxide reaction with red blood cells and hemoglobin under heterogeneous conditions. Proc Natl Acad Sci U S A 2002;99(11):7763–8.
25. Srinivasan S, Avadhani NG. Cytochrome c oxidase dysfunction in oxidative stress. Free Radic Biol Med 2012;53(6):1252–63.
26. Meng Q, Sun Y, Gao H. Cytochromes c constitute a layer of protection against nitric oxide but not nitrite. Appl Environ Microbiol 2018;84(17) [pii: e01255-18].
27. Swain DP, Pittman RN. Oxygen exchange in the microcirculation of hamster retractor muscle. Am J Physiol Heart Circ Physiol 1989;256(1):H247–55.
28. Kerger H, Torres Filho IP, Rivas M, et al. Systemic and subcutaneous microvascular oxygen tension in conscious Syrian golden hamsters. Am J Physiol Heart Circ Physiol 1995;268(2):H802–10.
29. Duling Brian R, Berne Robert M. Longitudinal gradients in periarteriolar oxygen tension. Circ Res 1970;27(5):669–78.
30. Shibata M, Ichioka S, Ando J, et al. Microvascular and interstitial Po 2measurements in rat skeletal muscle by phosphorescence quenching. J Appl Physiol 2001;91(1):321–7.
31. Cabrales P, Intaglietta M, Tsai AG. Transfusion restores blood viscosity and reinstates microvascular conditions from hemorrhagic shock independent of oxygen carrying capacity. Resuscitation 2007;75(1):124–34.
32. Pittman RN. Oxygen transport and exchange in the microcirculation. Microcirculation 2005;12(1):59–70.
33. Secomb TW, Hsu R, Pries AR. A model for red blood cell motion in glycocalyx-lined capillaries. Am J Physiol Heart Circ Physiol 1998;274(3):H1016–22.
34. Alberts B, Johnson A, Lewis J, et al. Blood vessels and endothelial cells. Mol Biol Cell 2002. 4th edition. Available at: https://www.ncbi.nlm.nih.gov/books/NBK26848/. Accessed July 23, 2019.
35. Baez S, Lamport H, Baez A. Pressure effects in living microscopic vessels. In: Copley A, Stainsby G, editors. Flow Properties of Blood and Other Biological Systems. London: Pergamon; 1960. p. 122–36.
36. Fung YC, Zweifach BW, Intaglietta M. Elastic environment of the capillary bed. Circ Res 1966;19(2):441–61.
37. Sobin SS, Fung YC, Tremer HM, et al. Elasticity of the pulmonary alveolar microvascular sheet in the cat. Circ Res 1972;30(4):440–50.
38. Sobin SS, Tremer HM, Fung YC. Morphometric basis of the sheet-flow concept of the pulmonary alveolar microcirculation in the cat. Circ Res 1970;26(3):397–414.
39. Krogh A. The anatomy and physiology of capillaries. Vol. 18. Yale University Press; 1922.
40. Altura BM. Chemical and humoral regulation of blood flow through the precapillary sphincter. Microvasc Res 1971;3(4):361–84.
41. Baker M, Wayland H. On-line volume flow rate and velocity profile measurement for blood in microvessels. Microvasc Res 1974;7(1):131–43.

42. Gaehtgens P, Meiselman HJ, Wayland H. Velocity profiles of human blood at normal and reduced hematocrit in glass tubes up to 130 μ diameter. Microvasc Res 1970;2(1):13–23.
43. Schmid-Schoenbein GW, Zweifach BW. RBC velocity profiles in arterioles and venules of the rabbit omentum. Microvasc Res 1975;10(2):153–64.
44. Segre G, Silberberg A. Behaviour of macroscopic rigid spheres in Poiseuille flow. Part 2. Experimental results and interpretation. J Fluid Mech 1962;14: 136–57.
45. Wang S-K, Hwang NHC. On transport of suspended particulates in tube flow. Biorheology 1992;29(2–3):353–77.
46. Munn LL, Dupin MM. Blood cell interactions and segregation in flow. Ann Biomed Eng 2008;36(4):534–44.
47. Lew HS, Fung YC. On the low-reynolds-number entry flow into a circular cylindrical tube. J Biomech 1969;2(1):105–19.
48. Lew HS, Fung YC. The motion of the plasma between the red cells in the bolus flow. Biorheology 1969;6(2):109–19.
49. Prothero J, Burton AC. The physics of blood flow in capillaries: I. The nature of the motion. Biophys J 1961;1(7):565–79.
50. Fung YC. Blood flow in the capillary bed. J Biomech 1969;2(4):353–72.
51. Fitz-Gerald JM. Implications of a theory of erythrocyte motion in narrow capillaries. J Appl Physiol 1969;27(6):912–8.
52. Lighthill MJ. Pressure-forcing of tightly fitting pellets along fluid-filled elastic tubes. J Fluid Mech 1968;34:113–43.
53. Fung Y-C. Stochastic flow in capillary blood vessels. Microvasc Res 1973;5(1): 34–48.
54. Trzeciak S, Dellinger RP, Parrillo JE, et al. Early microcirculatory perfusion derangements in patients with severe sepsis and septic shock: relationship to hemodynamics, oxygen transport, and survival. Ann Emerg Med 2007;49(1): 88–98.e2.
55. Cabrales P, Tsai AG, Intaglietta M. Microvascular pressure and functional capillary density in extreme hemodilution with low- and high-viscosity dextran and a low-viscosity Hb-based O2 carrier. Am J Physiol Heart Circ Physiol 2004; 287(1):H363–73.
56. Rahbar E, Cardenas JC, Baimukanova G, et al. Endothelial glycocalyx shedding and vascular permeability in severely injured trauma patients. J Transl Med 2015; 13(1):117.
57. Cabrales P, Tsai AG, Intaglietta M. Increased plasma viscosity prolongs microhemodynamic conditions during small volume resuscitation from hemorrhagic shock. Resuscitation 2008;77(3):379–86.
58. Cannon JW. Hemorrhagic shock. N Engl J Med 2018;378(4):370–9.
59. Cabrales P, Intaglietta M. Blood substitutes: evolution from non-carrying to oxygen and gas carrying fluids. ASAIO J 1992;59(4):337–54.
60. Groner W, Winkelman JW, Harris AG, et al. Orthogonal polarization spectral imaging: a new method for study of the microcirculation. Nat Med 1999;5(10):1209.
61. Endrich B, Asaishi K, Götz A, et al. Technical report—a new chamber technique for microvascular studies in unanesthetized hamsters. Res Exp Med (Berl) 1980; 177(2):125–34.
62. Intaglietta M, Silverman NR, Tompkins WR. Capillary flow velocity measurements in vivo and in situ by television methods. Microvasc Res 1975;10(2): 165–79.

63. Wayland H, Johnson PC. Erythrocyte velocity measurement in microvessels by a two-slit photometric method. J Appl Physiol 1967;22(2):333–7.
64. Lipowsky HH, Zweifach BW. Application of the "two-slit" photometric technique to the measurement of microvascular volumetric flow rates. Microvasc Res 1978; 15(1):93–101.
65. Torres Filho IP, Intaglietta M. Microvessel PO2 measurements by phosphorescence decay method. Am J Physiol Heart Circ Physiol 1993;265(4):H1434–8.

Nitric Oxide and Endothelial Dysfunction

Anthony R. Cyr, MD, PhD[a], Lauren V. Huckaby, MD[a], Sruti S. Shiva, PhD[b],
Brian S. Zuckerbraun, MD[c],*

KEYWORDS

- Nitric oxide • Endothelial dysfunction • Nitric oxide synthase

KEY POINTS

- Nitric oxide is a small highly reactive signaling molecule that is a primary determinant of vascular homeostasis.
- Nitric oxide production is tightly regulated through transcriptional and post-translational control of 3 main nitric oxide synthase isoforms.
- Endothelial nitric oxide synthase is constitutively expressed in platelets and endothelial cells and is associated with maintenance of appropriate vascular tone, regulation of angiogenesis, and regulation of platelet function.
- In disease states nitric oxide production can be deleterious through production of reactive oxygen and nitrogen species, and nitric oxide signaling plays a major role in the pathophysiology of numerous systemic illnesses including sepsis.
- Nitric oxide and its effect on endothelial function continues to be a promising target for pharmacologic manipulation in a diverse number of critical illnesses.

INTRODUCTION

The vascular endothelium is composed of a monolayer of specialized cells (endothelial cells), which form the interface between the underlying smooth muscle cells from the vascular lumen. Endothelial cells may exhibit significant plasticity in function depending on the milieu in which they exist; for example, the endothelium comprising the blood–brain barrier has significantly different functional characteristics than that lining the aorta. However, all endothelial cells share a common set of functions, including the regulation of hemostasis, maintenance of vascular permeability, mediation of both

[a] Department of Surgery, University of Pittsburgh Medical Center, F679 Presbyterian University Hospital, 200 Lothrop Street, Pittsburgh, PA 15213, USA; [b] Vascular Medicine Institute, University of Pittsburgh, E1240 BST, 200 Lothrop Street, Pittsburgh, PA 15261, USA; [c] Department of Surgery, University of Pittsburgh Medical Center, F1281 Presbyterian University Hospital, 200 Lothrop Street, Pittsburgh, PA 15213, USA
* Corresponding author.
E-mail address: zuckerbraunbs@upmc.edu
Twitter: @TonyCyr (A.R.C.); @zuckerbraun (B.S.Z.)

Crit Care Clin 36 (2020) 307–321
https://doi.org/10.1016/j.ccc.2019.12.009
0749-0704/20/Published by Elsevier Inc.
criticalcare.theclinics.com

acute and chronic immune responses to various types of injury, and control of vascular tone.[1] There are several molecular mechanisms that govern these critical processes, but none are as critical as the nitric oxide (NO) signaling pathway.[2] NO is a small, soluble gas with strong vasodilatory, anti-inflammatory, and antioxidant properties that plays a central role in the maintenance of vascular homeostasis.[3] Highlighting this, the concept of endothelial dysfunction (ED) is centrally linked to decreased NO production and sensitivity, which ultimately results in an imbalance in vascular homeostasis leading to a prothrombotic, proinflammatory, and less compliant blood vessel wall.[2,4] In the present review, we highlight the mechanisms underpinning the regulatory effects of NO on ED and link these to currently understood clinical phenomena.

NITRIC OXIDE IN NORMAL ENDOTHELIAL FUNCTION
Nitric Oxide Synthesis and Nitric Oxide Synthase Enzyme Isoforms

NO is a highly reactive, readily diffusible gaseous free radical with strong intrinsic oxidant properties. It is synthesized by 3 distinct subtypes of the NO synthase (NOS) enzyme, each with unique expression patterns and functional properties: neuronal NOS (nNOS, NOS1), inducible NOS (iNOS, NOS2), and endothelial NOS (eNOS, NOS3).[5,6] Broadly, these proteins catalyze the production of NO and L-citrulline from L-arginine and O_2, using electrons donated from dihydronicotinamide-adenine dinucleotide phosphate (NADPH). This process is tightly regulated requiring several key protein–protein interactions and multiple prosthetic groups and cofactors. In monomeric form, the NOS subtypes are incapable of binding to L-arginine, and subsequently can function primarily as weak NADPH oxidases resulting in the production of harmful superoxide radical anion ($O_2^{\bullet-}$). When bound by the calcium signaling protein calmodulin (CaM), the transfer of electrons through a flavin adenine mononucleotide and flavin adenine dinucleotide domain is enhanced. Finally, in the presence of heme and tetrahydrobiopterin (BH_4), NOS monomers form homodimers capable of using the donated NADPH electrons to catalyze the 2-step oxidation of L-arginine to L-citrulline and NO. In the first step, NOS promotes the hydroxylation of L-arginine to Nω-hydroxy-L-arginine, which remains bound by the enzyme. In the second step, NOS catalyzes the oxidation of Nω-hydroxy-L-arginine to L-citrulline, thereby releasing NO (**Fig. 1**).

NOS isoforms are differentially regulated through post-translational modifications as well as interactions with the associated scaffolding proteins. nNOS and eNOS, for example, are highly dependent on Ca^{2+}-activated CaM for homodimerization and activity, whereas iNOS is minimally dependent on calcium concentration.[6] These nuances have critical functional effects. In neurons, NO produced by nNOS signaling functions to modulate longer term synaptic transmission, leading to critical involvement in learning, memory, and neurogenesis.[7] Additionally, some data suggest that nNOS may play a significant role in the maintenance of vascular tone through effects of nNOS-expressing end neurons that innervate smooth muscle in microvasculature.[8] In contrast, iNOS is strongly induced in activated macrophages, in which it creates an NO burst representing the sentinel event in the acute inflammatory cascade. This often leads to significant collateral damage to bystander healthy tissue through the generation of downstream reactive oxygen species (ROS) and reactive nitrogen species.[9] Herein, we focus on the regulation and function of eNOS, the native NOS of vascular endothelial cells.

Endothelial Nitric Oxide Synthase Regulation and Function

eNOS is predominantly expressed in vascular endothelial cells, although its expression has been detected in other specialized groups of cells with important circulatory roles. These include cardiac myocytes, platelets, certain neurons in the

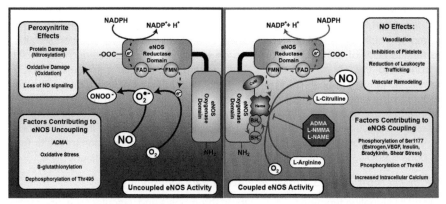

Fig. 1. eNOS regulation, coupling, and uncoupling. During coupled eNOS activity (*blue side*), in the presence of heme and tetrahydrobiopterin, electrons from NADPH are passed through a core of flavin adenine dinucleotide–flavin adenine mononucleotide in the reductase domain to the Heme prosthetic group on the oxygenase domain. Here, L-arginine and O_2 are consumed to create L-citrulline and NO. In the uncoupled state (*red side*), electrons are passed directly from the flavin adenine dinucleotide (FAD)–flavin adenine mononucleotide (FMN) core of the reductase domain to O_2, generating superoxide ($O_2^{•-}$), which can ultimately combine with locally produced NO to make peroxynitrite ($ONOO^-$). Several of the effects of $ONOO^-$ and NO are listed here, as well as factors contributing to both coupling and uncoupling of eNOS activity. These are explained in greater detail in the body of the text. VEGF, vascular endothelial growth factor.

brain, placental cells, and kidney tubular epithelium.[10] Nominally, NO production by eNOS increases substantially with increasing calcium concentrations secondary to its dependence on CaM. However, there are several alternative mechanisms for eNOS activation that lessen the importance of sustained increases in intracellular calcium for enzyme activity. The most well-studied of these is phosphorylation of the Ser1177 residue in the eNOS reductase domain, which leads to a higher flux of electrons and increased calcium sensitivity.[6,11,12] This modification is the end result of multiple signaling cascades associated with a variety of different protein kinase activation pathways. Signals include estrogen and vascular endothelial growth factor, which activate protein kinase B (Akt); insulin, which is thought to function through both Akt and AMP-activated protein kinase; bradykinin, which signals via $Ca^{2+}/$ CaM-dependent protein kinase II; and mechanical shear stress, which activates protein kinase A as well as Akt.[6,11,13] Another important residue is Thr495, which is phosphorylated by protein kinase C under resting conditions in endothelial cells. Phosphorylation of Thr495 limits CaM binding to eNOS, slowing electron transfer, and studies have demonstrated that Thr495 becomes dephosphorylated under stimuli that promote increases in intracellular Ca^{2+}.[11] However, this may be deleterious under certain circumstances, as dephosphorylated Thr495 also seems to favor uncoupling of eNOS activity.[14] Several other sites of post-translational modification have been identified, and are reviewed elsewhere.[15]

eNOS function is critical for maintenance of appropriate vascular homeostasis. NO signaling directly leads to blood vessel dilation by stimulating soluble guanylyl cyclase, leading to an increase in cyclic guanosine monophosphate and subsequent relaxation of vascular smooth muscle.[16–18] However, NO has multiple other distinct roles in vascular physiology. NO exerts antiplatelet effects through inhibition of platelet aggregation and adhesion; furthermore, eNOS-derived NO from platelets likely has both autocrine and paracrine inhibitory effects in a developing thrombus to limit pathologic clot formation.[5] NO decreases the expression of macrophage chemoattractant protein-1, which limits leukocyte trafficking to endothelium.[19] NO additionally alters the functionality of CD11/CD18 proteins on leukocytes, further altering their ability to adhere to the endothelial wall.[20] With regard to vascular remodeling, eNOS-derived NO plays a critical role in angiogenesis, and NO production is one of the final products of angiogenic signaling cascades. Studies have shown roles for eNOS in early neonatal lung capillary development, as well as for the appropriate development of collateral circulation and neovascularization following ischemic insult.[21] Broadly, this may be associated with the mobilization of appropriate progenitor cells from the bone marrow, as demonstrated by murine studies in eNOS-deficient mice.[22]

Endothelial Nitric Oxide Synthase in Vascular Pathophysiology

NO and its signaling functions, particularly in thrombosis and vascular tone, are central to the maintenance of vascular homeostasis. Highlighting this, ED is defined biochemically as a decreased amount of bioavailable NO in the vasculature. Broadly, the mechanisms underpinning ED can be placed into 2 basic categories: consumptive processes that transform bioavailable NO into other species and deficiencies in production of NO in the endothelium (**Fig. 2**).

Because NO is a highly diffusible and reactive species with an unpaired electron, there are a variety of chemical fates that prevent appropriate signaling. A primary driver of this deficiency is ROS, and $O_2^{\bullet-}$ in particular. $O_2^{\bullet-}$ reacts readily with NO, forming peroxynitrite ($ONOO^-$), a deleterious reactive nitrogen species that itself reacts readily with biological molecules both as a potent oxidant as well as a nitrating agent. Myriad acute and chronic pathologic states can potentiate the overproduction of ROS and subsequent $ONOO^-$ formation; a full discussion of these reactions is beyond the scope of this review.

In addition to the consumption of bioavailable NO as a mechanism to reduce NO signaling in ED, modifications to eNOS itself can also alter the production of NO at the source. As mentioned elsewhere in this article, eNOS requires dimerization in the presence of heme and BH_4 for effective electron movement to L-arginine. If this relationship is disrupted, the end result is that eNOS functions as a weak NADPH oxidase, producing $O_2^{\bullet-}$ instead of NO—a situation referred to as eNOS uncoupling. Multiple mechanisms contribute to eNOS uncoupling, which enhances local oxidative stress in addition to eliminating the vasoprotective effects of NO signaling. One such pathway involves $ONOO^-$ produced by initial oxidative stressors and functional eNOS. $ONOO^-$ both disrupts a key zinc-thiolate cluster in eNOS and oxidizes BH_4 to $BH_3^{\bullet}$, which is biologically inactive and leads to eNOS uncoupling—creating a vicious cycle in which more ROS are produced instead of NO.[23,24]

Another potential mechanism for eNOS uncoupling involves the bioavailability of L-arginine or its inhibitor, asymmetric dimethyl-L-arginine (ADMA). L-Arginine supplementation has been shown to partially alleviate ED in various animal and human subject models.[25-28] This does not seem to be associated with substantially altered global L-arginine levels, but instead with relative bioavailability at the endothelium. Endothelial cells and acute inflammatory cells such as macrophages can express arginases that locally decrease L-arginine pools and effectively starve eNOS of substrate.[29-31] ADMA, in contrast, is an endogenous inhibitor of eNOS and its production is strongly governed by redox status. Both the production of ADMA by protein arginine N-methyltransferase type 1 and its subsequent degradation by dimethylarginine dimethylaminohydrolase are altered by oxidative stress. Protein arginine N-methyltransferase type 1 is more active under oxidative conditions and dimethylarginine

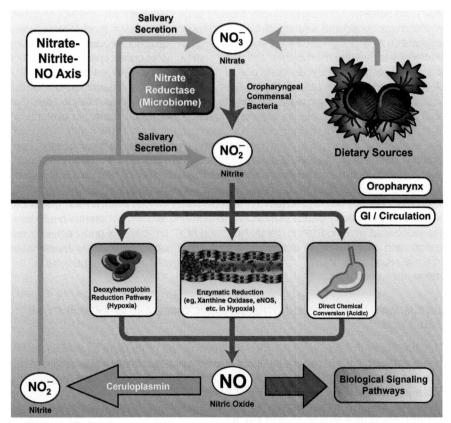

Fig. 2. The nitrate–nitrite–NO pathway. Increasingly, research is demonstrating that dietary nitrates and nitrites serve as an endogenous reservoir for noncanonically produced NO, particularly in hypoxic conditions when NOS may be less functional or predisposed to being uncoupled. A detailed explanation of this pathway can be found in the body of the text.

dimethylaminohydrolase is less active, leading to increased steady-state concentrations of ADMA and eNOS inhibition and uncoupling.[32]

Post-translational modifications of eNOS may also contribute to pathologic uncoupling and reduction of NO production. As mentioned elsewhere in this article, dephosphorylation of Thr495 may lead to uncoupling and production of deleterious ROS. Another increasingly well-characterized modification is S-glutathionylation, which is involved in signaling under conditions of oxidative stress and may serve to protect redox-sensitive cysteine residues in the eNOS protein. S-glutathionylation, which is reversible under reducing conditions, is associated with reduced eNOS activity and enhanced production of $O_2^{\bullet-}$.[33,34]

ALTERNATIVE NITRIC OXIDE NO PRODUCTION: NITRATE–NITRITE–NITRIC OXIDE PATHWAY

NO produced enzymatically from L-arginine by NOS isoforms may not always be sufficient to maintain appropriate endothelial homeostasis, particularly under hypoxic conditions. Recently, more research has focused on the contributions of alternative routes to NO production—namely, from the reduction of dietary nitrates and nitrites to NO.[35–38] Nitrate

(NO_3^-) and nitrite (NO_2^-) were previously thought to be inert metabolites of NO, and their detection was considered a surrogate for NO production.[38] However, more recent studies suggest that NO_3^-, NO_2^-, and NO all exist in a complex equilibrium mediated by microenvironmental stimuli, the microbiome, and dietary nitrate/nitrite consumption. A full discussion of this pathway is beyond the scope of the present review, but a summary of the relevant material can be seen in **Fig. 2**. Briefly, dietary NO_3^- is reduced by oral nitrate reductase-expressing commensal bacteria to NO_2^-. NO_2^- then has multiple fates that result in NO production, both via enzymatic and nonenzymatic means. For example, in the acidic environment of the stomach, NO_2^- is nonenzymatically converted to NO, which then exerts local effects. NO_2^- may also enter the bloodstream via gastrointestinal absorption. Here, under relative hypoxia, NO_2^- can be reduced by deoxyhemoglobin, releasing NO in local microcirculation. Xanthine oxidase and eNOS itself also likely reduce NO_2^- to NO under acidic or hypoxic conditions, such as tissue ischemia. Critically, circulating NO_2^- also may be oxidized to NO_3^-, approximately 25% of which is recirculated into the saliva by the salivary glands to maintain the signaling axis.[36] The potential health benefits associated with modulating dietary NO_2^- and NO_3^- are currently under active investigation, and recent studies demonstrate that NO_3^- supplementation is beneficial in ischemia–reperfusion injury,[39,40] pulmonary hypertension,[41–43] and hypertension,[44–46] among other conditions.

CLINICAL IMPLICATIONS OF ENDOTHELIAL NITRIC OXIDE AND NITRIC OXIDE REGULATION

NO signaling pathways, involving the regulation of NO production as well as downstream activation of second messengers, are heavily associated with a variety of pathologies. Here, we discuss broadly how the NO axis plays a role in both the multisystem organ dysfunction of critical illness and sepsis, as well as provide brief summaries of some of the data regarding NO signaling in specific organ pathology. This process is also summarized in **Fig. 3**.

Sepsis and Infectious Disease

Sepsis is characterized by a dysregulated immune response to an initial infectious insult, and has gained significant attention owing to its emergence as a leading cause of in-hospital mortality.[47] ED is a key feature of sepsis and septic shock, resulting in microcirculatory dysfunction and end-organ hypoperfusion. Subsequently, NO has been studied extensively as a potential therapeutic target in treating sepsis.

NO mediates the inflammatory response to host pathogens through various mechanisms. Endogenous NO from iNOS expressed during the acute inflammatory response has been identified as a regulator of the NLRP3 inflammasome via stabilization of mitochondria.[48] Using either genetic knockout ($iNOS^{-/-}$) or pharmacologic inhibition of iNOS in a murine endotoxemia model, inflammatory cytokine production was significantly enhanced and associated with increased mortality.[48] In another study, supplementation with L-arginine decreased neutrophil adhesion and increased rolling velocity, which was reversed with a nonselective NOS inhibitor but not a selective iNOS inhibitor.[49] This result suggests that eNOS mediates these effects, although it is unclear what the relative contributions of endothelium-derived eNOS versus platelet-derived eNOS are in the regulation of the inflammatory response. Nevertheless, selective regulation of eNOS in relation to the deleterious impact of iNOS may attenuate the negative effects on microvascular tone.[49]

Despite its vasodilatory properties, administration of inhaled NO (iNO) has not been demonstrated to cause systemic hypotension. However, this treatment does increase

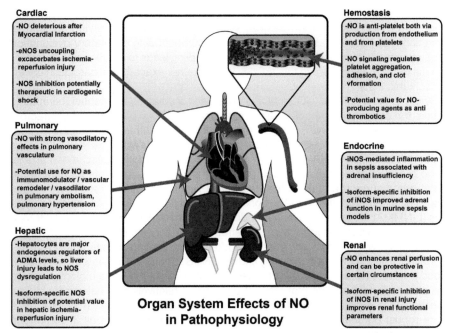

Cardiac
- NO deleterious after Myocardial Infarction
- eNOS uncoupling excacerbates ischemia-reperfusion injury
- NOS inhibition potentially therapeutic in cardiogenic shock

Pulmonary
- NO with strong vasodilatory effects in pulmonary vasculature
- Potential use for NO as immunomodulator / vascular remodeler / vasodilator in pulmonary embolism, pulmonary hypertension

Hepatic
- Hepatocytes are major endogenous regulators of ADMA levels, so liver injury leads to NOS dysregulation
- Isoform-specific NOS inhibition of potential value in hepatic ischemia-reperfusion injury

Hemostasis
- NO is anti-platelet both via production from endothelium and from platelets
- NO signaling regulates platelet aggregation, adhesion, and clot vformation
- Potential value for NO-producing agents as anti thrombotics

Endocrine
- iNOS-mediated inflammation in sepsis associated with adrenal insufficiency
- Isoform-specific inhibition of iNOS improved adrenal function in murine sepsis models

Renal
- NO enhances renal perfusion and can be protective in certain circumstances
- Isoform-specific inhibition of iNOS in renal injury improves renal functional parameters

Organ System Effects of NO in Pathophysiology

Fig. 3. A brief overview of NO signaling in specific organ system pathophysiology. For more specific details and references, please refer to the body of the text.

nitrite levels, which might supply NO and promote beneficial vasodilatation in targeted microcirculatory beds. Because local shunting and imbalance in regional flow may contribute to sepsis-induced organ dysfunction, this paradigm has remained a therapeutic target. A randomized controlled trial of iNO compared with a sham treatment in severe sepsis was designed to address this issue. However, on evaluation the authors found no differences in microcirculatory flow, lactate clearance, or organ dysfunction, suggesting little value for NO in the later stages of sepsis.[50]

Methylene blue has also been studied for its potential therapeutic value in NO-mediated vasodilatation. In addition to being a powerful reducing agent, methylene blue inhibits guanylate cyclase and has been demonstrated to increase systemic vascular resistance in patients with shock. Its widespread use is currently limited owing to associations with renal failure and hyperbilirubinemia, in addition to broader questions about its efficacy.[51]

Although multisystem organ dysfunction is a deadly consequence of sepsis, isolated organ dysfunction can occur secondary to a wide array of noninfectious critical illnesses. Global tissue hypoperfusion results in hypoxia, accumulation of toxic metabolites, and subsequent ischemia–reperfusion injury, all of which may result in permanent organ damage or compound preexisting injuries to other organ systems. Regulation of microvascular flow mediated by NO in these circumstances may thus determine outcomes in critically ill patients. Several specific studied roles for NO and ED in the in the pathophysiology of various organ systems are discussed in the subsequent sections.

Cardiovascular System

NO has demonstrable direct inotropic effects in addition to its role in peripheral vasodilatation. Cardiomyocytes express both nNOS and eNOS constitutively, whereas iNOS expression can be induced by inflammatory mediators. Abnormally high amounts of NO produced in response to acute inflammation following myocardial infarction may have negative inotropic effects, compounding circulatory dysfunction after myocardial infarction. Moreover, NOS uncoupling leads to additional ROS formation (as detailed elsewhere in this article), which further exacerbates cardiac injury after ischemic insult.[52]

Owing to these effects, NOS inhibition has been studied as a potential therapeutic option for cardiogenic shock.[53] In a randomized trial in patients with refractory cardiogenic shock, N-γ-nitro-L-arginine methyl ester (L-NAME), a nonspecific NOS inhibitor, was associated with significantly improved mortality at 30 days (27% vs 67%).[53] Additionally, L-NAME therapy was associated with increased mean arterial blood pressure, increased urine output, and decreased requirements for intra-aortic blood pump support and need for mechanical ventilation. Similar results were seen in a small exploratory trial with the nonspecific NOS inhibitor N^G-monomethyl-L-arginine (L-NMMA).[54] However, a larger randomized controlled trial evaluating L-NMMA in patients with myocardial infarction and refractory cardiogenic shock (TRIUMPH) was terminated early owing to a lack of efficacy after demonstrating no difference in 30-day mortality.[55] Despite these conflicting findings, NOS inhibition-associated increases in blood pressure were present in all treated patients suggesting some biological effect. It is also important to note that these drugs carry a relatively safe risk profile.[55] One question that remains is whether isoform-specific NOS inhibition may provide a more robust outcome, given the confluence of NO signaling from all 3 isoforms in cardiomyocytes.

Pulmonary Function and Nitric Oxide

iNO has theoretic benefit in the lungs owing to its ability induce selective pulmonary vasodilatation and improve ventilation–perfusion mismatch.[56] Studies have demonstrated that iNO exerts a vasodilatory effect only in conditions of elevated pulmonary vascular tone and has little effect in normal pulmonary vasculature.[57] The US Food and Drug Administration has approved iNO administration for neonatal hypoxic respiratory failure; at present, there is no US Food and Drug Administration approval for treatment in adults. However, there are several lung pathologies for which iNO is presently being investigated as a potential therapy.

The theoretic benefit of iNO in adult acute respiratory distress syndrome is 2-fold: immune modulation in the setting of exuberant inflammation, as well as alleviation pulmonary vasoconstriction. However, a Cochrane review from 2010 found no benefit to iNO administration in acute respiratory distress syndrome, despite the theoretic benefit of direct pulmonary administration.[56] Indeed, iNO administration in acute respiratory distress syndrome was associated with harmful effects, most notably renal impairment.

In pulmonary arterial hypertension (PAH) with associated right ventricular dysfunction, localized ED of the pulmonary vasculature is a known entity. In PAH, pulmonary arterial eNOS is frequently uncoupled, favoring $O_2^{\bullet-}$ generation and leading to less production of NO.[57] The NO pathway is 1 of 3 well-characterized molecular pathways in PAH, alongside prostacyclin and endothelin-1 signaling.[58] Several therapies in current clinical use target downstream elements of the NO signaling pathway, including phosphodiesterase type 5 inhibitors (sildenafil) as well as direct soluble guanylate cyclase stimulators (riociguat).[59] Collectively, these agents enhance cyclic guanosine monophosphate-based signaling, which comprises the second message portion of the NO signaling cascade. Other approaches have examined the production of NO itself: the PHACeT trial was designed as a phase I clinical trial to deliver eNOS-overexpressing endothelial progenitor cells to patients with refractory PAH.[60] Endothelial cells were delivered via pulmonary artery catheter to 5 patients resulting in a transient improvement in pulmonary resistance with a sustained increase in 6-minute walk distance even at 6 months.[60] This promising approach requires further study to examine efficacy.

Given the vasodilatory effect of iNO on the pulmonary vasculature and potential to alter shunt fraction, iNO therapy has theoretic benefit in patients with acute pulmonary embolism. In the recently published iNOPE trial, patients with submassive pulmonary embolism and right ventricular dysfunction were randomized to receive either iNO or O_2. The authors demonstrated that iNO failed to normalize troponin or echocardiogram endpoints, but patients receiving iNO were more likely to display improvements in right ventricular hypokinesis and dilation on echocardiography.[61] This area is another that demands additional study for the delineation of exact benefits of iNO on pulmonary physiology.

Hepatic Function and Nitric Oxide

NO has been implicated in the hyperdynamic circulation seen in acute liver failure, subsequent to presumed overproduction of NO in splanchnic circulation.[62] In a devascularized porcine model of acute liver failure, Sharma and colleagues[62] measured plasma levels of L-arginine, citrulline, ornithine, NO, and ADMA, as well as plasma arginase activities in both sham and injured animals. Plasma arginine was significantly depleted 6 hours after injury, concomitant with an increase in plasma ADMA as well as enhanced plasma arginase activity. Despite this, systemic levels of NO were not significantly decreased, suggesting that in this model of acute liver failure NO production was not limited by plasma substrate or inhibitor bioavailability. However, other data suggest that hepatic clearance of ADMA may play a central role in the propagation of multiorgan failure in shock states. Hepatocytes are the primary expressors of dimethylarginine dimethylaminohydrolase, which metabolize ADMA, and liver dysfunction through a variety of means leads to increasing plasma ADMA levels. Increasing ADMA concentration, in turn, is an independent risk factor for multiorgan failure in critically ill patients, highlighting the importance of this NOS regulatory capacity.[63]

Hepatic ischemia–reperfusion injury studies have similarly provided a wealth of data that could be extrapolated to whole organism shock states and global hypoperfusion. These studies have been recently reviewed elsewhere by Zhang and colleagues.[64] In summary, NO has multiple complex functions in hepatic ischemia–reperfusion injury, depending on the source of production and depending on the downstream pathways favored. For example, eNOS expression in hepatic vasculature is protective against hepatic ischemia–reperfusion injury, but overexpression can be detrimental. In contrast, inhibition of iNOS induced during the inflammatory cascade after reperfusion is also protective, suggesting that overproduction of NO leads to detrimental downstream effects. Clearly, NOS regulation involves a delicate homeostasis, and extreme overproduction or underproduction of NO after liver injury can lead to harmful downstream effects.

Renal Function and Nitric Oxide

NO broadly regulates renal hemodynamics and function, which has been extensively reviewed elsewhere.[65] In shock states, as modeled by ischemic models of acute renal failure, targeting the NO pathway seems to be beneficial.[66] In addition to its direct vasodilatory effects, NO also suppresses production of endothelin-1, a potent vasoconstrictor. In a rat model of renal ischemia-reperfusion injury, a key pathologic driver of acute kidney injury, pretreatment with the NO donor FK409 attenuated renal dysfunction, histologic damage, and endothelin-1 overproduction. Conversely, pretreatment with the NOS inhibitor L-NAME resulted in increased endothelin-1 production, demonstrating that the inhibition of NO production led to deleterious effects.[66] The effects of NOS inhibition seems to be isoform specific, similar to what is seen in the liver. In a similar model system, selective iNOS inhibition attenuated the decrease in renal oxygen delivery and microvascular oxygen pressure seen with reperfusion injury; it also improved renal oxygen extraction and consumption.[67] Taken together, these findings suggest that iNOS may be contributing to harmful pathways in ischemia–reperfusion events and that inhibition of iNOS in selected scenarios may be of clinical value.

Nitric Oxide and Coagulation

Studies in human patients have demonstrated activation of coagulation factors as well as platelets in severe sepsis and septic shock.[68] This may represent a protective mechanism to contain pathogen spread that is exhausted in severe sepsis and septic shock. However, overexuberant coagulation with platelet activation leads to the consumptive pathology of disseminated intravascular coagulation, a devastating condition that is associated with significantly increased mortality.[69] NO signaling plays a major role in regulating platelet aggregation, adhesion, and clot formation overall.[5] NO produced by healthy endothelium nominally serves a local antiplatelet role by limiting platelet adhesion and activation through activation of the NO-soluble guanylate cyclase axis in platelets themselves. There is additionally a substantial amount of eNOS expressed by platelets, suggesting that both autocrine and paracrine NO signaling occurs within developing clots, thereby limiting progression. Indeed, there is some consideration that NO-enhancing drugs may provide both cardiovascular and antiplatelet benefit, and this area of research is constantly evolving.[5]

Endocrine Signaling and Nitric Oxide

Sepsis is marked by low cortisol levels and blunted response to adrenocorticotrophic hormone stimulation, which together lead to adrenal insufficiency. Because NO has been linked to organ dysfunction in various other tissues, studies have focused on NO-mediated effects in the adrenal glands. In an experimental endotoxemia model, both iNOS expression and NO production were increased in the adrenal glands of mice.[70] This was associated with the development of an adrenal insufficiency phenotype in these animals, as well as enhanced mitochondrial superoxide production in adrenal cortical cells. This effect was mitigated by iNOS inhibition, but was exacerbated by treatment with a systemic NO donor. Notably, increased expression of iNOS was localized to the endothelium and resident macrophages rather than adrenocortical cells, suggesting that some degree of ED contributes to adrenal insufficiency in sepsis.[70]

SUMMARY

NO is a critically important gaseous transmitter with a large number of context-dependent functions, and its production and consumption are tightly regulated to limit potential damage. The endothelium is a major source of NO, as it constitutively expresses eNOS and modifies NO production profiles in response to a variety of endogenous and exogenous stressors. ED occurs when this signaling axis is perturbed, limiting the ability of the vasculature and local structures either to produce NO itself or to respond appropriately to its presence. This is a central pathologic process in a number of different acute and chronic conditions, and NO and its downstream signaling partners are thus a prime therapeutic target. Although enthusiasm regarding iNO as a therapy is partially hindered by its exorbitant cost, numerous pharmacologic approaches for NO delivery have been researched and more are certainly in development.

Underscoring this, there are currently 101 registered clinically trials in the United States involving NO that are actively recruiting subjects. These trials span a wide breadth of disease processes, echoing the diverse effects and widespread therapeutic potential of this gaseous mediator. With the increasing recognition of the roles of specific NOS isoforms in certain tissues and a focus on optimizing NO delivery given its intrinsic properties, future work stands poised to optimize this pharmacologic target and provide a helpful toolbox to mitigate ED associated with critical illness.

DISCLOSURE

The authors have nothing to disclose.

REFERENCES

1. Sturtzel C. Endothelial cells. In: Sattler S, Kennedy-Lydon T, editors. The Immunology of Cardiovascular Homeostasis and Pathology. Advances in Experimental Medicine and Biology, vol. 1003. Cham: Springer; 2017.
2. Incalza MA, D'Oria R, Natalicchio A, et al. Oxidative stress and reactive oxygen species in endothelial dysfunction associated with cardiovascular and metabolic diseases. Vascul Pharmacol 2018;100(June 2017):1–19.
3. Tousoulis D, Kampoli A-M, Tentolouris Nikolaos Papageorgiou C, et al. The role of nitric oxide on endothelial function. Curr Vasc Pharmacol 2012;10(1):4–18.
4. Vallet B. Bench-to-bedside review: endothelial cell dysfunction in severe sepsis: a role in organ dysfunction? Crit Care 2003;7(2):130–8.
5. Gresele P, Momi S, Guglielmini G. Nitric oxide-enhancing or -releasing agents as antithrombotic drugs. Biochem Pharmacol 2019;166(June):300–12.
6. Förstermann U, Sessa WC. Nitric oxide synthases: regulation and function. Eur Heart J 2012;33(7):829–37.
7. Zhou L, Zhu D-Y. Neuronal nitric oxide synthase: structure, subcellular localization, regulation, and clinical implications. Nitric Oxide 2009;20(4):223–30.
8. Melikian N, Seddon MD, Casadei B, et al. Neuronal nitric oxide synthase and human vascular regulation. Trends Cardiovasc Med 2009;19(8):256–62.
9. Lind M, Hayes A, Caprnda M, et al. Inducible nitric oxide synthase: good or bad? Biomed Pharmacother 2017;93:370–5.
10. Förstermann U, Closs EI, Pollock JS, et al. Nitric oxide synthase isozymes. Characterization, purification, molecular cloning, and functions. Hypertension 1994; 23(6_pt_2):1121–31.
11. Fleming I, Busse R. Molecular mechanisms involved in the regulation of the endothelial nitric oxide synthase. Am J Physiol Integr Comp Physiol 2003;284(1): R1–12.
12. Fulton D, Gratton J-P, McCabe TJ, et al. Regulation of endothelium-derived nitric oxide production by the protein kinase Akt. Nature 1999;399(6736):597–601.
13. Dixit M, Loot AE, Mohamed A, et al. Gab1, SHP2, and protein kinase a are crucial for the activation of the endothelial NO synthase by fluid shear stress. Circ Res 2005;97(12):1236–44.
14. Lin MI, Fulton D, Babbitt R, et al. Phosphorylation of threonine 497 in endothelial nitric-oxide synthase coordinates the coupling of L-arginine metabolism to efficient nitric oxide production. J Biol Chem 2003;278(45):44719–26.

15. Fleming I. Molecular mechanisms underlying the activation of eNOS. Pflugers Arch 2010;459(6):793–806.

16. Ignarro LJ, Harbison RG, Wood KS, et al. Activation of purified soluble guanylate cyclase by endothelium-derived relaxing factor from intrapulmonary artery and vein: stimulation by acetylcholine, bradykinin and arachidonic acid. J Pharmacol Exp Ther 1986;237(3):893–900. Available at: http://www.ncbi.nlm. nih.gov/pubmed/2872327.

17. Rapoport RM, Draznin MB, Murad F. Endothelium-dependent relaxation in rat aorta may be mediated through cyclic GMP-dependent protein phosphorylation. Nature 1983;306(5939):174–6.

18. Förstermann U, Mülsch A, Böhme E, et al. Stimulation of soluble guanylate cyclase by an acetylcholine-induced endothelium-derived factor from rabbit and canine arteries. Circ Res 1986;58(4):531–8.

19. Zeiher AM, Fisslthaler B, Schray-Utz B, et al. Nitric oxide modulates the expression of monocyte chemoattractant protein 1 in cultured human endothelial cells. Circ Res 1995;76(6):980–6.

20. Kubes P, Suzuki M, Granger DN. Nitric oxide: an endogenous modulator of leukocyte adhesion. Proc Natl Acad Sci U S A 1991;88(11):4651–5.

21. Murohara T, Asahara T, Silver M, et al. Nitric oxide synthase modulates angiogenesis in response to tissue ischemia. J Clin Invest 1998;101(11):2567–78.

22. Aicher A, Heeschen C, Mildner-Rihm C, et al. Essential role of endothelial nitric oxide synthase for mobilization of stem and progenitor cells. Nat Med 2003; 9(11):1370–6.

23. Landmesser U, Dikalov S, Price SR, et al. Oxidation of tetrahydrobiopterin leads to uncoupling of endothelial cell nitric oxide synthase in hypertension. J Clin Invest 2003;111(8):1201–9.

24. Kuzkaya N, Weissmann N, Harrison DG, et al. Interactions of peroxynitrite, tetrahydrobiopterin, ascorbic acid, and thiols: implications for uncoupling endothelial nitric-oxide synthase. J Biol Chem 2003;278(25):22546–54.

25. Hishikawa K, Nakaki T, Suzuki H, et al. Role of L-arginine-nitric oxide pathway in hypertension. J Hypertens 1993;11(6):639–45.

26. Ishikawa K, Calzavacca P, Bellomo R, et al. Effect of selective inhibition of renal inducible nitric oxide synthase on renal blood flow and function in experimental hyperdynamic sepsis. Crit Care Med 2012;40(8):2368–75.

27. Drexler H, Zeiher AM, Meinzer K, et al. Correction of endothelial dysfunction in coronary microcirculation of hypercholesterolaemic patients by L-arginine. Lancet 1991;338(8782–8783):1546–50.

28. Rossitch E, Alexander E, Black PM, et al. L-arginine normalizes endothelial function in cerebral vessels from hypercholesterolemic rabbits. J Clin Invest 1991; 87(4):1295–9.

29. Xu W, Kaneko FT, Zheng S, et al. Increased arginase II and decreased NO synthesis in endothelial cells of patients with pulmonary arterial hypertension. FASEB J 2004;18(14):1746–8.

30. Ming X-F, Barandier C, Viswambharan H, et al. Thrombin stimulates human endothelial arginase enzymatic activity via RhoA/ROCK pathway: implications for atherosclerotic endothelial dysfunction. Circulation 2004;110(24):3708–14.

31. Berkowitz DE, White R, Li D, et al. Arginase reciprocally regulates nitric oxide synthase activity and contributes to endothelial dysfunction in aging blood vessels. Circulation 2003;108(16):2000–6.

32. Karbach S, Wenzel P, Waisman A, et al. eNOS uncoupling in cardiovascular diseases–the role of oxidative stress and inflammation. Curr Pharm Des 2014;20(22): 3579–94.

33. Chen C-A, Wang T-Y, Varadharaj S, et al. S-glutathionylation uncouples eNOS and regulates its cellular and vascular function. Nature 2010;468(7327):1115–8.

34. Zweier JL, Chen C-A, Druhan LJ. S-glutathionylation reshapes our understanding of endothelial nitric oxide synthase uncoupling and nitric oxide/reactive oxygen species-mediated signaling. Antioxid Redox Signal 2011;14(10):1769–75.

35. Qu XM, Wu ZF, Pang BX, et al. From nitrate to nitric oxide: the role of salivary glands and oral bacteria. J Dent Res 2016;95(13):1452–6.

36. Ma L, Hu L, Feng X, et al. Nitrate and nitrite in health and disease. Aging Dis 2018;9(5):938.

37. DeMartino AW, Kim-Shapiro DB, Patel RP, et al. Nitrite and nitrate chemical biology and signalling. Br J Pharmacol 2019;176(2):228–45.

38. Carlstrom M, Montenegro MF. Therapeutic value of stimulating the nitrate-nitrite-nitric oxide pathway to attenuate oxidative stress and restore nitric oxide bioavailability in cardiorenal disease. J Intern Med 2019;285(1):2–18.

39. Yang T, Zhang X-M, Tarnawski L, et al. Dietary nitrate attenuates renal ischemia-reperfusion injuries by modulation of immune responses and reduction of oxidative stress. Redox Biol 2017;13:320–30.

40. Jeddi S, Khalifi S, Ghanbari M, et al. Effects of nitrate intake on myocardial ischemia-reperfusion injury in diabetic rats. Arq Bras Cardiol 2016;107(4): 339–47.

41. Malikova E, Carlström M, Kmecova Z, et al. Effects of inorganic nitrate in a rat model of monocrotaline-induced pulmonary arterial hypertension. Basic Clin Pharmacol Toxicol 2019. https://doi.org/10.1111/bcpt.13309.

42. Cortés-Puch I, Sun J, Schechter AN, et al. Inhaled nebulized nitrite and nitrate therapy in a canine model of hypoxia-induced pulmonary hypertension. Nitric Oxide 2019;91:1–14.

43. Koch CD, Gladwin MT, Freeman BA, et al. Enterosalivary nitrate metabolism and the microbiome: intersection of microbial metabolism, nitric oxide and diet in cardiac and pulmonary vascular health. Free Radic Biol Med 2017;105:48–67.

44. Lara J, Ashor AW, Oggioni C, et al. Effects of inorganic nitrate and beetroot supplementation on endothelial function: a systematic review and meta-analysis. Eur J Nutr 2016;55(2):451–9.

45. Ashor AW, Lara J, Siervo M. Medium-term effects of dietary nitrate supplementation on systolic and diastolic blood pressure in adults: a systematic review and meta-analysis. J Hypertens 2017;35(7):1353–9.

46. Kapil V, Khambata RS, Robertson A, et al. Dietary nitrate provides sustained blood pressure lowering in hypertensive patients: a randomized, phase 2, double-blind, placebo-controlled study. Hypertension 2015;65(2):320–7.

47. Hall MJ, Levant S, Defrances CJ. Trends in inpatient hospital deaths: national hospital discharge survey, 2000–2010. NCHS Data Brief 2013;(118):1–8.

48. Mao K, Chen S, Chen M, et al. Nitric oxide suppresses NLRP3 inflammasome activation and protects against LPS-induced septic shock. Cell Res 2013;23(2): 201–12.

49. Khan R, Kirschenbaum LA, Larow C, et al. Augmentation of platelet and endothelial cell enos activity decreases sepsis-related neutrophil-endothelial cell interactions. Shock 2010;33(3):242–6.

50. Trzeciak S, Glaspey LJ, Dellinger RP, et al. Randomized controlled trial of inhaled nitric oxide for the treatment of microcirculatory dysfunction in patients with sepsis. Crit Care Med 2014;42(12):2482–92.
51. Weiner MM, Lin H-M, Danforth D, et al. Methylene blue is associated with poor outcomes in vasoplegic shock. J Cardiothorac Vasc Anesth 2013;27(6):1233–8.
52. Umar S, Van Der Laarse A. Nitric oxide and nitric oxide synthase isoforms in the normal, hypertrophic, and failing heart. Mol Cell Biochem 2010;333(1–2):191–201.
53. Cotter G, Kaluski E, Milo O, et al. LINCS: L-NAME (a NO synthase inhibitor) in the treatment of refractory cardiogenic shock: a prospective randomized study. Eur Heart J 2003;24(14):1287–95.
54. Cotter G, Kaluski E, Blatt A, et al. L-NMMA (a nitric oxide synthase inhibitor) is effective in the treatment of cardiogenic shock. Circulation 2000;101(12): 1358–61. Available at: http://ovidsp.ovid.com/ovidweb.cgi?T=JS&PAGE= reference&D=emed5&NEWS=N&AN=2000114347.
55. The TRIUMPH Investigators. Effect of tilarginine acetate in patients with acute myocardial infarction and cardiogenic shock. JAMA 2007;297(15):1657.
56. Afshari A, Brok J, Møller AM, et al. Inhaled nitric oxide for acute respiratory distress syndrome and acute lung injury in adults and children. Cochrane Database Syst Rev 2010;7. https://doi.org/10.1097/sa.0b013e318242c0bc.
57. Klinger JR, Abman SH, Gladwin MT. Nitric oxide deficiency and endothelial dysfunction in pulmonary arterial hypertension. Am J Respir Crit Care Med 2013;188(6):639–46.
58. Huertas A, Tu L, Guignabert C. New targets for pulmonary arterial hypertension: going beyond the currently targeted three pathways. Curr Opin Pulm Med 2017; 23(5):377–85.
59. Watanabe H. Treatment selection in pulmonary arterial hypertension: phosphodiesterase type 5 inhibitors versus soluble guanylate cyclase stimulator. Eur Cardiol 2018;13(1):35–7.
60. Granton J, Langleben D, Kutryk MB, et al. Endothelial NO-synthase gene-enhanced progenitor cell therapy for pulmonary arterial hypertension: the PHACeT Trial. Circ Res 2015;117(7):645–54.
61. Kline JA, Puskarich MA, Jones AE, et al. Inhaled nitric oxide to treat intermediate risk pulmonary embolism: a multicenter randomized controlled trial. Nitric Oxide 2019;84:60–8.
62. Sharma V, Ten Have GAM, Ytrebo L, et al. Nitric oxide and l-arginine metabolism in a devascularized porcine model of acute liver failure. Am J Physiol Gastrointest Liver Physiol 2012;303(3):G435–41.
63. Ferrigno A, Di Pasqua LG, Berardo C, et al. Liver plays a central role in asymmetric dimethylarginine-mediated organ injury. World J Gastroenterol 2015; 21(17):5131–7.
64. Zhang Y-Q, Ding N, Zeng Y-F, et al. New progress in roles of nitric oxide during hepatic ischemia reperfusion injury. World J Gastroenterol 2017;23(14):2505–10.
65. Krishnan SM, Kraehling JR, Eitner F, et al. The impact of the Nitric Oxide (NO)/Soluble Guanylyl Cyclase (sGC) signaling cascade on kidney health and disease: a preclinical perspective. Int J Mol Sci 2018;19(6). https://doi.org/10.3390/ijms19061712.
66. Kurata H, Takaoka M, Kubo Y, et al. Protective effect of nitric oxide on ischemia/reperfusion-induced renal injury and endothelin-1 overproduction. Eur J Pharmacol 2005;517(3):232–9.

67. Legrand M, Almac E, Mik EG, et al. I -NIL prevents renal microvascular hypoxia and increase of renal oxygen consumption after ischemia-reperfusion in rats. Am J Physiol Renal Physiol 2009;296(5):F1109–17.
68. Mavrommatis AC, Roussos C, Zakynthinos S, et al. Coagulation system and platelets are fully activated in uncomplicated sepsis. Crit Care Med 2000;28(2): 451–7.
69. Iba T, Levi M, Levy JH. Sepsis-induced coagulopathy and disseminated intravascular coagulation. Semin Thromb Hemost 2019. https://doi.org/10.1055/s-0039-1694995.
70. Wang CN, Duan GL, Liu YJ, et al. Overproduction of nitric oxide by endothelial cells and macrophages contributes to mitochondrial oxidative stress in adrenocortical cells and adrenal insufficiency during endotoxemia. Free Radic Biol Med 2015;83:31–40.

Microvascular Dysfunction in the Critically Ill

Can Ince, PhD[a], Daniel De Backer, MD, PhD[b], Philip R. Mayeux, PhD[c],*

KEYWORDS

- Microcirculation • Lymphatics • Endothelium • Critical illness • Aging

KEY POINTS

- Microvascular dysfunction may occur as a result of direct endothelial injury or by mediators released as a result of inadequate perfusion or trauma.
- Preservation of endothelial function and rapid restoration of microcirculatory perfusion should be the goals of resuscitation efforts.
- Effects of aging on the microvasculature could make resuscitation and recovery in the critically ill more difficult and less predictable.
- Advances in imaging technology and analysis have made it possible to assess the effectiveness of resuscitative strategies in real time and at the bedside.

INTRODUCTION

Microvascular dysfunction contributes to the pathogenesis of chronic conditions such as diabetes and cardiovascular disease and acute critical illnesses such as trauma, hemorrhagic shock, ischemia, and sepsis. The elderly is especially at risk due to aging of the microvasculature, which can sensitize the microvasculature to injury and hinder recovery.[1,2] Oxygen and nutrient delivery and the removal of metabolic waste are critical functions of the microcirculation to maintain organ function and promote recovery following organ injury. Indeed, it is well established that the severity of microvascular dysfunction is associated with the development of organ dysfunction and ultimately poorer patient outcomes.[3,4] The goal of resuscitative therapies must be correction of tissue perfusion and oxygen delivery. Thus, measured improvements in the microcirculation would be a valuable readout to assess effective resuscitative efforts. This review summarizes briefly these concepts in the context of the importance of targeting the microcirculation and the difficulties encountered in the clinical setting.

[a] Department of Intensive Care, Laboratory of Translational Intensive Care, Erasmus MC, University Medical Center, Dr Molewaterplein 40, 3015 GD Rotterdam, the Netherlands; [b] Department of Intensive Care, CHIREC Hospitals and Université Libre de Bruxelles, Bd du Triomphe 201, 1160 Brussels, Belgium; [c] Department of Pharmacology and Toxicology, University of Arkansas for Medical Sciences, 4301 West Markham Street, #611, Little Rock, AR 72212, USA
* Corresponding author.
E-mail address: prmayeux@uams.edu

Crit Care Clin 36 (2020) 323–331
https://doi.org/10.1016/j.ccc.2019.11.003
0749-0704/20/© 2019 Elsevier Inc. All rights reserved.

criticalcare.theclinics.com

THE MICROCIRCULATION

The microcirculation can be defined broadly as a branching network of small-diameter ($\sim$5–100 µm) blood vessels including arterioles, capillaries, and venules. The microcirculation is responsible for functions critical to tissue and organ preservation and recovery in the critically ill. These include delivery of oxygen and nutrients, removal of carbon dioxide and metabolic waste, conveyance of immune cells, and tissue/organ fluid balance. Impairment of the microcirculation is common in chronic illnesses such as diabetes, neurodegenerative, and cardiovascular disorders[5–9] and in acute critical illness such as blunt trauma, hemorrhagic shock, ischemia/reperfusion, and sepsis.[10–13] Systemic complications such as acute respiratory distress syndrome and multiple organ dysfunction syndrome are relatively common in these patients due to release of inflammatory (and other) mediators. In these patients, microcirculatory dysfunction likely contributes significantly to morbidity and mortality.[12,14] However, the blood microcirculation is not the only microvasculature regulating tissue/organ oxygen delivery, fluid balance, and delivery of immune cells.

THE LYMPHATICS

The lymphatic microvasculature is a pump and valve system, which runs essentially parallel to the blood microvasculature.[15] It functions as a conduit for interstitial fluid and immune cell transport. The discontinuous endothelial layer allows movement of fluid and cells from the interstitial space to move into the lymphatic system and ultimately into the systemic circulation. Lymph propulsion is accomplished via synchronized contraction waves of the lymphatic muscle present in larger collecting lymphatics and one-way valves.[16] Functioning lymphatic vessels prevent accumulation of interstitial fluid, thereby reducing edema. Dysfunction of the lymphatic endothelium, muscle, or valves can disrupt fluid homeostasis and increase intraorgan pressure.[17–20] Changes in lymphatic function are associated with some chronic diseases such as metabolic syndrome, congestive heart failure, chronic renal failure, and hypertension.[18–21] In the critically ill, lymphatic dysfunction could exacerbate edema formation, impair oxygen deliver to tissues, and weaken the immune response.

THE ENDOTHELIUM

All blood and lymph vessels are lined with endothelial cells. The endothelium mediates and regulates many crucial physiologic functions of the microvasculature, including perfusion, permeability, local coagulation, and immune responses. Endothelial injury and shedding of the endothelial glycocalyx are associated with microvascular dysfunction and increased coagulation following traumatic hemorrhagic shock and sepsis.[11,13,22] It is well established that endothelial dysfunction contributes to the microvascular dysfunction in critically ill patients, especially. Microvascular dysfunction may occur as a result of direct endothelial injury (sepsis or eclampsia) or due to ischemia/reperfusion injury (trauma or cardiogenic shock). Chronic critically illness as well as certain causes of acute illness such as sepsis are prevalent in the elderly,[23,24] and in this population, especially, a functioning endothelial barrier is critical for proper microvascular function.[25] Preservation of endothelial function and rapid restoration of microcirculatory perfusion should be the goals of resuscitation efforts.[26]

AGING OF THE MICROVASCULATURE

An aged microvasculature likely contributes to poorer outcomes observed in the critically ill elderly.[23,27] Endothelial dysfunction, including impaired endothelium-dependent vasodilation, increased endothelial reactive oxygen species (ROS) production, a diminished glycocalyx, and a reduced endothelial barrier integrity, increases with age.[5,7,25,28] Although the mechanisms are not well understood, reduced nitric oxide (NO) production by the endothelium coupled with reduced NO availability due to increases in superoxide generation is thought to shift the balance between the beneficial effects of NO toward the generation of reactive nitrogen species (RNS) and the injurious effects of nitrosative and nitrative stress.[2] This can injure not only the endothelium but also the underlying vessel structures and adjacent parenchyma.

Endothelial senescence is also considered a contributor to vascular aging associated with a sedentary lifestyle[29] and to reduced recovery of the microcirculation in the elderly following disease or trauma.[1,25,27] Endothelial oxidative stress and an inflammatory microenvironment are thought to drive endothelial senescence.[1] Aging also reduces angiogenesis, which is necessary for revascularization following acute injury such as myocardial infarction, ischemia, and stroke.[30–32] Although age-related endothelial dysfunction is recognized as a key contributor to processes leading to atherosclerosis of larger vessels and hyperpermeability of the microvasculature, the role of endothelial dysfunction in impaired angiogenesis is still unclear, especially in humans. Also unclear is whether impaired angiogenesis is causally linked to microvascular dysfunction.[2,25,33] Regardless, merely increasing microvessel angiogenesis through pharmacologic means would not necessarily be enough to restore the microcirculation. Neovascularization must integrate into the existing perfusion networks.[34] A great deal more research is needed in this area to help identify potential therapeutic targets, which could speed recovery of the endothelium and the microcirculation.

There is also growing interest in how aging contributes to lymphatic dysfunction. Studies in rodents show that aging weakens lymphatic contractility, alters the endothelial glycocalyx, and decreases junctional proteins.[35,36] NO, ROS, and RNS can disrupt lymphatic contraction and barrier function. This may be especially important in high NO/ROS states such as chronic inflammation and the more acute systemic inflammatory response syndrome.[15,21,37] Also, lymphatic function can be influenced by metabolites released in the aged tissue microenvironment.[38] Given the close proximity of the blood and lymphatic microvasculature, it is not surprising that both microvasculatures are affected by a prooxidant and proinflammatory microenvironment, which often occurs during critical illness.

MONITORING THE MICROVASCULATURE

Although experimental studies have amply demonstrated that microvascular dysfunction is occurring in all organs that have been investigated, the demonstration of microvascular dysfunction in humans has been more laborious. In 2002, De Backer and colleagues[39] demonstrated that the sublingual microcirculation is altered in septic patients, compared with healthy and intensive care unit controls. The microvascular alterations were characterized by a decrease in perfused vascular density, with absence of intermittent flow in some capillaries while others were still adequately perfused. One of the most important features noted was the heterogeneity of perfusion in areas within a few microns in proximity.[40] These features nicely illustrated the distributive aspect of septic shock. The severity of microvascular alterations was associated with a poor outcome and development of organ dysfunction.[3,4,39,40] These data have now been reproduced more than 30 times around the globe.

Still, an important question is whether the sublingual area is representative of other organs. From experimental studies it can be assumed that microvascular alterations occur simultaneously in the various organs and have similar severity. However, microvascular alterations may be more severe in areas with increased interstitial pressure such as in abdominal compartment syndrome. Also, some organs with specific anatomic features such as the kidney or gut villi may be more sensitive and may also present more severe microvascular alterations.[41]

Specialized handheld vital microscopes introduced clinically more than 20 years ago[42] have allowed direct observation of the microcirculation at the bedside, providing much insight into the efficacy of various resuscitation procedures to improve tissue red blood cell (RBC) perfusion at the bedside.[43] However, the absence of automated analysis software to extract physiologic parameters related to the functional state of the microcirculation from the complex microcirculatory images has hindered the use of this technology more widely in the clinic setting. Recently, a validated automated microcirculatory analysis software platform called MicroTools was introduced, which now allows instantaneous quantitative calculation of all relevant microcirculatory variables[44] required by the international consensus on the bedside assessment of sublingual microcirculation.[43] The ability to obtain these physiologic variables instantaneously at the bedside will make microcirculatory-guided resuscitation targeting tissue RBC perfusion as a point of care, a reality.

In severe heart failure and cardiogenic shock, alterations in microvascular perfusion are also reported.[45] The severity of microvascular dysfunction and its persistence is associated with a poor outcome.[45,46] Interestingly, these are very similar in nature to those observed in sepsis, even though often less severe. In cardiogenic shock also there is some dissociation between microvascular and systemic perfusion. Interestingly, in patients with cardiogenic shock supported with extracorporeal membrane oxygenation, the onset of microvascular alterations during the weaning attempt was predictive of weaning failure.[47]

Microvascular dysfunction has also been reported in other conditions affecting the endothelium, such as eclampsia,[48] or circulating cells, such as hematological diseases.[49] In trauma, detectable microvascular alterations have also been reported.[50] Patients with more severe alterations at initial evaluation suffer from more severe organ dysfunction in the following days. Importantly, the first microvascular imaging was obtained only after bleeding control. Hence, these alterations were more typical of the reperfusion phase than of the ischemic phase.

RESUSCITATIVE THERAPY

There is general agreement in the literature that the ultimate goal of resuscitation must be the correction of tissue perfusion with the aim of correction of oxygen availability in the microcirculation following microcirculatory hypoperfusion in states of shock.[51] In accepting this target of resuscitation, it should be clear what is precisely meant by tissue perfusion. In this context, adequate tissue perfusion should mean ensuring adequate oxygen delivery to the tissue cells. To accomplish this, resuscitation should achieve the availability in the microcirculation of sufficient number of hemoglobin (Hb)-loaded RBC entering the microcirculation to meet the metabolic demands of the parenchymal cells because Hb concentration is the predominant determinant of oxygen availability.[52] Thus, the concept of adequate tissue perfusion should encapsulate the convection of RBC entering the microcirculation as well as achieving an adequate density of RBC-filled capillaries to ensure the equally important diffusion of oxygen from the RBCs to the parenchymal cells.[53] These two aspects of tissue perfusion would be more correctly integrated into one variable, which we call tissue RBC perfusion. This concept considers the need to have an adequate capillary hematocrit and functional capillary density (diffusive capacity) combined with a sufficient convection or the flow of the RBCs in the microcirculation. It is clear that under this definition the only technique that offers quantification of these parameters is a technique that can directly observe the microcirculation in combination with algorithms to automatically evaluate the diffusive and convective component of tissue RBC perfusion.

It is now possible to actually evaluate the efficacy of different resuscitation procedures to promote tissue RBC perfusion in different states of shock. Although vasopressors are a corner stone and are certainly important in maintain cerebral perfusion, studies have shown the impact of vasopressors to have variable effects on improving tissue RBC perfusion depending on baseline conditions.[54,55] More effective recruitment has been shown by use of inodilators (agents with both positive inotropic and vasodilator actions) such as dobutamine[56] and enoximone[57] and vasodilators such as nitroglycerin.[58] Nitroglycerin has also been applied sublingually as a methodology to identify the maximum amount of recruitable capillaries,[59,60] an important microcirculatory variable that may signal that further resuscitation may be futile. Thus, it is important to target the microcirculation rather than just the systemic circulation because there is often a clear dissociation between systemic hemodynamics, often maintained within targets, and microvascular dysfunction.[3] In addition, the response of the microcirculation and systemic circulation often diverged during therapeutic interventions due to heterogeneity in the types of microcirculatory alterations.[56,61,62]

Fluids, as all resuscitation procedures, present themselves as a double-edged sword. On the one hand fluid therapy promotes blood flow by increasing stroke volume and reducing viscosity and can improve the microcirculation if given timely and in appropriate amounts.[63,64] However, fluid administration can also reduce the oxygen carrying capacity of blood by dilution of Hb, thus ultimately having a marginal effect on tissue RBC perfusion. The dilutional effect of fluid administration has been estimated at giving a reduction of 1 g/dL of Hb for every 500 mL of fluid administered.[65] Studies have shown that administration of excessive amounts of fluids is a common occurrence; a condition potentially imposing anemia on patients must be considered as potentially creating iatrogenic harm.[66] Indeed several studies have shown a reduction of RBC availability in the microcirculation following fluid resuscitation.[67] Conversely transfusion of RBCs[68] or deescalation procedures such as the administration of diuretics[69] are methodologies that have been shown to improve tissue RBC perfusion by increasing the diffusive capacity of the microcirculation by increasing its functional capillary density. In summary, achieving optimal tissue RBC perfusion by resuscitation must target an optimal convection with sufficient number of RBC flowing into the microcirculation as well as filling previously empty capillaries to maximize functional capillary density of the microcirculation and reduce the diffusion distance between the RBCs and the respiring parenchymal cells.[70]

SUMMARY

In addition to treating the underlying causes of critical illness, physicians must understand how endothelial and microvascular dysfunction not only contributes to organ damage but also may hinder effective therapeutic strategies. Moreover, there is growing evidence that, similar to the blood microcirculation, a dysfunctional lymphatic microvasculature can contribute significantly to organ injury. Clearly, additional basic research is needed to better understand the causes of endothelial and microvascular dysfunction in the setting of critical illness and especially with aging. Basic research is the most direct approach to uncovering new therapeutic targets. However, the complexities and heterogeneity of critical illness, especially in the elderly patient, requires more mechanistically oriented clinical trials that monitor the effectiveness of existing therapies and of those to come. Being able to directly observe and quantify microcirculatory function at the bedside using handheld vital microscopes allows translational application of the results of such basic research to the benefit of patients.

DISCLOSURE

Dr Ince and his team provide training and educational services related to performing clinical sublingual microcirculation measurements described in this paper. To this purpose, he runs an Internet site called https://www.microcirculationacademy.org, where also the automatic software for analysis of microcirculation images called MicroTools is made available. The Internet site and its activities are run by a company called Active Medical BV of which he owns shares. Dr De Backer and Dr Mayeux have nothing to disclose.

REFERENCES

1. Liu Y, Bloom SI, Donato AJ. The role of senescence, telomere dysfunction and shelterin in vascular aging. Microcirculation 2019;26(2):e12487.
2. Ungvari Z, Tarantini S, Kiss T, et al. Endothelial dysfunction and angiogenesis impairment in the ageing vasculature. Nat Rev Cardiol 2018;15(9):555–65.
3. De Backer D, Donadello K, Sakr Y, et al. Microcirculatory alterations in patients with severe sepsis: impact of time of assessment and relationship with outcome. Crit Care Med 2013;41:791–9.
4. Sakr Y, Dubois MJ, De Backer D, et al. Persistent microcirculatory alterations are associated with organ failure and death in patients with septic shock. Crit Care Med 2004;32(9):1825–31.
5. Barrett EJ, Liu Z, Khamaisi M, et al. Diabetic microvascular disease: an Endocrine Society scientific statement. J Clin Endocrinol Metab 2017;102(12):4343–410.
6. Burrage E, Marshall KL, Santanam N, et al. Cerebrovascular dysfunction with stress and depression. Brain Circ 2018;4(2):43–53.
7. Izzo C, Carrizzo A, Alfano A, et al. The impact of aging on cardio and cerebrovascular diseases. Int J Mol Sci 2018;19(2).
8. Zhao Z, Nelson AR, Betsholtz C, et al. Establishment and dysfunction of the blood-brain barrier. Cell 2015;163(5):1064–78.
9. Delaney C, Campbell M. The blood brain barrier: insights from development and ageing. Tissue Barriers 2017;5(4):e1373897.
10. Amtul Z, Yang J, Lee TY, et al. Pathological changes in microvascular morphology, density, size and responses following comorbid cerebral injury. Front Aging Neurosci 2019;11:47.
11. Naumann DN, Hazeldine J, Midwinter MJ, et al. Poor microcirculatory flow dynamics are associated with endothelial cell damage and glycocalyx shedding after traumatic hemorrhagic shock. J Trauma Acute Care Surg 2018;84(1):81–8.
12. Qiao Z, Horst K, Teuben M, et al. Analysis of skeletal muscle microcirculation in a porcine polytrauma model with haemorrhagic shock. J Orthop Res 2018;36(5):1377–82.
13. Ince C, Mayeux PR, Nguyen T, et al. The endothelium in sepsis. Shock 2016;45(3):259–70.
14. Domizi R, Damiani E, Scorcella C, et al. Association between sublingual microcirculation, tissue perfusion and organ failure in major trauma: a subgroup analysis of a prospective observational study. PLoS One 2019;14(3):e0213085.
15. Scallan JP, Zawieja SD, Castorena-Gonzalez JA, et al. Lymphatic pumping: mechanics, mechanisms and malfunction. J Physiol 2016;594(20):5749–68.

16. Negrini D, Moriondo A. Lymphatic anatomy and biomechanics. J Physiol 2011; 589(Pt 12):2927–34.

17. Krouwer VJ, Hekking LH, Langelaar-Makkinje M, et al. Endothelial cell senescence is associated with disrupted cell-cell junctions and increased monolayer permeability. Vasc Cell 2012;4(1):12.

18. Russell PS, Hong J, Windsor JA, et al. Renal lymphatics: anatomy, physiology, and clinical implications. Front Physiol 2019;10:251.

19. Stolarczyk J, Carone FA. Effects of renal lymphatic occlusion and venous constriction on renal function. Am J Pathol 1975;78(2):285–96.

20. Zawieja SD, Wang W, Wu X, et al. Impairments in the intrinsic contractility of mesenteric collecting lymphatics in a rat model of metabolic syndrome. Am J Physiol Heart Circ Physiol 2012;302(3):H643–53.

21. Kneedler SC, Phillips LE, Hudson KR, et al. Renal inflammation and injury are associated with lymphangiogenesis in hypertension. Am J Physiol Renal Physiol 2017;312(5):F861–9.

22. Tuma M, Canestrini S, Alwahab Z, et al. Trauma and endothelial glycocalyx: the microcirculation helmet? Shock 2016;46(4):352–7.

23. Kahn JM, Le T, Angus DC, et al. The epidemiology of chronic critical illness in the United States. Crit Care Med 2015;43(2):282–7.

24. Rhee C, Dantes R, Epstein L, et al. Incidence and trends of sepsis in US hospitals using clinical vs claims data, 2009-2014. JAMA 2017;318(13):1241–9.

25. Oakley R, Tharakan B. Vascular hyperpermeability and aging. Aging Dis 2014; 5(2):114–25.

26. Hutchings SD, Naumann DN, Watts S, et al. Microcirculatory perfusion shows wide inter-individual variation and is important in determining shock reversal during resuscitation in a porcine experimental model of complex traumatic hemorrhagic shock. Intensive Care Med Exp 2016;4(1):17.

27. Gates PE, Strain WD, Shore AC. Human endothelial function and microvascular ageing. Exp Physiol 2009;94(3):311–6.

28. Machin DR, Bloom SI, Campbell RA, et al. Advanced age results in a diminished endothelial glycocalyx. Am J Physiol Heart Circ Physiol 2018;315(3):H531–9.

29. Rossman MJ, Kaplon RE, Hill SD, et al. Endothelial cell senescence with aging in healthy humans: prevention by habitual exercise and relation to vascular endothelial function. Am J Physiol Heart Circ Physiol 2017;313(5):H890–5.

30. Edelberg JM, Tang L, Hattori K, et al. Young adult bone marrow-derived endothelial precursor cells restore aging-impaired cardiac angiogenic function. Circ Res 2002;90(10):E89–93.

31. Faber JE, Zhang H, Lassance-Soares RM, et al. Aging causes collateral rarefaction and increased severity of ischemic injury in multiple tissues. Arterioscler Thromb Vasc Biol 2011;31(8):1748–56.

32. Tang Y, Wang L, Wang J, et al. Ischemia-induced angiogenesis is attenuated in aged rats. Aging Dis 2016;7(4):326–35.

33. Hodges NA, Suarez-Martinez AD, Murfee WL. Understanding angiogenesis during aging: opportunities for discoveries and new models. J Appl Physiol (1985) 2018;125(6):1843–50.

34. LeBlanc AJ, Krishnan L, Sullivan CJ, et al. Microvascular repair: postangiogenesis vascular dynamics. Microcirculation 2012;19(8):676–95.

35. Nagai T, Bridenbaugh EA, Gashev AA. Aging-associated alterations in contractility of rat mesenteric lymphatic vessels. Microcirculation 2011;18(6):463–73.

36. Zolla V, Nizamutdinova IT, Scharf B, et al. Aging-related anatomical and biochemical changes in lymphatic collectors impair lymph transport, fluid homeostasis, and pathogen clearance. Aging Cell 2015;14(4):582–94.

37. Zawieja DC, Greiner ST, Davis KL, et al. Reactive oxygen metabolites inhibit spontaneous lymphatic contractions. Am J Physiol 1991;260(6 Pt 2):H1935–43.

38. Akl TJ, Nagai T, Cote GL, et al. Mesenteric lymph flow in adult and aged rats. Am J Physiol Heart Circ Physiol 2011;301(5):H1828–40.

39. De Backer D, Creteur J, Preiser JC, et al. Microvascular blood flow is altered in patients with sepsis. Am J Respir Crit Care Med 2002;166(1):98–104.

40. Edul VS, Enrico C, Laviolle B, et al. Quantitative assessment of the microcirculation in healthy volunteers and in patients with septic shock. Crit Care Med 2012; 40(5):1443–8.

41. Boerma EC, Kuiper MA, Kingma WP, et al. Disparity between skin perfusion and sublingual microcirculatory alterations in severe sepsis and septic shock: a prospective observational study. Intensive Care Med 2008;34(7):1294–8.

42. Groner W, Winkelman JW, Harris AG, et al. Orthogonal polarization spectral imaging: a new method for study of the microcirculation. Nat Med 1999;5(10): 1209–12.

43. Ince C, Boerma EC, Cecconi M, et al. Second consensus on the assessment of sublingual microcirculation in critically ill patients: results from a task force of the European Society of Intensive Care Medicine. Intensive Care Med 2018;44(3): 281–99.

44. Hilty MP, Guerci P, Ince Y, et al. MicroTools enables automated quantification of capillary density and red blood cell velocity in handheld vital microscopy. Commun Biol 2019;2:217.

45. De Backer D, Creteur J, Dubois MJ, et al. Microvascular alterations in patients with acute severe heart failure and cardiogenic shock. Am Heart J 2004; 147(1):91–9.

46. den Uil CA, Lagrand WK, van der Ent M, et al. Impaired microcirculation predicts poor outcome of patients with acute myocardial infarction complicated by cardiogenic shock. Eur Heart J 2010;31(24):3032–9.

47. Akin S, Dos Reis Miranda D, Caliskan K, et al. Functional evaluation of sublingual microcirculation indicates successful weaning from VA-ECMO in cardiogenic shock. Crit Care 2017;21(1):265.

48. Ospina-Tascon GA, Nieto Calvache AJ, Quinones E, et al. Microcirculatory blood flow derangements during severe preeclampsia and HELLP syndrome. Pregnancy Hypertens 2017;10:124–30.

49. Meinders AJ, Elbers P. Images in clinical medicine. Leukocytosis and sublingual microvascular blood flow. N Engl J Med 2009;360(7):e9.

50. Tachon G, Harrois A, Tanaka S, et al. Microcirculatory alterations in traumatic hemorrhagic shock. Crit Care Med 2014;42(6):1433–41.

51. Cecconi M, Hernandez G, Dunser M, et al. Fluid administration for acute circulatory dysfunction using basic monitoring: narrative review and expert panel recommendations from an ESICM task force. Intensive Care Med 2019;45(1):21–32.

52. Siam J, Kadan M, Flaishon R, et al. Blood flow versus hematocrit in optimization of oxygen transfer to tissue during fluid resuscitation. Cardiovasc Eng Technol 2015;6(4):474–84.

53. Bateman RM, Sharpe MD, Ellis CG. Bench-to-bedside review: microvascular dysfunction in sepsis–hemodynamics, oxygen transport, and nitric oxide. Crit Care 2003;7(5):359–73.

54. Dubin A, Pozo MO, Casabella CA, et al. Increasing arterial blood pressure with norepinephrine does not improve microcirculatory blood flow: a prospective study. Crit Care 2009;13(3):R92.
55. Jhanji S, Stirling S, Patel N, et al. The effect of increasing doses of norepinephrine on tissue oxygenation and microvascular flow in patients with septic shock. Crit Care Med 2009;37(6):1961–6.
56. De Backer D, Creteur J, Dubois MJ, et al. The effects of dobutamine on microcirculatory alterations in patients with septic shock are independent of its systemic effects. Crit Care Med 2006;34(2):403–8.
57. den Uil CA, Lagrand WK, van der Ent M, et al. Conventional hemodynamic resuscitation may fail to optimize tissue perfusion: an observational study on the effects of dobutamine, enoximone, and norepinephrine in patients with acute myocardial infarction complicated by cardiogenic shock. PLoS One 2014;9(8):e103978.
58. Spronk PE, Ince C, Gardien MJ, et al. Nitroglycerin in septic shock after intravascular volume resuscitation. Lancet 2002;360(9343):1395–6.
59. Hilty MP, Merz TM, Hefti U, et al. Recruitment of non-perfused sublingual capillaries increases microcirculatory oxygen extraction capacity throughout ascent to 7126 m. J Physiol 2019;597(10):2623–38.
60. Hilty MP, Pichler J, Ergin B, et al. Assessment of endothelial cell function and physiological microcirculatory reserve by video microscopy using a topical acetylcholine and nitroglycerin challenge. Intensive Care Med Exp 2017;5(1):26.
61. Ince C. Hemodynamic coherence and the rationale for monitoring the microcirculation. Crit Care 2015;19(Suppl 3):S8.
62. Stenberg TA, Kildal AB, Sanden E, et al. The acute phase of experimental cardiogenic shock is counteracted by microcirculatory and mitochondrial adaptations. PLoS One 2014;9(9):e105213.
63. Pottecher J, Deruddre S, Teboul JL, et al. Both passive leg raising and intravascular volume expansion improve sublingual microcirculatory perfusion in severe sepsis and septic shock patients. Intensive Care Med 2010;36(11):1867–74.
64. Ospina-Tascon G, Neves AP, Occhipinti G, et al. Effects of fluids on microvascular perfusion in patients with severe sepsis. Intensive Care Med 2010;36(6): 949–55.
65. Perel A, Javidroozi M, Shander A. Blood transfusion in sepsis and iatrogenic hemodilution. Am J Crit Care 2018;27(6):442–3.
66. Marik PE, Linde-Zwirble WT, Bittner EA, et al. Fluid administration in severe sepsis and septic shock, patterns and outcomes: an analysis of a large national database. Intensive Care Med 2017;43(5):625–32.
67. Atasever B, van der Kuil M, Boer C, et al. Red blood cell transfusion compared with gelatin solution and no infusion after cardiac surgery: effect on microvascular perfusion, vascular density, hemoglobin, and oxygen saturation. Transfusion 2012;52(11):2452–8.
68. Tanaka S, Escudier E, Hamada S, et al. Effect of RBC transfusion on sublingual microcirculation in hemorrhagic shock patients: a pilot study. Crit Care Med 2017;45(2):e154–60.
69. Uz Z, Ince C, Guerci P, et al. Recruitment of sublingual microcirculation using handheld incident dark field imaging as a routine measurement tool during the postoperative de-escalation phase-a pilot study in post ICU cardiac surgery patients. Perioper Med (Lond) 2018;7:18.
70. Ince C. The rationale for microcirculatory guided fluid therapy. Curr Opin Crit Care 2014;20(3):301–8.

Typical and Atypical Hemolytic Uremic Syndrome in the Critically Ill

Carlos L. Manrique-Caballero, MD[a,b],
Sadudee Peerapornratana, MD[a,b,c,d], Cassandra Formeck, MD[a,b,e],
Gaspar Del Rio-Pertuz, MD[a,b],
Hernando Gomez Danies, MD, MPH[a,b],
John A. Kellum, MD, MCCM[a,b,*]

KEYWORDS

- Atypical HUS • Critically ill • Microangiopathy • Complement-mediated HUS

KEY POINTS

- Hemolytic uremic syndrome is a thrombotic microangiopathy, clinically defined by the triad of thrombocytopenia, microangiopathic hemolytic anemia, and acute kidney injury.
- Hemolytic uremic syndrome may result from inherited or acquired genetic mutations or can be associated with disease-driven or environmental triggers. Classification systems are based on etiology and pathophysiologic mechanisms.
- Shiga toxin-associated hemolytic uremic syndrome and atypical hemolytic uremic syndrome constitute the most common presentations in children and adults respectively.
- Other subtypes of hemolytic uremic syndrome such as diacylglycerol kinase epsilon mutations or cobalamin C deficiency are extremely rare.
- It is crucial to consider hemolytic uremic syndrome in the patient with thrombotic microangiopathy manifestations, because specific therapeutic strategies are available for some forms of hemolytic uremic syndrome.

Funding: Supported by NIH (NIGMS) grant 1K08GM117310-01A.
[a] Center for Critical Care Nephrology, Department of Critical Care Medicine, University of Pittsburgh School of Medicine, 3347 Forbes Avenue Suite 220, Pittsburgh, PA 15213, USA; [b] The CRISMA (Clinical Research, Investigation and Systems Modeling of Acute Illness) Center, Department of Critical Care Medicine, University of Pittsburgh School of Medicine, 3550 Terrace Street, Scaife Hall, Suite 600, Pittsburgh, PA 15213, USA; [c] Excellence Center for Critical Care Nephrology, Division of Nephrology, Department of Medicine, Chulalongkorn University, 1873 Rama 4 Road, Pathumwan, Bangkok 10330, Thailand; [d] Department of Laboratory Medicine, Chulalongkorn University, 1873 Rama 4 Road, Pathumwan, Bangkok 10330, Thailand; [e] Department of Nephrology, Children's Hospital of Pittsburgh of UPMC, 4401 Penn Avenue, Floor 3, Pittsburgh, PA 15224, USA
* Corresponding author. Center for Critical Care Nephrology, Department of Critical Care Medicine, University of Pittsburgh School of Medicine, 3347 Forbes Avenue Suite 220, Pittsburgh, PA 15213.
E-mail address: kellum@pitt.edu

INTRODUCTION

Hemolytic uremic syndrome (HUS) is a thrombotic microangiopathy (TMA) defined by the clinical triad of thrombocytopenia, microangiopathic hemolytic anemia (MAHA) and renal dysfunction.[1] TMA is a histopathologic term used to describe a variety of thrombotic vascular lesions that characterize a group of diseases that include HUS, thrombotic thrombocytopenic purpura (TTP), and the hemolysis, elevated liver enzymes and low platelets (HELLP) syndrome.[2] Despite having different etiologies, TMAs share similar pathologic features, and clinically manifest with consumptive thrombocytopenia, MAHA and organ dysfunction. Earliest reports of TMAs date back to the 1920s. However, it was not until 1955 that Gasser and colleagues[3] proposed the term "hemolytic uremic syndrome" to describe those patients who presented with this clinical triad. Although renal injury is a major feature of HUS, owing to susceptibility of renal vasculature endothelial injury, other organs such as the brain, intestines, pancreas, and heart may also be involved.

In the last few decades, experimental, genetic, and clinical studies have contributed to the understanding of HUS by elucidating many of the pathophysiologic mechanisms involved in each of the HUS subtypes, but also describing the clinical features that characterize each of these syndromes. The increased understanding and amount of available evidence have permitted the development of new specific targeted therapies for some subtypes of HUS such as atypical HUS (aHUS). These targeted therapies have had a significant impact in morbidity and mortality. However, therapies for other HUS variants remain reactive and nonspecific. We review recent concepts related to the classification, epidemiology, pathophysiologic mechanisms, and clinical presentation of HUS. We also propose a practical diagnostic algorithm to approach the critically ill patient with suspicion of TMA. Finally, we will review some of the current management strategies for HUS in the intensive care unit (ICU) setting.

CLASSIFICATION

The classification of HUS is rapidly evolving based on knowledge of underlying mechanisms and at least 7 classification systems have been proposed to differentiate HUS from other TMAs, and to delineate the differences between the diverse subtypes of HUS.[1,2] Current classification systems are based on etiology and primary driving mechanisms involved in each HUS subtype (**Fig. 1**).[1,4–8] Shiga toxin-associated HUS (STEC-HUS), also known as typical HUS, is caused by Shiga toxin (Stx)-producing pathogens such as enterohemorrhagic strains of *Escherichia coli*. aHUS, also known as complement-mediated HUS, encompasses HUS cases resulting from genetic variants in the complement system and acquired alterations.[5] All other causes of HUS such as inborn errors of metabolism (eg, cobalamin C deficiency, diacylglycerol kinase epsilon deficiency), infections (eg, *Streptococcus pneumoniae*-associated HUS [SP-HUS]), drugs, cancer, transplants, pregnancy-associated and autoimmune disorders are included under the category of secondary HUS.[5]

EPIDEMIOLOGY

HUS is an extremely rare disease that occurs most frequently in children, primarily affecting those younger than 5 years of age (overall annual incidence of 5–6 per 100,000 children), with equal distribution by gender.[8] It is one of the leading causes of severe acute kidney injury (AKI) in children.[9] HUS in adults is even less common, and most cases are reported during epidemics and outbreaks.[10] Although the epidemiology in this group of the population is not well-documented because of the scarce case reports,

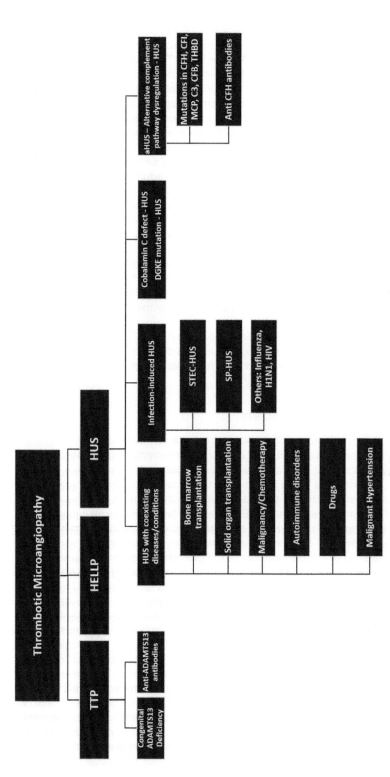

Fig. 1. Classification of HUS. In 2016, the International Consensus for Hemolytic Uremic Syndrome proposed a new etiology-based classification system. ADAMTS13, A disintegrin and metalloproteinase with a thrombospondin type 1 motif, member 13; CFB, complement factor B; DGKE, diacylglycerol kinase epsilon; HIV, human immunodeficiency virus; MCP, membrane cofactor protein (CD46); SP-HUS, *Streptococcus pneumoniae*-associated HUS; STEC-HUS, Shiga toxin-associated HUS; THBD, thrombomodulin. (*Data from* Loirat C, Fakhouri F, Ariceta G, et al. An international consensus approach to the management of atypical hemolytic uremic syndrome in children. Pediatric Nephrology. 2016;31(1):15-39 and Fakhouri F, Zuber J, Fremeaux-Bacchi V, et al. Haemolytic uraemic syndrome. Lancet. 2017;390(10095):681-96.)

some studies calculate an overall annual incidence of 0.5 to 2.0 per 100,000 people.[11–13] STEC-HUS constitutes the most frequent presentation in children, accounting for 85% to 95% of cases in the United States and Europe.[6,11,14–16] Annual incidence reports in Europe and North America estimate 1.9 to 2.9 cases per 100,000 children less than 5 years of age, and 0.6 to 0.8 cases per 100,000 children less than 15 to 18 years of age.[6] Approximately 20% of children younger than 5 years and 5% of adults older than 60 years will develop HUS in the presence of an enterohemorrhagic E coli (EHEC) infection.[8–10,17,18] Moreover, approximately 25% of these cases will have long-term sequelae or develop chronic conditions such as chronic kidney disease.[9,19,20]

By contrast, aHUS accounts for 5% to 10% of HUS cases in children,[21–28] but constitutes the most frequent presentation of HUS in adults; although the overall incidence remains lower in adults than in children (about 1 per million adults vs 3.5–7.0 per million children).[23,25,26,29,30] Low incidence reports are somehow attributed to the clinical presentation similarities that HUS shares with different TMA syndromes and other more prevalent diseases such as sepsis and disseminated intravascular coagulation (DIC). Emerging evidence and increased understanding of the pathophysiologic mechanisms suggest that the incidence of HUS may be higher than currently reported. SP-HUS accounts for only 5% of cases in children (annual incidence of 0.06 cases per 100,000 children).[31] Other subtypes of HUS (which are not associated with infectious diseases or complement factors dysregulations) are extremely rare.

Although the overall mortality rates are around 3% to 5% in STEC-HUS,[8] these rates can increase substantially in the presence of disease complications (eg, neurologic, cardiovascular, and intra-abdominal) and the rates can be higher or some specific complement gene mutations in aHUS.[14,32–34]

GENERAL PATHOPHYSIOLOGIC CONCEPTS

HUS may result from a variety of etiologies that include genetic mutations, secondary to a systemic disease or as a result of an external environmental trigger. Despite varying in etiology, all forms of HUS along with other types of TMA arise from an initial endothelial injury that leads to the formation of thrombotic and nonthrombotic microvascular lesions characterized by fibrin and platelet-rich thrombi formation, affecting arterioles and capillaries predominantly. Endotheliosis (eg, endothelium and subendothelial space swelling and accumulation of protein and debris, and detachment from the glomerular basement membrane), mesangiolysis, thickening of the vascular wall, and appearance of double contours of the glomerular base membrane arise as well.[6,35,36] However, some studies have shown that some cases of aHUS do not present with thrombotic lesions, giving rise to the debate as to whether aHUS is a truly TMA or if it is better to refer to a HUS just as a microangiopathy.[5]

Complement system activation also plays a key role in the development of HUS along with endothelial injury. However, the specific mechanisms of how these events occur in each subtype of HUS are not well-understood.[37] Vascular pathologic lesions and thrombi formation eventually lead to thrombocytopenia owing to increased platelet aggregation. Furthermore, hemolytic anemia is caused by the excessive shearing stress forces that the erythrocytes undergo when running through these vessels with thrombotic lesions. Finally, microvascular thrombosis may result in decreased oxygen delivery, leading to ischemic organ injury. These pathologic changes manifest clinically as the classic clinical triad of thrombocytopenia, MAHA, and organ injury. Specific pathophysiologic mechanistic details of each HUS subtype are described.

DIAGNOSTIC APPROACH TO THE CRITICALLY ILL PATIENT WITH SUSPECTED THROMBOTIC MICROANGIOPATHY

Patients with TTP and HUS develop organ dysfunction and often require management in the ICU. Therefore, the diagnosis of TMAs is challenging because many syndromes within the scope of critical illness, like sepsis, DIC, and malignant hypertension, mimic the clinical presentation of TMAs. These syndromes share the proinflammatory, endothelialopathy, and complement activation features of TMAs, which also lead to platelet aggregation and thrombus formation.[38] Thrombocytopenia with MAHA are common signs that should trigger clinicians to search for these life-threatening conditions.[39] Early recognition of the etiology can also allow of prescription of specific treatments (see **Fig. 1** and **Fig. 2**).

DIC, TTP, and HUS can share common clinical features and laboratory results as seen in **Table 1**.[35,40] In patients without MAHA, other causes of thrombocytopenia such as drug-induced thrombocytopenia, immune thrombocytopenic purpura, vasculitis, liver failure, and even laboratory artifacts should be considered and excluded.[39] AKI is found to be more common in patient with HUS,[8] whereas TTP is more associated with central nervous system abnormalities.[41] The presence of coagulopathy is

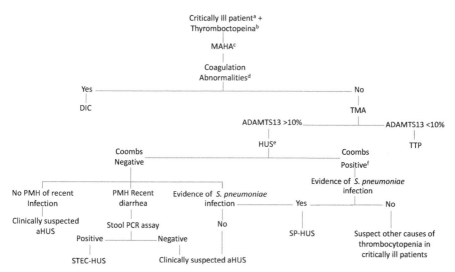

Fig. 2. Algorithm to approach a critically ill patient with suspected TMA. [a] Critically ill patient is defined as a patient with any sign of organ damage. [b] Thrombocytopenia* less than 150×10^9/L or greater than 25% decrease from baseline. [c] MAHA defined by the presence of any of the following: elevated indirect bilirubin and lactate dehydrogenase (LDH), decreased hemoglobin and haptoglobin, presence of schistocytes in peripheral blood smear. [d] Coagulation abnormalities: prolonged prothrombin time or elevated fibrinogen or any fibrin marker. Other causes of thrombocytopenia in critically ill patients: pulmonary embolism (PE), heparin-induced thrombocytopenia (HIT), immune thrombocytopenic purpura (ITP), post-transfusion purpura, hemodilution, splenic sequestration, decreased production of platelets (chemotherapy, radiotherapy, bone marrow disorder, hematinic deficiency), laboratory artifacts. [e] In pregnant women suspect HELLP syndrome, before continue approach. [f] Coombs test has shown to be positive in 85% of the cases of SP-HUS 121,122. ADAMTS13, A disintegrin and metalloproteinase with a thrombospondin type 1 motif, member 13; DIC, disseminated intravascular coagulation; PCR, polymerase chain reaction; PMH, past medical history; SP-HUS, *Streptococcus pneumoniae*-associated HUS; STEC-HUS, Shiga toxin-associated HUS.

Table 1
Laboratory profile in patient with suspected TMA

Disease/ Condition	Platelet Count	MAHA[a]	PT (INR)	PTT	Fibrinogen	Fibrin Marker[b]	ADAMTS13 Activity
HUS	↓	+	↔	↔	↔	↔[c]	↔
DIC	↓	+	↓	↓	↓	↓	↔
TTP	↓	+	↔	↔	↔	↔	↓[d]

↓, decreased level; ↔, normal level; +, present.

Abbreviations: ADAMTS13, A disintegrin and metalloproteinase with a ThromboSpondin type 1 motif, member 13; DIC, disseminated intravascular coagulation; INR, international normalized ratio; LDH, lactate dehydrogenase; PT, prothrombin time; PTT, partial thromboplastin time.

[a] Presence of any of the following: elevated indirect bilirubin and LDH, decreased hemoglobin and haptoglobin, presence of schistocytes in peripheral blood smear.

[b] Include D-dimer and fibrin degradation products.

[c] There can be activation of the fibrinolytic pathway with increased circulating levels of fibrin degradation products.

[d] Less than 10% activity of ADAMTS13 is indicated for TTP.

key to differentiate DIC from TTP and HUS (see **Fig. 2**). Although DIC is a systemic disorder of the coagulation system resulting in a consumptive coagulopathy and pathologic thrombosis,[40] TTP and HUS are associated with normal coagulation profiles.[42]

The most critical and urgent step is to distinguish TTP from HUS, because the earlier specific therapy is initiated, the greater the chance is for renal functional recovery.[43] Many scoring systems using clinical and laboratory data have been proposed to predict TTP.[44–47] Platelet count, serum creatinine, antinuclear antibodies, D-dimer, reticulocytes, and indirect bilirubin are included in those risk scores. The PLASMIC score[45] is a 7-component prediction tool that has shown a sensitivity of 90%, and specificity of 92% to predict the presence of TTP.[48] These scoring systems should be complemented by measurement of ADAMTS13 activity, as an activity of less than 10% is the gold standard for TTP.[35,41,49]

As soon as TTP has been ruled out, we have to think about HUS. Unlike TTP, there are no validated scoring systems to predict it. The diagnostic approach is thus based on clinical features and laboratory findings. STEC-HUS should be suspected in a patient with history of recent gastrointestinal infection and then an STEC stool culture or stool polymerase chain reaction should be performed to confirm diagnosis.[35,49] Stool polymerase chain reaction assay has shown a sensitivity and specificity of 100% to detect STEC.[50] A diagnosis of SP-HUS should be suspected in patients with recent pneumonia or meningitis, and have the evidence of pneumococcal infection from the blood or other body fluids[51] together with a positive direct Coombs test.[22] Other secondary causes of aHUS should be excluded, starting by conducting a thorough medical history, which may include history of underlying malignancy, autoimmune disease, related medication use, pregnancy, infection, a family history of TMA, or a history of kidney injury. In addition, laboratory testing including, but not limited to HIV, pregnancy, hepatitis, Epstein-Barr virus, cytomegalovirus, influenza, antinuclear antibodies, and anti-DNA antibodies, as well as imaging such as brain and lung computed tomography scans based on the medical history, should provide the grounds to establish a diagnosis.[5,52]

No specific diagnostic test for aHUS exists to date. Ultimately, the diagnosis of aHUS can be made by exclusion of other secondary causes, and in the ICU setting, by exclusion of TTP, other related TMAs, and DIC is recommended.[52] Performing screening of the following set of genes: CD46, CHF, CFI, C3, CFB, CFHR1, THBD, CFHR5, and diacylglycerol kinase epsilon,[5] provides prognostic information, but it has several limitations. For instance, genetic testing may take weeks, which means that it is impractical in the acute setting and for the rapid diagnosis of aHUS.[52] Furthermore, mutations are only identified in 30% to 50% of patients with aHUS,[26] and thus a negative genetic result does not necessarily exclude aHUS.

SHIGA TOXIN-ASSOCIATED HEMOLYTIC UREMIC SYNDROME
Pathophysiology

Enterocolitis from Stx-producing E coli (STEC) is the most common cause of HUS in children in the United States and Europe.[16] Shiga-toxin producing serotype 0157:H7 is the most frequent causing strain. However, other EHEC serotypes have also been reported to cause HUS, such as O26, O45, O103, O111, O113, O121 and O145.[8,14,53–55] Conversely, in developing countries, Shigella dysenteriae type 1 remains the predominant cause.[8,54,56]

Infection begins with ingestion of contaminated food or water. Once the pathogen reaches the intestines, it enters the cell by binding to specific receptors expressed on the cell surface of enterocytes. Stx released into the cytoplasm will initiate an inflammatory response, causing effacement of the luminal brush border of the gut epithelia resulting in malabsorption and diarrhea. Additionally, Stx is secreted into the vascular compartment, where it needs to bind surface receptors present on neutrophils, monocytes, erythrocytes, and platelets to be transported. Once it reaches the renal vasculature, Stx may irrupt into the renal endothelial cells by binding to globotriaosylceramide receptors present on the endothelial surface or by direct entry. Globotriaosylceramides are glycolipid surface receptors that are highly expressed in the kidney and are also found in the intestines, pancreas, heart, and brain. Stx initiates a cascade of signals that induce upregulation and gene expression of prothrombotic and proinflammatory factors such as von Willebrand Factor, P-selectin, cellular adhesion molecules (eg, vascular cell adhesion molecule, intracellular adhesion molecules, and platelet endothelial cell adhesion molecule) and chemokines receptors (eg, CXCR4/CSCR7/SDF1) on the cell surface. Moreover, Stx may halt protein synthesis by impairing ribosomal activity, by affecting the 60s subunit, resulting in cellular dysfunction and cell death (**Fig. 3**).[2,14,57–60]

Complement factors can be activated when they come into contact with prothrombotic factors. Hence, augmented expression of adhesion molecules and selectins, especially P-selectin, on the endothelial surface results in a complement hyperactivation owing to the formation of C3 convertase that will cleave C3, resulting in increased C3a and shedding of the THBD (**Fig. 4**). Hyperactivation of the alternative complement pathway may also result from the binding of Stx to the complement regulator factor CFH.[57] Additionally, increased Bb and sC5b-9 plasma levels have been detected in some patients during acute phases of STEC-HUS.[37] Furthermore, some studies have shown that, in some specific cases C3 and factor B plasma levels remain elevated after the resolution of the disease.[61] However, further studies are needed to clarify the specific roles of Stx and complement system in the development of STEC-HUS.

Clinical Manifestation and Risk Factors

Symptoms of STEC infection usually begin with watery diarrhea that starts 2 to 12 days after pathogen exposure,[11,14] progressing to bloody diarrhea, nausea, vomiting, abdominal pain, and cramping within 1 to 3 days thereafter.[14,56] As the gastrointestinal symptoms begin to improve, the sequelae of HUS develop, typically 2 to 14 days after the initial onset of diarrhea.[56] Clinical manifestations of HUS are

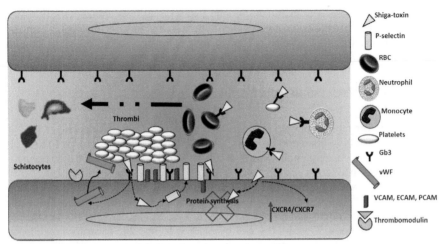

Fig. 3. Molecular pathogenesis of STEC-HUS. Stx is transported in the blood stream attached to receptors present on the surface of neutrophils, monocytes, erythrocytes and platelets. When it reaches the renal vasculature, it binds globotriaosylceramide (Gb3) receptors expressed on the endothelial cell surfaces. Then, some receptor conformational changes begin letting the toxin enter the cell. Once inside the cell, the toxin initiates a cascade of signals that will stimulate expression of proinflammatory (CXCR4/CXCR7/SDF1) and prothrombotic mediators (eg, P-Selectin, von Willebrand Factor [vWF], cellular adhesion molecules, etc). Furthermore, it will exert proapoptotic effects by hindering ribosomal activity and therefore inhibiting protein synthesis. ECAM, endothelial cell adhesion molecule; PCAM, platelet cell adhesion molecule; RBC, red blood cells; VACM, vascular cell adhesion molecule.

generally nonspecific and can include pallor, jaundice, fatigue, shortness of breath, oliguria, and edema,[6,9] most without fever during the initial assessment.[11] Factors that have been associated with evolution from STEC infection to STEC-HUS include bloody diarrhea, young age, female sex, antimotility agents, and leukocytosis.[14,17] Acute neurologic symptoms occur in up to 20% of children and 50% of adults,[6,62] and can include altered mental status, diplopia, dysphasia, facial palsy, coma, seizures, and pyramidal and extrapyramidal syndromes.[62] Other extrarenal manifestations, which can manifest in 8% to 29% of patients, include perforating colitis, cholecystitis, pancreatitis, diabetes mellitus, myocardial dysfunction, rhabdomyolysis, and ulcerative-necrotic skin lesions.[6,9,62] Severe hypertension, when present, is usually associated with neurologic involvement or renal failure.[14]

Diagnosis

In children, the clinical diagnosis of HUS is also based on the triad of anemia (hemoglobin <8 g/dL or packed cell volume <30%), thrombocytopenia (platelet count <150 × 10^9/L), and evidence of renal dysfunction, including hematuria, proteinuria, or an elevated serum creatinine level for age and height.[11] The presence of STEC or Stx in the stool should be evaluated by stool culture using sorbitol-MacConkey agar or using Shiga-toxin detection assays.[11] STEC-HUS is characterized by a nonimmune hemolytic anemia; therefore, the direct Coombs test should be negative.[63] MAHA should be confirmed on peripheral blood smear by the presence of schistocytes, burr cells, or helmet cells.[8] This finding is key in differentiating STEC-HUS from other forms of Coombs-negative hemolytic anemia, including other rare disorders such as paroxysmal nocturnal hemoglobinuria.[64] Testing for ADAMTS13 activity level can

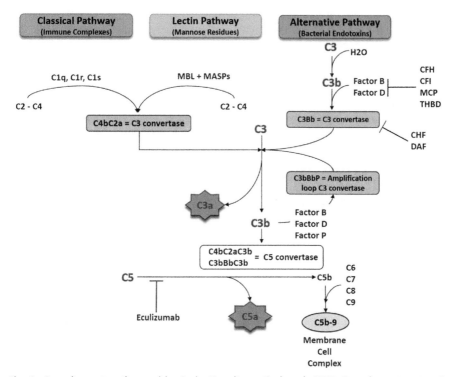

Fig. 4. Complement pathways (classic, lectin, alternative) and aHUS. Complement system is an essential component of the immune system, which pathways are activated through several mechanisms such as immune complexes (ie, classic pathway), mannose binding (ie, lectin pathway), and bacterial endotoxins (ie, alternative pathway). Activation of the complement alternative pathway is initiated by bacterial endotoxins and binding of preformed C3b to pathogens and cell membranes. The initial step in the activation of the alternative pathway is the spontaneous hydrolysis of C3 into C3b, also known as complement tickover. C3b facilitates binding of Factor B to C3b generating factor Ba and Bb. Factor Bb with C3b will give rise to factor C3bBb or mostly known as C3 convertase. CFH is a complement controlling factor that competes with Factor B for C3b inhibiting C3 convertase formation. It also prevents complement activation on the surface of cells by its cofactor activity with factor I. Finally, C3 convertase will mediate C3 cleavage into C3a and C3b. C3b is essential for all complement pathways to produce C5 convertase. Complement pathways (ie, classic, lectin, and alternative) converge at the terminal complement protein C5.[139] Factor P along with factor B and D keep stimulating the production of C3 and C5 convertases. C5 cleavage will result in C5a and C5b. C5b with C6, C7, C8, and C9 will lead to the formation of the membrane attack complex (C5b-9). Complement membrane attack complex injures the vascular endothelium enhancing the microvascular thrombotic lesions. The alternative complement pathway is regulated by numerous proteins such as CFH, CFI, membrane cofactor (MCP) and thrombomodulin (THBD). Eculizumab is a monoclonal antibody binds to C5 blocking the cleavage of C5 into C5a and C5b. CHF, DAF, (*Data from* Walport, M.J., Complement. First of two parts. N Engl J Med, 2001. 344(14): p. 1058-66.)

further distinguish STEC-HUS from TTP, with an activity level of less than 10% typically observed in patients with TTP.[65] If STEC testing is negative, further evaluation for other infectious causes of HUS should also be undertaken. Laboratory studies consistent with hemolysis may include elevated serum lactate dehydrogenase and free hemoglobin levels, and low serum haptoglobin levels. Evidence of DIC or other forms of coagulopathy should not be present; fibrinogen concentrations will be normal or high, and prothrombin time and partial thromboplastin time will be normal or slightly elevated in most cases of STEC-HUS.11 Additional stool studies may show leukocytes, which are present in approximately one-half of the patients.[56]

Treatment

Treatment of STEC-HUS is primarily supportive care consisting of volume expansion, antihypertensive therapy and renal replacement therapy. Early volume expansion during the diarrhea phase of STEC-associated illness has been associated with a lower frequency of oligoanuric AKI in patients who develop HUS.[66] In a cohort of 50 children with diarrhea-positive HUS in North America, patients were 1.6 times more likely to become oligoanuric if no intravenous fluids were given in the 4 days leading up to the onset of HUS.[66] Close monitoring of fluid balance is paramount to maintaining adequate renal perfusion while avoiding potentially harmful fluid overload. If symptoms of volume overload become evident, including hypertension, pulmonary edema, and increase in heart size, fluid restriction should be undertaken. Diuretics should be used judiciously in patients with oliguria owing to the risk for intravascular volume depletion and exacerbation of microvascular thrombi formation. Antibiotic therapy for treatment of EHEC diarrhea or STEC-HUS remains controversial. Early data indicated that treatment of EHEC infection with bactericidal antibiotics was associated with the subsequent development of HUS.[67,68] However, data from a 2002 meta-analysis did not show a difference in the risk of developing HUS in patients with or without antibiotic exposure,[33] and recent data from the STEC O104:H4 outbreak in Germany indicate that azithromycin use in patients with STEC-HUS may decrease the duration of bacterial shedding.[10] Similarly, platelet transfusions have historically been avoided in patients with HUS, owing to concern for propagation of microthrombi and worsening of end-organ damage. Recent evidence has demonstrated that patients with STEC-HUS receiving platelet transfusions do not have an increase in major complications, thrombotic events or mortality compared with patients who did not receive platelets.[69,70] However, platelet administration does not reduce bleeding complications in this population either,[71,72] thus questioning the role of platelets as a therapeutic strategy.

The efficacy of therapeutic plasma exchange (PE) for the management of STEC-HUS also remains unclear. No randomized controlled trial to evaluate the effectiveness of PE in STEC-HUS has been performed to date. In a review by Keenswijk and colleagues,[73] evidence suggests that early PE may decrease mortality and improve outcomes in patients with STEC-HUS over the age of 60 or in select pediatric patients with severe disease. However, no definite recommendations can be made based on the current body of evidence.

Although the role of complement activation in STEC-HUS is a topic of active research, the use of eculizumab, a humanized monoclonal antibody against C5, has not been shown to improve short-term or midterm outcomes in patients with STEC-HUS.[74] However, like many of the proposed treatment modalities for HUS, clinical trials to evaluate the efficacy of eculizumab in patients with STEC-HUS are lacking.

Prognosis

The long-term renal prognosis in patients with STEC-HUS is most strongly associated with the severity of renal injury sustained during the acute phase of illness. Patients with anuria for more than 10 days and those requiring renal replacement therapy are at greater risk for developing chronic kidney disease.[75] Chronic kidney disease occurs in 9% to 28% of patients with STEC-HUS, increasing up to 69% in patients with anuria for more than 11 days. End-stage renal disease occurs in approximately 3% of patients.[75–78] Other chronic renal sequelae, including hypertension and proteinuria, have been found in 5% to 15% and 15% to 30% of patients with STEC-HUS, respectively.[75] Extrarenal complications of HUS can persist after the acute phase. In patients with severe colitis, colonic strictures may develop,[9] and bowel resection in patients with hemorrhagic colitis is not uncommon.[79] Acute pancreatitis and pancreatic thromboses can lead to pancreatic necrosis and fibrosis, resulting in type 1 diabetes mellitus, which has been reported in up to one-third of patients who survive STEC-HUS.[80] Neurologic deficits are not frequently observed in the long term.[62,81,82] Mortality rates from STEC-HUS in children and young adults are estimated at 3% to 5%, but have been reported to be as high as 30% in the elderly.[9,17] Mortality is most often observed during the acute phase and in patients with severe extrarenal manifestations, especially in those with central nervous system involvement.[75]

ATYPICAL HEMOLYTIC UREMIC SYNDROME
Pathophysiology

Atypical HUS is primarily caused by a dysregulation of the complement system. Approximately 50% to 70% cases of aHUS have an underlying inherited or acquired complement genetic abnormality. However, no mutations are identified in 30% to 50% of patients,[5,26,83] and despite having known related heterozygous gene mutations, some patients never develop aHUS, suggesting that associated at-risk polymorphisms in the various complement genes, disease modifiers, or precipitating events are necessary to develop the syndrome (second hit).[1,4,29,36,84–88] However, the fact that a complement genetic abnormality is not detectable in these cases does not exclude the possible role of complement in these diseases. Common environmental triggers include nonenteric bacterial or viral infection, drugs, autoimmune conditions, malignancies, transplantation, and pregnancy.[4]

Complement genetic abnormalities can be characterized as a loss of function mutation of regulator factors or a gain of function mutation of effector factors. The list of extensively reported genes involved in complement related and non–complement-related aHUS include complement factor H (CFH) (20%–30%), membrane cofactor protein (MCP or CD46) (10%–15%), C3, complement factor I (CFI), complement factor B, THBD (encoding thrombomodulin), and diacylglycerol kinase epsilon. Acquired CFH deficiency (5%–10%)[5,89,90] causing inhibition of CFH function by autoantibodies also has a genetic predisposition, which is strongly associated with a deletion of the CFHR1 and CFHR3 genes.[91] Furthermore, some of these gene mutations have also been identified in patients with sepsis.[92] Loss of function in complement regulator factors causes excessive C3b and C3 convertase production, resulting in an increase formation of membrane attack complex (C5b-C9). Membrane attack complex causes endothelial injury, exacerbating vascular thrombotic lesions. Thrombomodulin genetic abnormalities, along with DKGE loss of function, results in upregulation and expression of von Willebrand Factor and a decrease in vascular endothelial growth factor, exacerbating the prothrombotic effects of complement.[93] An understanding of the complement pathways and the documentation of genetic mutations have allowed investigators to predict progression of the disease and develop targeted mechanistic therapies.

Clinical Manifestations

Atypical HUS is rarely considered in the diagnostic differential in critically ill patients because more common conditions, such as sepsis, often result in unexplained AKI, thrombocytopenia, and multiorgan failure. It is important for critical care physicians to recognize this condition because it can resemble DIC and sepsis, which are more common in the ICU. It might also be unmasked by other conditions with enhanced complement activation. More important, this condition has a specific treatment and needs rapid action.

Atypical HUS is known to have incomplete genetic penetrance with only 40% to 50% among carriers of CFH, MCP, and CFI mutations.[85] Onset of the disease might follow trigger events (including viral gastroenteritis, influenza, vaccination, or childbirth) in approximately 50% of children and one-third of adults.[6] Age of onset varies between patients. AKI is a major organ dysfunction in aHUS; however, about 20% of the cases have normal renal function; conversely TTP may present with renal failure making it important to consider both diagnoses. Extrarenal manifestations are reported in approximately 20% of patients with aHUS and can include pulmonary, gastrointestinal, neurologic, cardiac, integumentary, and ocular involvement.[5]

Diagnosis

In children, the main differential diagnosis of aHUS is STEC-HUS, whereas in adults, ADAMTS13 deficiency TTP and secondary HUS are more common.[6] Pretreatment blood samples should be promptly obtained to measure ADAMTS13 activity to differentiate aHUS from TTP.[5,94] The test is typically available within a few hours and useful for guiding further treatment. When not available rapidly, it will sometimes be necessary to start presumptive treatment (eg, PE) in patients at high risk for TTP while awaiting the test results. Low C3 and normal C4 levels are found in about 40% of aHUS cases. However, normal complement concentrations do not rule out complement aHUS because low concentrations of circulating C3 have low sensitivity and high concentrations of circulating C5a and soluble C5b-9 might have insufficient specificity.[95] Culture-based assay (serology or polymerase chain reaction) should be routine in all patients suspected aHUS (5% of STEC-HUS cases have no prodromal diarrhea and 30% of patients with complement-mediated aHUS have concurrent gastroenteritis).[5,96] Coombs test and body fluid culture can help to differentiate in cases with suspected SP-HUS. As mentioned, genetic testing is not useful in the acute setting. The diagnosis of aHUS is based on exclusion of other possible causes of TMA.

Treatment

All patients with a clinical diagnosis of aHUS are eligible for treatment with a complement C5 inhibitor. Eculizumab has been demonstrated to be effective and well-tolerated in aHUS treatment.[43,97–99] Although the clinical benefits of eculizumab have been demonstrated by reduced rates of morbidity and mortality, further studies are needed to assess its effect at the vascular endothelium level.[100] Patients should receive meningococcal vaccine, but this should not delay the start of eculizumab. Antibiotic prophylaxis is mandated during the first 2 weeks of treatment.[5] If access to eculizumab is unavailable, PE can be used for critically ill patients with severe TMA and is often necessary while laboratory results are being determined,[52,101] even though there is no strong evidence for the efficacy of PE in aHUS.[6] Platelet transfusion should be avoided, and dialysis support should be used in cases with severe renal failure. Treatment duration remains controversial and based on expert opinion. Discontinuation of eculizumab therapy can be considered on a case-by-case basis after at least 6 to 12 months of treatment and at least 3 months of renal recovery.[5] Kidney transplantation can be considered by underlying genetic abnormality owing to variation in outcome and disease recurrence rates and should be delayed until at least 6 months after the start of dialysis and also require resolution of extrarenal manifestations.[5,97,102]

Prognosis

The clinical outcome of aHUS is unfavorable in which about 50% of cases progress to end-stage renal disease and up to 25% may die during the acute phase.[1] Progression to end-stage renal disease after the first aHUS episode was more frequent in adults than in children.[26] Different genetic abnormalities also account for different outcomes, response to therapy, and risk of recurrence after kidney transplantation. CFH and CFI mutations are associated with a very poor outcome, with 80% of cases presenting with recurrent disease, whereas MCP mutations are usually associated with good outcome with less recurrence after kidney transplantation.[1]

SECONDARY HEMOLYTIC UREMIC SYNDROME

The pathophysiologic mechanisms of secondary HUS are incompletely understood and the role of the complement system is not well established. Despite the absence of genetic complement abnormalities, a second-hit theory has been proposed to explain the role of complement in secondary HUS. Endothelial injury and activation lead to an increase in the expression and secretion of proinflammatory and procoagulant mediators that indirectly induce complement activation. Specific mechanisms for some forms of secondary HUS have been identified.[6]

Management of secondary HUS relies on treatment and withdrawal of the triggering condition and supportive care. PE is often empirically used whenever TTP cannot be excluded despite the lack of established benefit.[6] Eculizumab has been used in cases of secondary HUS with worsening renal function and persistence of TMA despite treatment with PE[50,103] and may be a potential second-line treatment. Specific details of the most frequent types of secondary HUS are described in detail.

STREPTOCOCCUS PNEUMONIAE–ASSOCIATED HEMOLYTIC UREMIC SYNDROME
Pathophysiology

Although the pathogenesis of SP-HUS is not fully understood, evidence suggests that Thomsen-Freidenreich antigen (T-antigen) may play an important role in the development of the disease. After exposure to neuraminidase-producing S pneumoniae, N-acetylneuraminic acid is cleaved from glycoproteins on the cell membranes of glomeruli, erythrocytes, and platelets, exposing the underlying T-antigen to the plasma environment.[104] T-antigen reacts with circulating anti–T-antigen IgM antibodies present in the plasma (T-antigen activation). This process is thought to lead to damage of the glomerular endothelial cells, red blood cells, and platelets, thereby causing AKI, anemia, and thrombocytopenia.[105] T-antigen activation testing for neuraminidase activity has been demonstrated to be higher in patients with acute SP-HUS compared with patients with other forms of HUS[106]; however, T-antigen activation can also occur in patients with invasive pneumococcal infection who do not develop HUS.[107] Specific alleles of neuraminidase subtypes expressed by S pneumoniae, and neuraminidase A, B, and C have not been associated with the occurrence of SP-HUS.[108] Therefore, the role of neuraminidase in the pathogenesis of SP-HUS remains unclear. Recent research has also demonstrated another mechanism that may underlie the pathogenesis of SP-HUS. Meinel and colleagues[109] demonstrated plasminogen binding by S pneumoniae isolates obtained from 2 patients with SP-HUS. This mechanism results in damage to endothelial cells and exposure of the underlying matrix, leading to thrombosis and the other clinical features of HUS.[50] Limited data are available on complement activation in patients with SP-HUS. In a recent case series by Bitzan and colleagues,[110] low levels of C3 and C4 were observed in 2 of the 3 patients. In another case series by Szilagyi and colleagues,[111] 5 of 5 patients with SP-HUS had low C3 and C4 levels during their initial admission to the hospital. Three patients survived and were followed for at least 2 months after hospital discharge. Of these 3 patients, 1 had persistently low C3 levels at time of follow-up. CH50 and AH50 levels may also be reduced in some patients with SP-HUS.[110]

A variety of S pneumoniae serotypes have been associated with SP-HUS cases and, of those reported, serotype 19A is the most common.[21,22,51,110,112] The proportion of S pneumoniae with serotype 19A notably increased in frequency after the introduction of the Prevnar 7 vaccine, which covers serotypes 4, 6B, 9V, 14, 18C, 19F, and 23F.[21] Although the newest pneumococcal polysaccharide vaccine, Pneumovax 23, now covers a wider range of serotypes, including 19A, this vaccine is not recommended for children under the age of 2.

Clinical Manifestations

SP-HUS is rare, occurring in approximately 0.4% to 0.6% of patients with invasive S pneumoniae infection[113–115] and accounts for 5% to 15% of HUS cases.[21,115,116] SP-HUS is most often observed in pediatric patients, with the incidence highest among children less than 2 years of age.[22,113,116] The onset of HUS typically occurs 3 to 14 days after the presenting symptoms of the associated S pneumoniae infection.[23,111,115,117] Compared with patients with STEC-HUS, patients with SP-HUS usually have a higher severity of illness at the time of presentation, frequently exhibiting clinical symptoms of sepsis with cardiopulmonary compromise and altered mental status.[110,113,118,119] Patients with SP-HUS also tend to have a longer duration of oliguria and thrombocytopenia, and need more transfusions.[21] SP-HUS most frequently occurs in the setting of S pneumoniae pneumonia with or without empyema or meningitis, and less commonly in the setting of mastoiditis, pericarditis, peritonitis, or spontaneous bacteremia.[116] In a cohort of children from the United Kingdom with SP-HUS,[22] pneumonia was the source of infection in 35 of 43 cases (81%); of the 35 patients with pneumonia, 23 cases (66%) were complicated by empyema. Thirteen patients in the cohort (30%) were diagnosed with meningitis. Similarly, in a case series by Cabrera and colleagues,[113] among 7 children presenting with SP-HUS over a 3-year period, 5 patients (71%) had pneumonia and 2 patients (29%) had meningitis. Of those 7 patients, 3 with pneumonia and 1 with meningitis had concurrent otitis media, and 1 child with meningitis and otitis media was also diagnosed with mastoiditis.

Diagnosis

The diagnosis of SP-HUS is based on a combination of clinical and laboratory findings, in association with S pneumoniae infection. Cases are divided into definite and suspected, based on those with proven versus suspected invasive S pneumoniae infection.[51] S pneumoniae infection can be confirmed by bacterial culture or by antigen or nucleic acid detection assays.[105] Laboratory findings must then demonstrate the triad of HUS. In cases of SP-HUS, fibrinogen levels should remain normal, compared with cases of DIC with associated renal injury where fibrinogen levels will be decreased. Furthermore, the prothrombin time and partial thromboplastin time will be normal or slightly elevated in most cases of SP-HUS, and significantly prolonged in cases of DIC.[51,116] T-antigen activation may be suspected if minor cross-match of patient's red blood cells with donor serum reveals agglutination or inconsistencies in a patient's blood group and type occurs over time.[120] Direct Coombs testing may also be helpful in differentiating cases of SP-HUS from aHUS and STEC-HUS. Of patients with SP-HUS, 58% to 89% will have positive direct Coombs test,[121,122] likely secondary to the interaction of T-antigen and anti–T-antigen IgM antibodies on the surface of red blood cells.[122] T-antigen activation can be confirmed by lectin agglutination methods,[123] which result positive in 50% to 69% of patients with SP-HUS or *S pneumoniae*–associated hemolytic anemia without uremia.[104,105] Neuraminidase activity may also be measured directly using a rapid fluorogenic neuraminidase assay.[106]

Treatment

The mainstay of treatment in patients with SP-HUS is supportive care and treatment of the underlying bacterial infection. Broad-spectrum antibiotic coverage for *S pneumoniae* directed by regional antimicrobial susceptibility and resistance patterns until final culture susceptibility is reported is recommended. Although the clinical significance of neuraminidase in the pathogenesis of SP-HUS is not fully understood, avoidance of plasma and unwashed blood products, which contain anti–T-antigen antibodies, is generally recommended.[78,107] In critically ill patients and in patients with persistent hemolysis and renal dysfunction despite treatment of the underlying *S pneumoniae* infection, PE may be considered.[107,124] In patients with T-antigen activation, 5% albumin is the preferred replacement solution for PE, unless clinically significant coagulopathy and clotting factor deficiency develops.[107] Renal replacement therapy is required in 43% to 92% of patients with SP-HUS for the management of fluid overload and electrolyte abnormalities.[21,112,115]

Prognosis

The prognosis of patients with SP-HUS has improved in recent years; however, morbidity and mortality remain high in this patient population. Progression to end-stage renal disease and renal transplantation occurs in 8% to 10% of patients,[21,115] and hypertension, proteinuria, and chronic kidney disease are observed in an additional 5% to 37% of patients.[21,22,112] Extrarenal sequelae, including neurologic injury, cardiac dysfunction, pancreatitis, cholestasis, and liver dysfunction, have been reported.[51,115,125] In a review of 43 children with SP-HUS in the United Kingdom by Waters and colleagues,[22] 4 patients required ventriculoperitoneal shunt insertion for obstructive hydrocephalus, 3 patients had hearing loss, 6 patients had significant neurologic deficits, and only 2 of 13 patients presenting with meningitis has normal neurodevelopmental status at follow-up. Overall, long-term complications are reported in 26% to 40% of patients.[21] Mortality associated with SP-HUS ranges from 2% to 26%[21,22,112,115] and is highest among patients presenting with meningitis.

PREGNANCY-ASSOCIATED ATYPICAL HEMOLYTIC UREMIC SYNDROME

During pregnancy, many types of TMA can be triggered including ADAMTS13 deficiency TTP (during the second and third trimesters), aHUS (mostly in postpartum women), and HELLP syndrome, which is a severe variant of pre-eclampsia.[6] Pregnancy-associated aHUS occurs in approximately 20% of adult female patients with aHUS, with 80% presenting postpartum, and is associated with severe AKI requiring dialysis.[126] Complement abnormalities are identified in the majority of the patients, including mutations in CFH, CFI, MCP, and C3, which are thought to be only predisposing factor.[1,126] Clinical diagnosis might be difficult and should be based on history, and laboratory findings. Low ADAMTS13 activity and elevation of liver enzymes help to distinguish aHUS from TTP and HELLP syndrome, respectively. Although preeclampsia/HELLP is commonly associated with new-onset hypertension and proteinuria after 20 weeks of gestation, TTP and aHUS may also exhibit these features.[127] Pre-eclampsia and HELLP syndrome usually subside after delivery and is often characterized by complete remission, whereas PE is required if TTP/aHUS is diagnosed.[127] Eculizumab has been found remarkably efficient and safe to control pregnancy-associated aHUS.[128–130]

De Novo Posttransplant Hemolytic Uremic Syndrome

De novo HUS has been reported in patients receiving kidney transplants or other organs, including hematopoietic stem cell transplantation.[131–133] In kidney transplant recipients treated with cyclosporine, the incidence of de novo HUS is 4% to 15% with 43% graft survival.[134] The onset of the disease is usually in the first weeks after transplantation, when patients are treated with high doses of immunosuppressive agents. The mechanism is unclear and seems to be multifactorial, including calcineurin inhibitor toxicity, humoral rejection, and infection.[6] Some gene mutations have been reported in patients with de novo posttransplant HUS (CFH [15%] and CFI [16%]).[1]

Drug-Associated Hemolytic Uremic Syndrome

Recognition of drug-associated causes in a patient with HUS is important to avoid reexposure and recurrent illness. Many drugs have been reported to cause HUS including anticancer drugs (eg, mitomycin, cisplatin, bleomycin, and gemcitabine), immunotherapeutic agents (eg, cyclosporine, tacrolimus, muromonab-CD3, interferon, and quinine), and antiplatelet agents (eg, ticlopidine and clopidogrel).[135] Underlying mechanism of TMA is thought to be either immune mediated or dose dependent toxicity mediated or both.[135,136] The role of PE in the setting is uncertain.[137,138]

SUMMARY

HUS is characterized by MAHA, thrombocytopenia, and AKI. DIC, TTP, and HUS have similar clinical presentations. The diagnostic approach to a patient with suspect TMA should be implemented promptly to decrease mortality, because identifying the different disorders can help to tailor specific and effective therapies. However, diagnosis is challenging and morbidity and mortality remain high, especially in the critically ill patient population. The development of clinical prediction scores and rapid diagnostic tests for HUS based on mechanistic knowledge are needed to facilitate early diagnosis and assign timely specific treatments to patients with HUS variants.

REFERENCES

1. Noris M, Remuzzi G. Atypical hemolytic-uremic syndrome. N Engl J Med 2009; 361(17):1676–87.
2. George JN, Nester CM. Syndromes of thrombotic microangiopathy. N Engl J Med 2014;371(7):654–66.
3. Gasser C, Gautier E, Steck A, et al. Hemolytic-uremic syndrome: bilateral necrosis of the renal cortex in acute acquired hemolytic anemia. Schweiz Med Wochenschr 1955;85(38–39):905–9 [in German].
4. Kavanagh D, Goodship TH, Richards A. Atypical haemolytic uraemic syndrome. Br Med Bull 2006;77-78:5–22.
5. Goodship TH, Cook HT, Fakhouri F, et al. Atypical hemolytic uremic syndrome and C3 glomerulopathy: conclusions from a "Kidney Disease: Improving Global Outcomes" (KDIGO) controversies conference. Kidney Int 2017;91(3):539–51.
6. Fakhouri F, Zuber J, Fremeaux-Bacchi V, et al. Haemolytic uraemic syndrome. Lancet 2017;390(10095):681–96.

7. Loirat C, Fakhouri F, Ariceta G, et al. An international consensus approach to the management of atypical hemolytic uremic syndrome in children. Pediatr Nephrol 2016;31(1):15–39.

8. Noris M, Remuzzi G. Hemolytic uremic syndrome. J Am Soc Nephrol 2005; 16(4):1035–50.

9. Scheiring J, Andreoli SP, Zimmerhackl LB. Treatment and outcome of Shiga-toxin-associated hemolytic uremic syndrome (HUS). Pediatr Nephrol 2008; 23(10):1749–60.

10. Buchholz U, Bernard H, Werber D, et al. German outbreak of Escherichia coli O104:H4 associated with sprouts. N Engl J Med 2011;365(19):1763–70.

11. Tarr PI, Gordon CA, Chandler WL. Shiga-toxin-producing Escherichia coli and haemolytic uraemic syndrome. Lancet 2005;365(9464):1073–86.

12. Zoufaly A, Cramer JP, Vettorazzi E, et al. Risk factors for development of hemolytic uremic syndrome in a cohort of adult patients with STEC 0104:H4 infection. PLoS One 2013;8(3):e59209.

13. Ko H, Maymani H, Rojas-Hernandez C. Hemolytic uremic syndrome associated with Escherichia coli O157:H7 infection in older adults: a case report and review of the literature. J Med Case Rep 2016;10:175.

14. Salvadori M, Bertoni E. Update on hemolytic uremic syndrome: diagnostic and therapeutic recommendations. World J Nephrol 2013;2(3):56–76.

15. Kottke-Marchant K. Diagnostic approach to microangiopathic hemolytic disorders. Int J Lab Hematol 2017;39(Suppl 1):69–75.

16. Ardissino G, Salardi S, Colombo E, et al. Epidemiology of haemolytic uremic syndrome in children. Data from the North Italian HUS network. Eur J Pediatr 2016;175(4):465–73.

17. Gould LH, Demma L, Jones TF, et al. Hemolytic uremic syndrome and death in persons with Escherichia coli O157:H7 infection, foodborne diseases active surveillance network sites, 2000-2006. Clin Infect Dis 2009;49(10):1480–5.

18. Frank C, Werber D, Cramer JP, et al. Epidemic profile of Shiga-toxin-producing Escherichia coli O104:H4 outbreak in Germany. N Engl J Med 2011;365(19): 1771–80.

19. Ake JA, Jelacic S, Ciol MA, et al. Relative nephroprotection during Escherichia coli O157:H7 infections: association with intravenous volume expansion. Pediatrics 2005;115(6):e673–80.

20. Garg AX, Suri RS, Barrowman N, et al. Long-term renal prognosis of diarrhea-associated hemolytic uremic syndrome: a systematic review, meta-analysis, and meta-regression. JAMA 2003;290(10):1360–70.

21. Spinale JM, Ruebner RL, Kaplan BS, et al. Update on Streptococcus pneumoniae associated hemolytic uremic syndrome. Curr Opin Pediatr 2013;25(2): 203–8.

22. Waters AM, Kerecuk L, Luk D, et al. Hemolytic uremic syndrome associated with invasive pneumococcal disease: the United Kingdom experience. J Pediatr 2007;151(2):140–4.

23. Constantinescu AR, Bitzan M, Weiss LS, et al. Non-enteropathic hemolytic uremic syndrome: causes and short-term course. Am J Kidney Dis 2004;43(6): 976–82.

24. Shimizu M, Yokoyama T, Sakashita N, et al. Thomsen-Friedenreich antigen exposure as a cause of Streptococcus pyogenes-associated hemolytic-uremic syndrome. Clin Nephrol 2012;78(4):328–31.

25. Zimmerhackl LB, Besbas N, Jungraithmayr T, et al. Epidemiology, clinical presentation, and pathophysiology of atypical and recurrent hemolytic uremic syndrome. Semin Thromb Hemost 2006;32(2):113–20.

26. Fremeaux-Bacchi V, Fakhouri F, Garnier A, et al. Genetics and outcome of atypical hemolytic uremic syndrome: a nationwide French series comparing children and adults. Clin J Am Soc Nephrol 2013;8(4):554–62.

27. Sheerin NS, Kavanagh D, Goodship TH, et al. A national specialized service in England for atypical haemolytic uraemic syndrome-the first year's experience. QJM 2016;109(1):27–33.

28. Johnson S, Stojanovic J, Ariceta G, et al. An audit analysis of a guideline for the investigation and initial therapy of diarrhea negative (atypical) hemolytic uremic syndrome. Pediatr Nephrol 2014;29(10):1967–78.

29. Loirat C, Fremeaux-Bacchi V. Atypical hemolytic uremic syndrome. Orphanet J Rare Dis 2011;6:60.

30. Taylor CM, Machin S, Wigmore SJ, et al. Clinical practice guidelines for the management of atypical haemolytic uraemic syndrome in the United Kingdom. Br J Haematol 2010;148(1):37–47.

31. Veesenmeyer AF, Edmonson MB. Trends in US hospital stays for Streptococcus pneumoniae-associated hemolytic uremic syndrome. Pediatr Infect Dis J 2013; 32(7):731–5.

32. Scallan E, Crim SM, Runkle A, et al. Bacterial enteric infections among older adults in the United States: foodborne diseases active surveillance network, 1996-2012. Foodborne Pathog Dis 2015;12(6):492–9.

33. Safdar N, Said A, Gangnon RE, et al. Risk of hemolytic uremic syndrome after antibiotic treatment of Escherichia coli O157:H7 enteritis: a meta-analysis. JAMA 2002;288(8):996–1001.

34. Ardissino G, Dacco V, Testa S, et al. Hemoconcentration: a major risk factor for neurological involvement in hemolytic uremic syndrome. Pediatr Nephrol 2015; 30(2):345–52.

35. Campistol JM, Arias M, Ariceta G, et al. An update for atypical haemolytic uraemic syndrome: diagnosis and treatment. A consensus document. Nefrologia 2015;35(5):421–47.

36. Franchini M. Atypical hemolytic uremic syndrome: from diagnosis to treatment. Clin Chem Lab Med 2015;53(11):1679–88.

37. Thurman JM, Marians R, Emlen W, et al. Alternative pathway of complement in children with diarrhea-associated hemolytic uremic syndrome. Clin J Am Soc Nephrol 2009;4(12):1920–4.

38. Masias C, Vasu S, Cataland SR. None of the above: thrombotic microangiopathy beyond TTP and HUS. Blood 2017;129(21):2857–63.

39. Thachil J, Warkentin TE. How do we approach thrombocytopenia in critically ill patients? Br J Haematol 2017;177(1):27–38.

40. Boral BM, Williams DJ, Boral LI. Disseminated intravascular coagulation. Am J Clin Pathol 2016;146(6):670–80.

41. Joly BS, Coppo P, Veyradier A. Thrombotic thrombocytopenic purpura. Blood 2017;129(21):2836–46.

42. Trachtman H. HUS and TTP in children. Pediatr Clin North Am 2013;60(6): 1513–26.

43. Legendre CM, Licht C, Muus P, et al. Terminal complement inhibitor eculizumab in atypical hemolytic-uremic syndrome. N Engl J Med 2013;368(23):2169–81.

44. Coppo P, Schwarzinger M, Buffet M, et al. Predictive features of severe acquired ADAMTS13 deficiency in idiopathic thrombotic microangiopathies: the French TMA reference center experience. PLoS One 2010;5(4):e10208.

45. Bentley MJ, Lehman CM, Blaylock RC, et al. The utility of patient characteristics in predicting severe ADAMTS13 deficiency and response to plasma exchange. Transfusion 2010;50(8):1654–64.

46. Bendapudi PK, Hurwitz S, Fry A, et al. Derivation and external validation of the PLASMIC score for rapid assessment of adults with thrombotic microangiopathies: a cohort study. Lancet Haematol 2017;4(4):e157–64.

47. Bentley MJ, Wilson AR, Rodgers GM. Performance of a clinical prediction score for thrombotic thrombocytopenic purpura in an independent cohort. Vox Sang 2013;105(4):313–8.

48. Li A, Khalighi PR, Wu Q, et al. External validation of the PLASMIC score: a clinical prediction tool for thrombotic thrombocytopenic purpura diagnosis and treatment. J Thromb Haemost 2018;16(1):164–9.

49. Laurence J, Haller H, Mannucci PM, et al. Atypical hemolytic uremic syndrome (aHUS): essential aspects of an accurate diagnosis. Clin Adv Hematol Oncol 2016;14 Suppl 11(11):2–15.

50. Grys TE, Sloan LM, Rosenblatt JE, et al. Rapid and sensitive detection of Shiga toxin-producing Escherichia coli from nonenriched stool specimens by real-time PCR in comparison to enzyme immunoassay and culture. J Clin Microbiol 2009; 47(7):2008–12.

51. Copelovitch L, Kaplan BS. Streptococcus pneumoniae–associated hemolytic uremic syndrome: classification and the emergence of serotype 19A. Pediatrics 2010;125(1):e174–82.

52. Azoulay E, Knoebl P, Garnacho-Montero J, et al. Expert statements on the standard of care in critically ill adult patients with atypical hemolytic uremic syndrome. Chest 2017;152(2):424–34.

53. Ohanian M, Cable C, Halka K. Eculizumab safely reverses neurologic impairment and eliminates need for dialysis in severe atypical hemolytic uremic syndrome. Clin Pharmacol 2011;3:5–12.

54. Castro VS, Figueiredo EES, Stanford K, et al. Shiga-toxin producing Escherichia coli in Brazil: a systematic review. Microorganisms 2019;7(5) [pii:E137].

55. Council of State and Territorial Epidemiologists. Public Health reporting and National Notification for Shiga toxin-producing Escherichia coli (STEC). Atlanta (Georgia): Council of State and Territorial Epidemiologists; 2017.

56. Cody EM, Dixon BP. Hemolytic uremic syndrome. Pediatr Clin North Am 2019; 66(1):235–46.

57. Orth D, Khan AB, Naim A, et al. Shiga toxin activates complement and binds factor H: evidence for an active role of complement in hemolytic uremic syndrome. J Immunol 2009;182(10):6394–400.

58. Liu F, Huang J, Sadler JE. Shiga toxin (Stx)1B and Stx2B induce von Willebrand factor secretion from human umbilical vein endothelial cells through different signaling pathways. Blood 2011;118(12):3392–8.

59. Petruzziello-Pellegrini TN, Marsden PA. Shiga toxin-associated hemolytic uremic syndrome: advances in pathogenesis and therapeutics. Curr Opin Nephrol Hypertens 2012;21(4):433–40.

60. Morigi M, Galbusera M, Gastoldi S, et al. Alternative pathway activation of complement by Shiga toxin promotes exuberant C3a formation that triggers microvascular thrombosis. J Immunol 2011;187(1):172–80.

61. Monnens L, Molenaar J, Lambert PH, et al. The complement system in hemolytic-uremic syndrome in childhood. Clin Nephrol 1980;13(4):168–71.

62. Nathanson S, Kwon T, Elmaleh M, et al. Acute neurological involvement in diarrhea-associated hemolytic uremic syndrome. Clin J Am Soc Nephrol 2010;5(7):1218–28.

63. Talarico V, Aloe M, Monzani A, et al. Hemolytic uremic syndrome in children. Minerva Pediatr 2016;68(6):441–55.

64. Borowitz MJ, Craig FE, Digiuseppe JA, et al. Guidelines for the diagnosis and monitoring of paroxysmal nocturnal hemoglobinuria and related disorders by flow cytometry. Cytometry B Clin Cytom 2010;78(4):211–30.

65. Shibagaki Y, Fujita T. Thrombotic microangiopathy in malignant hypertension and hemolytic uremic syndrome (HUS)/thrombotic thrombocytopenic purpura (TTP): can we differentiate one from the other? Hypertens Res 2005;28(1):89–95.

66. Hickey CA, Beattie TJ, Cowieson J, et al. Early volume expansion during diarrhea and relative nephroprotection during subsequent hemolytic uremic syndrome. Arch Pediatr Adolesc Med 2011;165(10):884–9.

67. Smith KE, Wilker PR, Reiter PL, et al. Antibiotic treatment of Escherichia coli O157 infection and the risk of hemolytic uremic syndrome, Minnesota. Pediatr Infect Dis J 2012;31(1):37–41.

68. Wong CS, Jelacic S, Habeeb RL, et al. The risk of the hemolytic-uremic syndrome after antibiotic treatment of Escherichia coli O157:H7 infections. N Engl J Med 2000;342(26):1930–6.

69. Beneke J, Sartison A, Kielstein JT, et al. Clinical and laboratory consequences of platelet transfusion in shiga toxin-mediated hemolytic uremic syndrome. Transfus Med Rev 2017;31(1):51–5.

70. Balestracci A, Martin SM, Toledo I, et al. Impact of platelet transfusions in children with post-diarrheal hemolytic uremic syndrome. Pediatr Nephrol 2013;28(6):919–25.

71. Balestracci A, Martin SM, Toledo I. Hemoconcentration in hemolytic uremic syndrome: time to review the standard case definition? Pediatr Nephrol 2015;30(2):361.

72. Weil BR, Andreoli SP, Billmire DF. Bleeding risk for surgical dialysis procedures in children with hemolytic uremic syndrome. Pediatr Nephrol 2010;25(9):1693–8.

73. Keenswijk W, Raes A, De Clerck M, et al. Is plasma exchange efficacious in shiga toxin-associated hemolytic uremic syndrome? A narrative review of current evidence. Ther Apher Dial 2019;23(2):118–25.

74. Menne J, Nitschke M, Stingele R, et al. Validation of treatment strategies for enterohaemorrhagic Escherichia coli O104:H4 induced haemolytic uraemic syndrome: case-control study. BMJ 2012;345:e4565.

75. Spinale JM, Ruebner RL, Copelovitch L, et al. Long-term outcomes of Shiga toxin hemolytic uremic syndrome. Pediatr Nephrol 2013;28(11):2097–105.

76. Spizzirri FD, Rahman RC, Bibiloni N, et al. Childhood hemolytic uremic syndrome in Argentina: long-term follow-up and prognostic features. Pediatr Nephrol 1997;11(2):156–60.

77. Small G, Watson AR, Evans JH, et al. Hemolytic uremic syndrome: defining the need for long-term follow-up. Clin Nephrol 1999;52(6):352–6.

78. Siegler R, Oakes R. Hemolytic uremic syndrome; pathogenesis, treatment, and outcome. Curr Opin Pediatr 2005;17(2):200–4.

79. Rahman RC, Cobenas CJ, Drut R, et al. Hemorrhagic colitis in postdiarrheal hemolytic uremic syndrome: retrospective analysis of 54 children. Pediatr Nephrol 2012;27(2):229–33.

80. Suri RS, Mahon JL, Clark WF, et al. Relationship between Escherichia coli O157:H7 and diabetes mellitus. Kidney Int Suppl 2009;(112):S44–6.

81. Theobald I, Kuwertz-Broking E, Schiborr M, et al. Central nervous system involvement in hemolytic uremic syndrome (HUS)–a retrospective analysis of cerebral CT and MRI studies. Clin Nephrol 2001;56(6):S3–8.

82. Bennett B, Booth T, Quan A. Late onset seizures, hemiparesis and blindness in hemolytic uremic syndrome. Clin Nephrol 2003;59(3):196–200.

83. Noris M, Caprioli J, Bresin E, et al. Relative role of genetic complement abnormalities in sporadic and familial aHUS and their impact on clinical phenotype. Clin J Am Soc Nephrol 2010;5(10):1844–59.

84. Mannucci PM. Understanding organ dysfunction in thrombotic thrombocytopenic purpura. Intensive Care Med 2015;41(4):715–8.

85. Caprioli J, Noris M, Brioschi S, et al. Genetics of HUS: the impact of MCP, CFH, and IF mutations on clinical presentation, response to treatment, and outcome. Blood 2006;108(4):1267–79.

86. Buddles MR, Donne RL, Richards A, et al. Complement factor H gene mutation associated with autosomal recessive atypical hemolytic uremic syndrome. Am J Hum Genet 2000;66(5):1721–2.

87. Fremeaux-Bacchi V, Miller EC, Liszewski MK, et al. Mutations in complement C3 predispose to development of atypical hemolytic uremic syndrome. Blood 2008; 112(13):4948–52.

88. Sansbury FH, Cordell HJ, Bingham C, et al. Factors determining penetrance in familial atypical haemolytic uraemic syndrome. J Med Genet 2014;51(11): 756–64.

89. Noris M, Remuzzi G. Genetic abnormalities of complement regulators in hemolytic uremic syndrome: how do they affect patient management? Nat Clin Pract Nephrol 2005;1(1):2–3.

90. Geerdink LM, Westra D, van Wijk JA, et al. Atypical hemolytic uremic syndrome in children: complement mutations and clinical characteristics. Pediatr Nephrol 2012;27(8):1283–91.

91. Dragon-Durey MA, Loirat C, Cloarec S, et al. Anti-Factor H autoantibodies associated with atypical hemolytic uremic syndrome. J Am Soc Nephrol 2005;16(2): 555–63.

92. Kernan KF, Ghaloul-Gonzalez L, Shakoory B, et al. Adults with septic shock and extreme hyperferritinemia exhibit pathogenic immune variation. Genes Immun 2019;20(6):520–6.

93. Lemaire M, Fremeaux-Bacchi V, Schaefer F, et al. Recessive mutations in DGKE cause atypical hemolytic-uremic syndrome. Nat Genet 2013;45(5):531–6.

94. Scully M, Hunt BJ, Benjamin S, et al. Guidelines on the diagnosis and management of thrombotic thrombocytopenic purpura and other thrombotic microangiopathies. Br J Haematol 2012;158(3):323–35.

95. Cataland SR, Holers VM, Geyer S, et al. Biomarkers of terminal complement activation confirm the diagnosis of aHUS and differentiate aHUS from TTP. Blood 2014;123(24):3733–8.

96. Gerber A, Karch H, Allerberger F, et al. Clinical course and the role of shiga toxin-producing Escherichia coli infection in the hemolytic-uremic syndrome in pediatric patients, 1997-2000, in Germany and Austria: a prospective study. J Infect Dis 2002;186(4):493–500.

97. Licht C, Greenbaum LA, Muus P, et al. Efficacy and safety of eculizumab in atypical hemolytic uremic syndrome from 2-year extensions of phase 2 studies. Kidney Int 2015;87(5):1061–73.

98. Greenbaum LA, Fila M, Ardissino G, et al. Eculizumab is a safe and effective treatment in pediatric patients with atypical hemolytic uremic syndrome. Kidney Int 2016;89(3):701–11.

99. Fakhouri F, Hourmant M, Campistol JM, et al. Terminal complement inhibitor eculizumab in adult patients with atypical hemolytic uremic syndrome: a single-arm, open-label trial. Am J Kidney Dis 2016;68(1):84–93.

100. Goodship THJ, Cook HT, Fakhouri F, et al. Atypical hemolytic uremic syndrome and C3 glomerulopathy: conclusions from a "Kidney Disease: Improving Global Outcomes" (KDIGO) Controversies Conference. Kidney Int 2017;91(3):539–51.

101. Cataland SR, Wu HM. How I treat: the clinical differentiation and initial treatment of adult patients with atypical hemolytic uremic syndrome. Blood 2014;123(16): 2478–84.

102. Povey H, Vundru R, Junglee N, et al. Renal recovery with eculizumab in atypical hemolytic uremic syndrome following prolonged dialysis. Clin Nephrol 2014; 82(5):326–31.

103. Cavero T, Rabasco C, Lopez A, et al. Eculizumab in secondary atypical haemolytic uraemic syndrome. Nephrol Dial Transpl 2017;32(3):466–74.

104. Cochran JB, Panzarino VM, Maes LY, et al. Pneumococcus-induced T-antigen activation in hemolytic uremic syndrome and anemia. Pediatr Nephrol 2004; 19(3):317–21.

105. Huang DT, Chi H, Lee HC, et al. T-antigen activation for prediction of pneumococcus-induced hemolytic uremic syndrome and hemolytic anemia. Pediatr Infect Dis J 2006;25(7):608–10.

106. Szilagyi A, Gyorke Z, Bereczki C, et al. The use of a rapid fluorogenic neuraminidase assay to differentiate acute Streptococcus pneumoniae-associated hemolytic uremic syndrome (HUS) from other forms of HUS. Clin Chem Lab Med 2015;53(4):e117–9.

107. Geary DF. Hemolytic uremic syndrome and streptococcus pneumoniae: improving our understanding. J Pediatr 2007;151(2):113–4.

108. Smith A, Johnston C, Inverarity D, et al. Investigating the role of pneumococcal neuraminidase A activity in isolates from pneumococcal haemolytic uraemic syndrome. J Med Microbiol 2013;62(Pt 11):1735–42.

109. Meinel C, Sparta G, Dahse HM, et al. Streptococcus pneumoniae from patients with hemolytic uremic syndrome binds human plasminogen via the surface protein PspC and uses plasmin to damage human endothelial cells. J Infect Dis 2018;217(3):358–70.

110. Bitzan M, AlKandari O, Whittemore B, et al. Complement depletion and Coombs positivity in pneumococcal hemolytic uremic syndrome (pnHUS). Case series and plea to revisit an old pathogenetic concept. Int J Med Microbiol 2018; 308(8):1096–104.

111. Szilagyi A, Kiss N, Bereczki C, et al. The role of complement in Streptococcus pneumoniae-associated haemolytic uraemic syndrome. Nephrol Dial Transpl 2013;28(9):2237–45.

112. Banerjee R, Hersh AL, Newland J, et al. Streptococcus pneumoniae-associated hemolytic uremic syndrome among children in North America. Pediatr Infect Dis J 2011;30(9):736–9.

113. Cabrera GR, Fortenberry JD, Warshaw BL, et al. Hemolytic uremic syndrome associated with invasive Streptococcus pneumoniae infection. Pediatrics 1998;101(4 Pt 1):699–703.

114. Kaplan SL, Mason EO Jr, Barson WJ, et al. Three-year multicenter surveillance of systemic pneumococcal infections in children. Pediatrics 1998;102(3 Pt 1): 538–45.

115. Krysan DJ, Flynn JT. Renal transplantation after Streptococcus pneumoniae-associated hemolytic uremic syndrome. Am J Kidney Dis 2001;37(2):E15.

116. Copelovitch L, Kaplan BS. Streptococcus pneumoniae-associated hemolytic uremic syndrome. Pediatr Nephrol 2008;23(11):1951–6.

117. Huang YH, Lin TY, Wong KS, et al. Hemolytic uremic syndrome associated with pneumococcal pneumonia in Taiwan. Eur J Pediatr 2006;165(5):332–5.

118. Brandt J, Wong C, Mihm S, et al. Invasive pneumococcal disease and hemolytic uremic syndrome. Pediatrics 2002;110(2 Pt 1):371–6.

119. Angurana SK, Mehta A, Agrawal T, et al. Streptococcus pneumoniae-associated hemolytic uremic syndrome. Indian J Pediatr 2018;85(9):797–9.

120. Kumar ND, Sethi S. T-transformed red cells–role of minor cross-match in patients with T antigen activation. Vox Sang 1993;64(2):129.

121. Lee CS, Chen MJ, Chiou YH, et al. Invasive pneumococcal pneumonia is the major cause of paediatric haemolytic-uraemic syndrome in Taiwan. Nephrology (Carlton) 2012;17(1):48–52.

122. von Vigier RO, Seibel K, Bianchetti MG. Positive Coombs test in pneumococcus-associated hemolytic uremic syndrome. A review of the literature. Nephron 1999;82(2):183–4.

123. Osborn DA, Lui K, Pussell P, et al. T and Tk antigen activation in necrotising enterocolitis: manifestations, severity of illness, and effectiveness of testing. Arch Dis Child Fetal Neonatal Ed 1999;80(3):F192–7.

124. Petras ML, Dunbar NM, Filiano JJ, et al. Therapeutic plasma exchange in Streptococcus pneumoniae-associated hemolytic uremic syndrome: a case report. J Clin Apher 2012;27(4):212–4.

125. Anastaze Stelle K, Cachat F, Perez MH, et al. Streptococcus pneumoniae-associated hemolytic and uremic syndrome with cholestasis: a case report and brief literature review. Clin Pediatr (Phila) 2016;55(2):189–91.

126. Fakhouri F, Roumenina L, Provot F, et al. Pregnancy-associated hemolytic uremic syndrome revisited in the era of complement gene mutations. J Am Soc Nephrol 2010;21(5):859–67.

127. Jim B, Garovic VD. Acute kidney injury in pregnancy. Semin Nephrol 2017;37(4): 378–85.

128. De Sousa Amorim E, Blasco M, Quintana L, et al. Eculizumab in pregnancy-associated atypical hemolytic uremic syndrome: insights for optimizing management. J Nephrol 2015;28(5):641–5.

129. Zschiedrich S, Prager EP, Kuehn EW. Successful treatment of the postpartum atypical hemolytic uremic syndrome with eculizumab. Ann Intern Med 2013; 159(1):76.

130. Ardissino G, Wally Ossola M, Baffero GM, et al. Eculizumab for atypical hemolytic uremic syndrome in pregnancy. Obstet Gynecol 2013;122(2 Pt 2):487–9.

131. Bonser RS, Adu D, Franklin I, et al. Cyclosporin-induced haemolytic uraemic syndrome in liver allograft recipient. Lancet 1984;2(8415):1337.

132. Young BA, Marsh CL, Alpers CE, et al. Cyclosporine-associated thrombotic microangiopathy/hemolytic uremic syndrome following kidney and kidney-pancreas transplantation. Am J Kidney Dis 1996;28(4):561–71.

133. Besbas N, Karpman D, Landau D, et al. A classification of hemolytic uremic syndrome and thrombotic thrombocytopenic purpura and related disorders. Kidney Int 2006;70(3):423–31.

134. Noris M, Remuzzi G. Thrombotic microangiopathy after kidney transplantation. Am J Transplant 2010;10(7):1517–23.

135. Al-Nouri ZL, Reese JA, Terrell DR, et al. Drug-induced thrombotic microangiopathy: a systematic review of published reports. Blood 2015;125(4):616–8.

136. Reese JA, Bougie DW, Curtis BR, et al. Drug-induced thrombotic microangiopathy: experience of the Oklahoma Registry and the BloodCenter of Wisconsin. Am J Hematol 2015;90(5):406–10.

137. Medina PJ, Sipols JM, George JN. Drug-associated thrombotic thrombocytopenic purpura-hemolytic uremic syndrome. Curr Opin Hematol 2001;8(5):286–93.

138. Page EE, Little DJ, Vesely SK, et al. Quinine-induced thrombotic microangiopathy: a report of 19 patients. Am J Kidney Dis 2017;70(5):686–95.

139. Walport MJ. Complement. First of two parts. N Engl J Med 2001;344(14):1058–66.

Thrombotic Thrombocytopenic Purpura, Heparin-Induced Thrombocytopenia, and Disseminated Intravascular Coagulation

Ram Kalpatthi, MD[a], Joseph E. Kiss, MD[b],*

KEYWORDS

- Thrombocytopenia • ICU • Heparin • Plasmapheresis
- Thrombotic microangiopathy • Microangiopathic hemolytic anemia • Rituximab
- Caplacizumab

KEY POINTS

- Coagulation abnormalities are common and associated with excess morbidity and mortality in critically ill patients.
- Thrombocytopenia, a common finding in critically ill patients, has many causes, including sepsis, drugs (heparin), and thrombotic microangiopathy syndromes including thrombotic thrombocytopenic purpura (TTP) and disseminated intravascular coagulation (DIC).
- Plasmapheresis remains the cornerstone of therapy for TTP. However, caplacizumab, a recent US Food and Drug Administration–approved von Willebrand factor/platelet inhibitor can be lifesaving when used along with plasmapheresis in these severely ill patients.
- Heparin-induced thrombocytopenia is likely both overdiagnosed and underdiagnosed because of unavailability of the gold standard serotonin-release assay in most laboratories and because thrombocytopenia has diverse causes.
- Supportive care and management of underlying cause is the mainstay of therapy for DIC because trials addressing the efficacy of biologically based therapies to reestablish hemostasis (eg, recombinant human activated protein C) have been largely inconclusive.

[a] Division of Pediatric Hematology Oncology, Department of Pediatrics, UPMC Children's Hospital of Pittsburgh, 4401 Penn Avenue, Suite 501A, Pittsburgh, PA 15224, USA; [b] Division of Hematology Oncology, Department of Medicine, Clinical Apheresis and Blood Services, Vitalant Northeast Division, University of Pittsburgh School of Medicine, 3636 Boulevard of the Allies, Pittsburgh, PA 15213, USA
* Corresponding author.
E-mail address: jkiss@itxm.org

Crit Care Clin 36 (2020) 357–377
https://doi.org/10.1016/j.ccc.2019.12.006
0749-0704/20/© 2020 Elsevier Inc. All rights reserved.

criticalcare.theclinics.com

INTRODUCTION

Coagulation abnormalities are extremely common among critically ill patients in the intensive care unit (ICU). Early recognition of the clinically important hematologic changes, identification of underlying causes, and prompt treatment interventions are crucial because these abnormalities are often associated with significant morbidity and mortality.[1] Thrombocytopenia is the most common hematological abnormality seen in ICU patients and can develop before, at the time of, or after admission to the ICU. The incidence of thrombocytopenia in critically ill patients ranges from 14% to 44% but it can vary depending on the type of patients (medical, surgical, or transplant) and the definition used.[2] Note that timing of onset of thrombocytopenia may help identifying its cause: was there a preexisting or chronic thrombocytopenia? The occurrence of thrombocytopenia after admission to ICU is commonly caused by therapeutic interventions (surgery, fluid resuscitation, or drugs such as heparin) or complications such as sepsis.

Besides its association with bleeding and/or thrombosis, thrombocytopenia has been shown to be an independent risk factor for mortality in ICU patients in several studies.[2–4] Other hemostatic derangements that are frequently seen in ICU patients include prolonged prothrombin time (PT) and activated partial thromboplastin time (aPTT), increased fibrin split products such as D-dimer, and decreased natural antico-agulants such as antithrombin III and protein C in 14% to 28%, 42% to 99%, and 40% to 90% respectively.[1,5,6] These coagulation derangements are not only associated with bleeding and/or thrombosis but also play a role in modulating the inflammatory response by release of proinflammatory cytokines and activation of the endothelium, thereby promoting proinflammatory state in critically ill patients. The common causes of these coagulation abnormalities are listed in **Box 1**. This article focuses on 3 important disease states whose cardinal feature is thrombocytopenia: thrombotic thrombo-cytopenic purpura (TTP), heparin-induced thrombocytopenia (HIT), and disseminated intravascular coagulation (DIC). This article discusses the epidemiology, pathogenesis, clinical features, and recent advances in the diagnosis and management of each of these disorders.

THROMBOTIC THROMBOCYTOPENIC PURPURA

Thrombotic microangiopathy (TMA) syndromes (TMAs) are heterogeneous disorders characterized by thrombocytopenia, a microangiopathic hemolytic anemia (MAHA), and acute organ dysfunction caused by visceral ischemia and injury.[7] TTP is a specific TMA that is characterized by ischemic end-organ damage resulting from widespread formation of platelet-rich microvascular thrombi primarily involving the brain but also involving the abdominal viscera, kidney, and heart.[8] The clinical subtypes of TMA syndromes, primary and secondary, are listed in **Box 2**. For a more detailed discussion of TMA syndromes other than TTP, readers are referred to George and Nester.[9]

Definition

The classic definition of TTP includes the pentad of clinical and laboratory manifestations: (1) fever, (2) microangiopathic hemolytic anemia, (3) thrombocytopenia, (4) renal failure, and (5) neurologic dysfunction.[10] However, this pentad of features present only in 7% of TTP cases.[11–17] Because the mortality of untreated TTP is extremely high (>90%), the presence of thrombocytopenia with microangiopathic hemolytic anemia (MAHA) should be considered as TTP until proved otherwise.[18] Skillful assistance, especially from the hematology service, is often needed to diagnose TTP because of the highly variable clinical features and overlap of laboratory features with many other TMA disorders.

Box 1
Hemostatic abnormalities and their causes in critically ill patients

1. Thrombocytopenia
   i. Hemodilution
      - Cardiopulmonary bypass
      - Massive transfusion of packed red blood cells
      - Large-volume infusion of fluids and plasma
   ii. Increased destruction/consumption
      - Immune thrombocytopenia
      - Drugs (eg, heparin, vancomycin)
      - Thrombotic thrombocytopenic purpura
      - Antiphospholipid antibody syndrome
      - Sepsis
      - Disseminated intravascular coagulation
      - Major venous thromboembolism
      - Massive tissue trauma
      - Acute promyelocytic leukemia
      - HELLP syndrome
      - ECMO
   iii. Decreased production
      - Viral infections (EBV, CMV, HIV, HCV)
      - Acute and chronic liver failure
      - Nutritional deficiency (folate, vitamin B_{12})
      - Acute leukemia
      - Aplastic anemia
      - Myelodysplastic syndromes
      - Metastatic bone marrow infiltration
      - Chemotherapy and radiation
      - Alcohol abuse
      - Chronic graft-versus-host disease
   iv. Increased sequestration
      - Splenic sequestration
      - Hypothermia

2. Coagulation disturbances
   i. Isolated prolongation of PT
      - Factor II, V, VII or X deficiency
      - Inhibitor to factor II, V, VII or X
      - Mild liver failure
      - Early vitamin K deficiency or warfarin therapy
      - Hypofibrinogenemia or dysfibrinogenemia
   ii. Isolated prolongation of aPTT
      - Deficiency of factors XII, XI, IX, VIII
      - von Willebrand disease
      - Antiphospholipid antibody
      - Unfractionated heparin therapy
   iii. Combined prolongation of PT and aPTT
      - Disseminated intravascular coagulation
      - Sepsis
      - Liver failure
      - Massive bleeding
      - Vitamin K deficiency, warfarin therapy
   iv. Increased fibrin degradation products
      - Surgery
      - Trauma
      - Disseminated intravascular coagulation
      - Liver failure
      - Venous or major arterial thromboembolism
      - Malignancy
      - Extracorporeal procedures (eg, hemodialysis)

Abbreviations: CMV, cytomegalovirus; EBV, Epstein-Barr virus; ECMO, extracorporeal membrane oxygenation; HCV, hepatitis C virus; HELLP, hemolysis, elevated liver-enzymes and low platelets; HIV, human immunodeficiency virus.

Etiopathogenesis

TTP is differentiated from other TMA syndromes (see **Box 2**) by the severe deficiency (<10% activity) of ADAMTS13 (a disintegrin and metalloproteinase with a thrombospondin type 1 repeats, member 13), which is a metalloproteinase responsible for cleavage of von Willebrand factor (VWF) multimers.[18,19] In the absence of ADAMTS13, ultralarge VWF accumulates and leads to platelet adhesion to endothelium and platelet aggregation, leading to the deposition of microvascular platelet thrombi with ischemic end-organ damage.[20] During this process, thrombocytopenia and MAHA ensues because of platelet consumption and mechanical destruction of circulating red blood cells (RBCs) as they pass through the occluded microvasculature.

Epidemiology and Natural History of Thrombotic Thrombocytopenic Purpura

National and international registries reported an estimated prevalence of 2 to 6 TTP cases per million population per year.[11,17,21] Deficiency of ADAMTS13 in TTP can be either acquired (more common) or congenital (rare). Congenital TTP (cTTP) caused by biallelic mutations in the ADAMTS13 gene results in severe ADAMTS13 deficiency, often presenting in infancy (Upshaw-Schulman syndrome).[22] With a few exceptions, TTP in adults is immune mediated (iTTP) with anti-ADAMTS13 autoantibodies that neutralize or increase the clearance of ADAMTS13. iTTP most often occurs in the fourth decade of life, with a female preponderance (female to male ratio of 3:1); black people have higher incidence than other races.[23] Pregnancy is one of the known predisposing factors for TTP. In the French TMA registry, 3% of adult patients with TTP were found to have mutations in the ADAMTS13 gene and all these cases were occurred during first pregnancy.[12] Their data showed nearly a quarter of French women who developed TTP during pregnancy carried molecular defects causing severe ADAMTS13 deficiency (cTTP). Thus, it is useful to screen for cTTP mutations in women who present with a first episode of TTP during pregnancy.

Box 2
Thrombotic microangiopathic syndromes

1. Primary
   - Immune TTP (ADAMTS13 deficiency)
   - Hemolytic uremic syndrome (Shiga toxin induced)
   - Complement-mediated TMA (atypical hemolytic uremic syndrome; mutations in complement alternate pathway)
   - Drug-related TMA (mitomycin, cyclosporine, tacrolimus, quinine)
   - Coagulation-related TMA (mutations in thrombomodulin, plasminogen, and diacylglycerol kinase ε)
   - Metabolism-related TMA (cyanocobalamin deficiency)

2. Secondary
   - Systemic infection
   - Connective tissue diseases (lupus, scleroderma)
   - Tumor-related TMA (lymphomas, pancreatic cancer)
   - Transplant associated TMA (HSCT, solid organ transplant)
   - Malignant hypertension
   - HELLP syndrome

Abbreviations: ADAMTS13, a disintegrin and metalloproteinase with a thrombospondin type 1 repeats, member 13; HSCT, hematopoietic stem cell transplant.

Data from George JN, Nester CM. Syndromes of thrombotic microangiopathy. N Engl J Med. 2014;371(7):654-666; with permission.

Untreated TTP has a high mortality of greater than 90%, but introduction of therapeutic plasma exchange (TPE) has dramatically decreased its mortality to 5% to 16%.[18] In contrast with other TMA syndromes, patients with iTTP with severe deficiency of ADAMTS13 (<10%) represent a clinically distinct cohort that responds well to TPE, and these patients have a more favorable prognosis, including shorter hospitalization, more rapid platelet count recovery, and higher overall survival.[15] However, refractory disease requiring extensive TPE may occur in 10%, and relapses occur in approximately 30% to 50% of patients despite standard treatment.[11,24] Although TTP relapses tend to be less severe and require fewer TPE treatments, the associated mortality remains high, similar to the initial episodes.[25]

Clinical Features

Clinical features suggesting organ dysfunction are highly variable, especially in early phases of TTP.[7] In addition to signs and symptoms of hemolytic anemia (fatigue, pallor, dyspnea, and jaundice) and thrombocytopenia (petechiae, purpuric lesions, and mucosal bleeding), central nervous system (CNS) and kidneys are the most commonly affected in TTP. CNS manifestations range from mild headache and transient confusion to seizures, neurologic deficits, and coma.[11,12] Renal dysfunction is usually mild in patients with TTP (serum creatinine level ≤2 mg/dL). The presence of more severe renal dysfunction or renal failure (more common in hemolytic uremic syndrome/atypical hemolytic uremic syndrome) and coagulopathy (suggesting DIC) is not characteristic of TTP and warrants additional investigations. Cardiac arrhythmias and myocardial infarction may occur because of electrolyte disturbances and microvascular infarction, respectively. Although troponin levels may be increased, chest pain is uncommon, likely because the thrombo-occlusive lesion involves the microvasculature and not the coronary arteries. Nonspecific gastrointestinal symptoms such as nausea, vomiting, abdominal pain, or diarrhea can also occur. Rarely, acute pancreatitis and bloody diarrhea from mesenteric ischemia are the presenting manifestations of TTP.[26,27]

Laboratory Evaluation

Patients with TTP have laboratory markers of MAHA (anemia, reticulocytosis, indirect hyperbilirubinemia, increased lactate dehydrogenase [LDH] level, decreased plasma haptoglobin level, and most importantly presence of schistocytes on the peripheral smear) and thrombocytopenia often less than 30×10^9/L. A basic metabolic panel including serum blood urea nitrogen and creatinine, coagulation screen (PT, aPTT), fibrinogen, and D-dimer/fibrin degradation products should be performed. Obtaining troponin-I level, electrocardiogram, and echocardiogram is important because cardiac involvement is associated with increased mortality and refractoriness to therapy.[28] Human immunodeficiency virus and antinuclear antibodies should also be obtained. A pregnancy screen should be performed in women of child-bearing potential who present with suspected TTP.

Undetectable ADAMTS13 activity (<10%) with an inhibitor confirms the diagnosis of iTTP and helps differentiate from other TMA syndromes that have higher levels of ADAMTS13 activity. Most patients with iTTP also have anti-ADAMTS13 antibodies. These tests should be drawn before initiation of TPE to avoid the confounding effects of plasma dilution and exogenous replenishment of ADAMTS13. However, results of ADAMTS13 testing may not be readily available because the assay is usually performed in specialized laboratories.

Because of the need to rapidly assess the likelihood of severe ADAMTS13-deficient TTP and initiate urgent TPE, clinical scoring systems have been developed to help identify patients likely to benefit from therapy and exclude those in whom TPE is likely to be ineffective and should not be initiated. Among these, the PLASMIC score is calculated based on 1 point for each of the following 7 criteria (score 0–7): thrombo-cytopenia less than 30×10^9/L, hemolysis, no history of active cancer, no history of organ transplant, mean corpuscular volume less than 90 fL, International Normalized Ratio less than 1.5, and serum creatinine level less than 2 mg/dL.[29] A high PLASMIC score of 6 or 7 has been shown to have high sensitivity and specificity greater than 90%, and a low score (0–4) has a very good negative predictive value of 98% for iTTP.[30] This tool helps identify which patients may and may not benefit from TPE; if there is doubt, prompt initiation of TPE and immunosuppression with corticosteroids should be initiated without delay while awaiting ADAMTS13 results.

Management

Initial treatment

TPE remains the treatment of choice for iTTP and should be started as soon as possible after a provisional diagnosis of TTP. The efficacy of TPE was unequivocally established in a randomized controlled trial that showed that TPE was associated with higher survival compared with simple high-dose plasma infusion.[31] Other advantages of TPE include delivery of larger doses of functional ADAMTS13 without circulatory overload and removal of anti-ADAMTS13 antibodies. Although not a proven benefit, TPE is also capable of removing ultralarge VWF multimers, which bind avidly to platelets and are considered pathogenic in mediating platelet-microvascular occlusion.[7] The standard TPE protocol includes 1.0 to 1.5 times plasma volume exchanges daily until platelet count recovery ($>150 \times 10^9$/L) for 2 consecutive days.[32,33]

Immunosuppression with systemic corticosteroids is frequently used as an initial therapy along with TPE for iTTP. The rationale for using corticosteroids is to control the autoimmune response and efficacy as a single-agent therapy for TTP in small studies before the era of TPE.[34] Corticosteroids are usually given as 1 mg/kg/d prednisone or equivalent. One small study reported improved responses using high-dose corticosteroids (10–15 mg/kg solumedrol daily for 3 days) then prednisone in standard doses.[35]

Supportive care measures for TTP include packed red blood cell transfusion, strict blood pressure control, prophylaxis for deep vein thrombosis, and control of bleeding manifestations. Serious hemorrhage is uncommon in patients with TTP. Prophylactic platelet transfusions (eg, before central line placement) can cause exacerbation of TTP.[36] Thus, it is recommended that platelet transfusions be reserved for severe bleeding complications.

Management of refractory/relapsing thrombotic thrombocytopenic purpura

Refractory TTP has been defined as persistent thrombocytopenia and increased LDH level after 5 to 7 TPEs.[37] In addition to patients with a delayed response, some patients develop new or worsening symptoms and more severe thrombocytopenia after an initial salutary response. Several strategies, including the use of additional immunosuppressive drugs, twice-daily TPE, and even splenectomy, have been used in these circumstances.[7] Rituximab, a monoclonal antibody against cluster of differentiation (CD) 20 antigen on B cells, suppresses the production of anti-ADAMTS13 antibodies, thus restoring the function of ADAMTS13 activity. Many observational studies reported improved outcomes of using rituximab for refractory iTTP with improved platelet recovery and lower relapse rate.[38,39] Similarly, the addition of rituximab to TPE and corticosteroids in relapsed iTTP (defined as recurrence of thrombocytopenia >30 days after stopping TPE) induced remission in almost all patients with no relapses over a median follow-up of 19 months.[40] Based on this experience, rituximab is frequently added to TPE and corticosteroids for refractory and relapsed iTTP despite the absence of evidence from randomized controlled trials.[41] A dosing regimen of 375 mg/m^2 weekly for 4 weeks is most commonly used, although lower doses of rituximab (100 mg, 200 mg, and 500 mg fixed doses) have been reported to be effective.[42,43]

Recent Advances: Targeted Therapy Directed at Von Willebrand Factor–Platelet Interactions

Caplacizumab (CABLIVI, Ablynx NV), a humanized anti-VWF antibody fragment, reduces the formation of microvascular thrombi by inhibiting the interaction between VWF multimers and platelets.[44,45] Based on its efficacy shown in a multicenter, phase 3 randomized, double-blind, placebo-controlled study, caplacizumab was approved by the US Food and Drug Administration in 2019 for adults (age >18 years) with acquired TTP along with TPE and immunosuppression.[45] Patients received a single intravenous bolus dose of 11 mg of caplacizumab (or placebo) before initial TPE followed by daily subcutaneous injection of 11 mg of caplacizumab (or placebo) after TPE for the duration of TPE and 30 days after the cessation of TPE. Compared with placebo, patients in the caplacizumab group had shorter time to platelet normalization (primary end point) and lower iTTP-related composite end point of death, recurrence, and major thromboembolic events (49% vs 12%; P<.001). In addition, patients who received caplacizumab had shorter median length of stay (9 vs 12 days), median duration of TPE (5 vs 7 days), mortality (0 vs 4%), and refractory disease (0 vs 4%) compared with the placebo group. Although bleeding (mostly epistaxis and gingival bleeding) was observed more in the caplacizumab group (65% vs 48%), it was mostly of mild to moderate severity and resolved without intervention. The disease recurrence rate after stopping caplacizumab was 8%; nearly all recurrences occurred in the patients whose ADAMTS13 activity remained deficient. Therefore, it was recommended to extend the use of this drug an additional 4 weeks for patients who had ADAMTS13 activity less than 10% at the end of the treatment period; however, a threshold level of ADAMTS13 activity for stopping the treatment was not studied. Despite its efficacy, a disadvantage of caplacizumab is its cost (estimated $7700 per dose) which can limit its practical use.[46] However, considering its novel, direct action in blocking VWF-platelet binding, this drug is considered a major advance and is most likely to provide the greatest benefit to patients who are critically ill in the ICU.[47] Early use of rituximab along with TPE has been associated with lower relapse rate in patients with newly diagnosed iTTP compared with historical controls (10% vs 57%).[38] A significant reduction in relapse rate has been confirmed in other studies.[48] Future studies of the combination of caplacizumab and rituximab along with TPE as an upfront therapy in newly diagnosed iTTP may achieve faster clinical recovery, reduced mortality, and lower relapse rates, and may lead to reduced health care costs overall.

HEPARIN-INDUCED THROMBOCYTOPENIA

HIT is an adverse drug reaction characterized by the development of thrombocytopenia shortly after exposure to either unfractionated heparin (UFH) or low-molecular-weight heparin (LMWH).[49] This disorder is mediated by antibodies (primarily immunoglobulin [Ig] G) binding to heparin–platelet factor 4 (PF4) complexes resulting in platelet activation.[50] A high index of suspicion and early recognition of HIT is crucial because of the associated prothrombotic state that can result in new arterial or venous thrombosis, limb loss, and death in critically ill patients.[49] Both the diagnosis and the treatment of HIT can be challenging, because critically ill patients often have underlying conditions that result in thrombocytopenia and/or an increased risk of thrombosis, and discontinuation of anticoagulation and use of alternative anticoagulants can increase the risk of thrombosis and bleeding, respectively.

Epidemiology

HIT is uncommon in critically ill patients, with a reported incidence of 0.2% to 5%.[51] However, it is likely that HIT is both overdiagnosed and underdiagnosed because thrombocytopenia is very common and often multifactorial in these patients (see **Box 1**). The risk of developing HIT is higher in women (odds ratio [OR] = 2.37), patients with an increased body mass index (BMI) (BMI 30–39, OR = 2.94; BMI>40, OR = 6.98), patients undergoing surgery (OR = 3.25), and patients who are exposed to UFH versus LMWH (OR = 5.29).[52,53] In the largest prospective Prophylaxis for Thromboembolism in Critical Care Trial (PROTECT), fewer patients receiving low molecular weight heparin (Dalteparin) had HIT compared with UFH (hazard ratio = 0.27; 95% confidence interval, 0.08, 0.98; P = .046).[3] This rate is substantially higher in patients undergoing cardiac and orthopedic surgeries and those that require major surgeries after trauma.[54,55] HIT is very rare in children; thus, the diagnosis and management of HIT is exclusively based on adult data.[56]

Pathogenesis

In HIT, IgG antibodies complexed with heparin/PF4 bind to the FcγRIIA receptors on the platelet surface, causing platelet activation.[50] This process leads to release of procoagulant platelet microparticles that accelerate thrombin generation, platelet consumption, and thrombotic complications of HIT.[57] In addition, these antibodies can cause activation of monocytes and endothelium, resulting in release of tissue factor, augmenting the prothrombotic state. This mechanism underlies the occurrence of both venous and arterial thrombosis, in some cases resulting in overt DIC, and the recurrence of thrombosis in patients with HIT who are treated with direct thrombin inhibitors.[58–60]

Clinical Features

Thrombocytopenia usually develops between 5 and 10 days after heparin exposure. Typically, platelet count decreases less than 150×10^9/L or greater than 50% from the baseline that preceded exposure to heparin. A decrease in platelet count less than 20×10^9/L is unusual unless there is concomitant DIC. Bleeding complications are unusual in patients with HIT. Thrombosis occurs in greater than 50% of patients with serologically confirmed HIT, with venous thrombosis more common than arterial (ratio of 4:1).[61,62] Thrombi can occur in atypical sites (adrenal veins, mesenteric veins) and may be unusually severe.[63] Other rare clinical manifestations include acute anaphylactoid reactions after heparin administration (sudden hypotension and CNS changes), pruritic necrotic lesions at the site of injection (especially with LMWH), and the development of skin necrosis and venous limb gangrene.[64–66]

Diagnostic Evaluation and Management

The diagnosis of HIT depends on the presence of a clinical picture consistent with HIT in association with detection of heparin-dependent platelet antibodies in the patient's serum or plasma. In order to enable consistent clinical assessment, the so-called 4Ts scoring system (timing from start of heparin therapy, extent of thrombocytopenia, onset of new thrombosis, and other potential causes of thrombocytopenia) was developed to guide diagnosis and management based on the pretest probability score (**Table 1**).[67] The main advantage of the scoring system, which permits risk stratification into low, intermediate, and high probability, is to avoid use of alternative anticoagulants in patients who are at low risk of having true HIT. Most laboratories

Table 1
Four Ts scoring system for suspected heparin-induced thrombocytopenia

Criteria	Points
Degree of thrombocytopenia	
>50% decrease and platelet nadir >20 × 10⁹/L	2
30%–50% decrease and platelet nadir 10–19 × 10⁹/L	1
Decrease <30% or platelet nadir <10 × 10⁹/L	0
Timing of thrombocytopenia	
Onset between days 5 and 10 of heparin or <1 d if recent heparin exposure	2
Consistent with days 5–10 decrease, but not clear or onset after day 10	1
Platelet count decrease <4 d and no recent heparin exposure	0
Presence of Thrombosis	
New thrombosis (confirmed)/skin necrosis/systemic reaction	2
Progressive/recurrent/suspected thrombosis	1
None	0
Presence of other causes for thrombocytopenia	
None	2
Possible	1
Definite	0

Low score, 0 to 3; intermediate score, 4 to 5; high score, 6 to 8.
Data from Lo GK, Juhl D, Warkentin TE, Sigouin CS, Eichler P, Greinacher A. Evaluation of pretest clinical score (4 T's) for the diagnosis of heparin-induced thrombocytopenia in two clinical settings. J Thromb Haemost. 2006;4(4):759-765.

perform an enzyme-linked immunosorbent assay (ELISA) test for detection of anti-PF4/heparin antibodies.[50] These tests have a high sensitivity (close to 100%) but a low specificity, which results in a higher number of false-positive results. Although rare, the immunoassay is negative in some patients who have high clinical suspicion for HIT.[68,69] In addition, these tests do not reveal whether the antibodies are pathologic (ie, whether they activate platelets). Platelet activation assays such as serotonin-release assay are the gold standard tests that provide more specific results, but they are performed in very few laboratories. A new test, the platelet factor 4-dependent platelet activation assay, has recently been developed and is reported to improve the diagnostic accuracy and timeliness of HIT testing.[70] An algorithm for the diagnosis and management of HIT combining the 4Ts scoring system and the laboratory studies is shown in **Fig. 1**.

The current treatment paradigm in cases with intermediate-probability to high-probability 4T score is immediate cessation of heparin, including discontinuation of heparin-bonded catheters, and institution of an alternative anticoagulant that does not cross react with HIT antibodies. Argatroban, a direct thrombin inhibitor (DTI), is currently the only approved drug to treat HIT in the United States.[71] It is also the recommended first-line treatment in patients with renal dysfunction because it is excreted through liver. Careful monitoring with dose adjustments using aPTT (target 1.5–3 times the baseline) is required. Its disadvantages include rebound hypercoagulability after cessation of the drug and prolongation of the PT during warfarin overlap.[63] Bivalirudin, another direct thrombin inhibitor with the shortest half-life, is recommended as first-line treatment of patients requiring percutaneous coronary intervention with a history of HIT.[63] Factor Xa inhibitors such as danaparoid (not available in the United States) and fondaparinux are useful treatment options because of their ease of administration

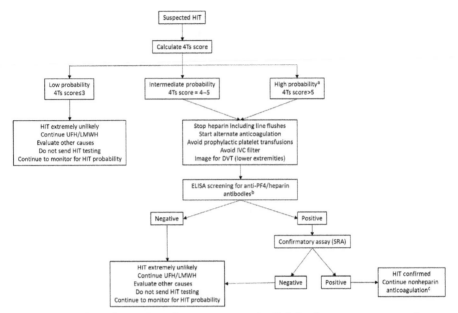

Fig. 1. Approach to diagnosis and management of HIT. [a] Confirmatory assay may be performed when pretest probability of HIT is high despite negative ELISA.[68,69] [b] Probability of positive serotonin-release assay (SRA; confirmed HIT) is related to strength of ELISA optical density (OD). Some centers opt to make decisions based on OD of ELISA tests; for example, OD greater than 2.0 (>90% SRA positive) do not routinely reflex to SRA. [c] Duration of anticoagulation therapy varies based on the presence of thrombosis. DVT, deep vein thrombosis; IVC, inferior vena cava.

and direct measurement of activity (anti–factor Xa level) rather than aPTT measurement, which is affected by patient comorbidities.[72,73] However, these drugs can only be used in patients with adequate renal function, which is often compromised in critically ill patients. Fondaparinux has been increasingly used as an off-label therapy for HIT and seems to be efficacious[74]; however, prospective studies should be performed to examine its true safety and efficacy.[75] In addition, because some patients develop severe outcomes despite use of alternate anticoagulants (so-called refractory HIT), additional therapeutic approaches have been advocated, including TPE for removal of pathogenic HPF4 antibodies[76] and use of intravenous Ig (IVIg).[77,78]

DISSEMINATED INTRAVASCULAR COAGULATION

DIC is a syndrome characterized by dysregulated systemic activation of coagulation and impairment in fibrinolysis, resulting in widespread deposition of fibrin thrombi in the microvasculature that is often associated with multiorgan dysfunction.[79] Consumption of platelets and plasma clotting factors often leads to a hemorrhagic state. Microangiopathic hemolytic anemia, variably present on the peripheral smear, results from mechanical injury to RBCs and consequent erythrocyte fragmentation. DIC is always secondary to an underlying condition, most commonly sepsis, and is associated with increased mortality. Because there is no reliable diagnostic test for DIC, a thorough search for an underlying cause and supportive treatment of coagulopathy remains the cornerstone of management of DIC.

Epidemiology and Cause

In a study in 1996, DIC was observed in approximately in 1% of university hospital admissions in Japan.[80] In subsequent studies, the incidence of DIC varied from 9% to 19% of ICU admissions.[81–84] The variation in the reported incidence of DIC depends on the presence of underlying conditions, diagnostic criteria used, time period, type of study (prospective vs retrospective), and location of patients treated (ward vs ICU). Common underlying conditions associated with higher rates of DIC are sepsis or infection (30%–51%), severe trauma (28%), or major surgery (45%).[85–87] The disease states that are associated with DIC are described in **Box 3**. Like its incidence, the reported mortality of DIC also depends on the abovementioned factors. The mortality

---

Box 3
Major disease states associated with disseminated intravascular coagulation

1. Sepsis
   - Meningococcemia (purpura fulminans)
   - Other gram-negative bacteria (*Haemophilus, Salmonella*)
   - Gram-positive bacteria (group B *Streptococcus*)
   - Dengue hemorrhagic fever
   - Rickettsia (Rocky Mountain spotted fever)
   - Malaria

2. Tissue injury
   - Massive head injury
   - Multiple fractures with fat emboli
   - Massive burns
   - Major surgery
   - Trauma/crush injuries

3. Malignancy
   - Acute promyelocytic leukemia
   - Solid tumors (eg, adenocarcinomas, neuroblastoma)

4. Obstetric conditions
   - Preeclampsia or eclampsia
   - Placental abruption
   - Amniotic fluid embolism
   - Septic abortion

5. Vascular anomalies
   - Giant hemangioma (Kasabach-Merritt syndrome)

6. Venoms or toxins
   - Snake bite
   - Recreational drugs

7. Gastrointestinal disorders
   - Fulminant hepatitis
   - Cirrhosis of liver
   - Severe inflammatory bowel disease

8. Pediatric conditions
   - Homozygous protein C deficiency (neonatal purpura fulminans)
   - Galactosemia
   - Reye syndrome

9. Miscellaneous
   - Heat stroke
   - Acute hemolytic transfusion reaction
   - Kawasaki disease

attributed to DIC in Japan (46% to 65%) and the United States (51% to 76%) is consistent with a decreasing trend in recent years.[84,88–90]

Pathogenesis

DIC is a form of consumptive coagulation characterized by an imbalance between coagulation and bleeding. The underlying conditions that predispose to DIC result in expression of tissue factor on endothelial cells and circulating monocytes because of high levels of inflammatory cytokines, bacterial endotoxins, and tissue damage.[91] This process in turn activates factor VII via an extrinsic pathway leading to excessive thrombin generation and widespread fibrin deposition in the microvasculature, leading to multiorgan dysfunction.[92] Thrombin activates platelets and other coagulation factors such as factor VIII, IX, XI, which further augments the formation of fibrin thrombi. In contrast, excessive thrombin generation is associated with a hyperfibrinolytic phase and severe bleeding, especially in the first 24 hours after massive trauma.[93] This phase is followed by a prothrombotic phase in which decreased levels of natural anticoagulants such as protein C and S and high circulating levels of plasma activator inhibitor-1 (physiologic inhibitor of fibrinolysis) lead to increased clotting.[93] Platelets and coagulation factors are depleted as a result of the consumptive coagulopathy. Recent evidence suggests that damage-associated molecular patterns such as histones and DNA play an important role in organ dysfunction in DIC because of a variety of mechanisms such as widespread dissemination of thrombin, platelet aggregation, vascular leakage, release of proinflammatory cytokines, and extracellular traps by neutrophils.[90]

Clinical Features

The clinical presentation of DIC reflects the underlying cause that eventuates in an imbalance of hypercoagulability and hyperfibrinolysis. DIC has been classified as several clinical subtypes: asymptomatic (pre-DIC), organ failure (thrombotic), bleeding (hyperfibrinolysis), and massive bleeding (consumptive) types.[94] However, these clinical subtypes can shift or change and sometimes can overlap. Asymptomatic DIC or pre-DIC is an early stage of DIC characterized by presence of abnormal laboratory studies in the absence of clinical symptoms. Treatment at this stage was reported to be effective in a retrospective study of patients with cancer; however, high index of suspicion and routine monitoring was necessary.[95] The thrombotic type is more common in patients with severe infection/sepsis wherein thrombosis of small and medium vessels leads to multiorgan dysfunction: digits (symmetric peripheral gangrene), kidneys (oliguria, anuria, hematuria), lungs (chest pain, dyspnea, tachypnea), liver (jaundice, coagulopathy), and brain (confusion, altered mental status, coma). Although early treatment of microthrombi-related organ impairment may improve outcome, its early recognition is often difficult because of the presence of comorbidities in these critically ill patients. Purpura fulminans, a severe form of DIC, is characterized by skin infarction and necrosis, which is commonly seen in patients with meningococcemia.[96] Neonatal purpura fulminans usually occurs in young infants with inherited protein C and/or S deficiency.[97] Bleeding manifestations include oozing from various sites, petechiae, ecchymosis, and sometimes internal hemorrhage. Bleeding-type DIC is often seen in patients with leukemias, especially acute promyelocytic leukemia (APML). DIC is the major cause of mortality in patients with APML because of increased risk of bleeding from enhanced fibrinolysis.[98,99] The consumptive-type DIC, which can be preceded by or can coexist with dilutional coagulopathy, is often associated with life-threatening massive bleeding that requires blood transfusions after major surgeries and in obstetric conditions.

Diagnostic Evaluation

Common laboratory abnormalities in DIC include thrombocytopenia, microangiopathic hemolytic anemia with increased reticulocytes (if erythropoiesis is not suppressed) and the presence of schistocytes on peripheral blood smear, prolonged PT and aPTT, increased fibrin degradation products and D-dimer, and reduced serum fibrinogen. Fibrinogen is an acute phase reactant; thus, its levels can be increased or normal during initial phases of DIC. Factor VIII levels can help differentiate DIC from liver disease because they are decreased in DIC but often increased in liver disease. However, no single clinical feature, examination finding, or laboratory test can establish or rule out the diagnosis of DIC.

The International Society of Thrombosis and Hemostasis (ISTH) introduced a composite scoring system to diagnose overt DIC.[79] The presence of an underlying pathologic condition that predisposes to DIC is a prerequisite to use this algorithm. The score is based on platelet count, prolonged PT, increased level of a fibrin-related marker such as D-dimer, and fibrinogen level. Total score greater than or equal to 5 is compatible with overt DIC; however, scores of less than 5 may still be consistent with nonovert or low-grade DIC. Diagnosis and treatment recommendations have been published by the ISTH.[100]

Management

The mainstay of therapy for DIC is the aggressive management of underlying pathologic conditions that predisposed to DIC, such as antibiotics for sepsis, chemotherapy for underlying malignancy, timely delivery for placental abruption, and early institution of all-trans retinoic acid (ATRA) for suspected APML. In addition, initiating and maintaining supportive care designed to treat DIC is crucial. Furthermore, serial evaluation of the ISTH DIC score aids diagnostic accuracy, guides supportive care, and may potentially improve outcomes.

Blood product replacement therapy

Transfusion of platelets, fresh frozen plasma (FFP), and cryoprecipitate should be administered in patients who have active bleeding or who are at high risk for bleeding, such as those requiring an invasive procedure, after surgery, or those receiving anticoagulation therapy. The threshold for platelet transfusions includes less than 50×10^9/L for patients with active bleeding and less than 20×10^9/L for those at higher risk of bleeding. FFP can be administered for patients with active bleeding and prolongation of either PT/aPTT (>1.5 times normal) and/or hypofibrinogenemia (eg, <150 mg/dL). Cryoprecipitate can also be used in patients with active bleeding or threatened bleeding with documented hypofibrinogenemia. Maintaining a higher fibrinogen threshold ($\geq$200 mg/dL) is recommended in certain clinical scenarios, such as obstetric patients with postpartum hemorrhage and patients with massive trauma, to avoid severe bleeding.[101,102] Off-label prothrombin complex concentrates and recombinant factor VIIa may be considered in patients with life-threatening bleeding refractory to standard blood products; however, these products have no established role in the treatment of DIC and concerns remain regarding thrombotic risk.

Anticoagulation therapy

Anticoagulation therapy is controversial in patients with DIC because of the evident bleeding risks. Therapeutic doses of UFH or LMWH can be considered in patients presenting with limb-threatening or life-threatening arterial thromboses, symptomatic venous thromboembolism (VTE), or purpura fulminans.[103] UFH is preferred because of its short life, although LMWH was shown to be superior in a small randomized controlled study.[104] If concerns regarding bleeding are present, low-dose UFH drip (, start 500 to 700 U/h without bolus, dose-adjusted upward by 100–200 U/h to low therapeutic anti-Xa level) may be effective in the authors' experience. Prophylactic anticoagulation for VTE using LMWH can be considered in patients with DIC who are critically ill without active bleeding. Anticoagulation therapy should be used cautiously in patients with DIC induced by trauma because it can lead to bleeding caused by hyperfibrinolysis.

Antifibrinolytic agents

Antifibrinolytic agents are generally contraindicated in patients with DIC, except in patients with hyperfibrinolysis, such as APML. However, a recent study showed no benefit with prophylactic use of tranexamic acid along with ATRA in patients with APML.[105] Fatal thrombosis can be caused by this combination therapy.[106]

Anticoagulant factor concentrates

Recombinant human activated protein C failed to show benefit in patients with DIC and was subsequently withdrawn from the market.[107] Infants presenting with purpura fulminans caused by congenital deficiency of protein C require FFP or human, plasma-derived, viral-inactivated protein C concentrate, if available. A Cochrane Review concluded that antithrombin concentrate did not reduce mortality but increased risk of bleeding in critically ill patients, including sepsis with DIC.[108] In addition, a phase 3 randomized trial of recombinant human soluble thrombomodulin (inhibition of thrombin formation) in severe sepsis and coagulopathy has just been completed and the results are pending (ClinicalTrials.gov Identifier: NCT01598831).

FUTURE CONSIDERATIONS

Thrombocytopenia has diverse causes in the ICU, and this article emphasizes recognizing and managing 3 of the most important disorders, namely iTTP, HIT, and DIC. Management of these entities continues to evolve as new diagnostics, therapies, and clinical paradigms are tested and implemented. In iTTP management, the availability of a true frontline VWF/platelet inhibitor, caplacizumab, has the potential to be lifesaving in patients who are severely affected by this disease. Immediate use of this antibody fragment, or nanobody, before the first TPE treatment, and continued daily, can prevent further microvascular thrombosis involving the heart, because cardiac involvement leading to asystole is the most common cause of death in the 10% to 20% of patients with iTTP who do not survive. The advent of recombinant ADAMTS13 holds the promise of further advances in iTTP outcomes. The treatment of HIT-associated thrombosis, although standardized with the current use of DTIs, is still problematic, with a high risk of composite adverse outcomes (death, new thrombosis, or limb loss) despite the use of alternative anticoagulants in most cases. In the meantime, trial results of newer direct oral anticoagulants, PLEX, and IVIg are awaited. In addition, the management of DIC continues to be based largely on empiricism tempered by clinical experience. In this regard, a controlled trial of heparin (UFH or LMWH) in DIC would be of great interest. Perhaps a close comparison is the ongoing trial of heparin in septic shock, because many of these patients have evidence of DIC (ClinicalTrials.gov Identifier: NCT03378466). However, at the present time in the management of DIC in the ICU, clinical judgment remains a necessary guide.

DISCLOSURE

R. Kalpatthi has nothing to disclose. J.E. Kiss reports service as a paid consultant on the medical advisory board for Sanofi, the maker of caplacizumab.

REFERENCES

1. Levi M, Opal SM. Coagulation abnormalities in critically ill patients. Crit Care 2006;10(4):222.
2. Williamson DR, Lesur O, Tetrault JP, et al. Thrombocytopenia in the critically ill: prevalence, incidence, risk factors, and clinical outcomes. Can J Anaesth 2013; 60(7):641–51.
3. PROTECT Investigators for the Canadian Critical Care Trials Group and the Australian and New Zealand Intensive Care Society Clinical Trials Group, Cook D, Meade M, Guyatt G, et al. Dalteparin versus unfractionated heparin in critically ill patients. N Engl J Med 2011;364(14):1305–14.
4. Vanderschueren S, De Weerdt A, Malbrain M, et al. Thrombocytopenia and prognosis in intensive care. Crit Care Med 2000;28(6):1871–6.
5. Shorr AF, Thomas SJ, Alkins SA, et al. D-dimer correlates with proinflammatory cytokine levels and outcomes in critically ill patients. Chest 2002;121(4):1262–8.
6. Bernard GR, Vincent JL, Laterre PF, et al. Efficacy and safety of recombinant human activated protein C for severe sepsis. N Engl J Med 2001;344(10):699–709.
7. Mariotte E, Veyradier A. Thrombotic thrombocytopenic purpura: from diagnosis to therapy. Curr Opin Crit Care 2015;21(6):593–601.
8. Moake JL. Thrombotic microangiopathies. N Engl J Med 2002;347(8):589–600.
9. George JN, Nester CM. Syndromes of thrombotic microangiopathy. N Engl J Med 2014;371(7):654–66.
10. George JN. Clinical practice. Thrombotic thrombocytopenic purpura. N Engl J Med 2006;354(18):1927–35.
11. Page EE, Kremer Hovinga JA, Terrell DR, et al. Thrombotic thrombocytopenic purpura: diagnostic criteria, clinical features, and long-term outcomes from 1995 through 2015. Blood Adv 2017;1(10):590–600.
12. Mariotte E, Azoulay E, Galicier L, et al. Epidemiology and pathophysiology of adulthood-onset thrombotic microangiopathy with severe ADAMTS13 deficiency (thrombotic thrombocytopenic purpura): a cross-sectional analysis of the French national registry for thrombotic microangiopathy. Lancet Haematol 2016;3(5):e237–45.
13. Matsumoto M, Bennett CL, Isonishi A, et al. Acquired idiopathic ADAMTS13 activity deficient thrombotic thrombocytopenic purpura in a population from Japan. PLoS One 2012;7(3):e33029.
14. Reese JA, Muthurajah DS, Kremer Hovinga JA, et al. Children and adults with thrombotic thrombocytopenic purpura associated with severe, acquired Adamts13 deficiency: comparison of incidence, demographic and clinical features. Pediatr Blood Cancer 2013;60(10):1676–82.
15. Bendapudi PK, Li A, Hamdan A, et al. Impact of severe ADAMTS13 deficiency on clinical presentation and outcomes in patients with thrombotic microangiopathies: the experience of the Harvard TMA Research Collaborative. Br J Haematol 2015;171(5):836–44.
16. Blombery P, Kivivali L, Pepperell D, et al. Diagnosis and management of thrombotic thrombocytopenic purpura (TTP) in Australia: findings from the first 5 years of the Australian TTP/thrombotic microangiopathy registry. Intern Med J 2016; 46(1):71–9.
17. Scully M, Yarranton H, Liesner R, et al. Regional UK TTP registry: correlation with laboratory ADAMTS 13 analysis and clinical features. Br J Haematol 2008; 142(5):819–26.

18. Chiasakul T, Cuker A. Clinical and laboratory diagnosis of TTP: an integrated approach. Hematology Am Soc Hematol Educ Program 2018;2018(1):530–8.
19. Sadler JE. Von Willebrand factor, ADAMTS13, and thrombotic thrombocytopenic purpura. Blood 2008;112(1):11–8.
20. Dane K, Chaturvedi S. Beyond plasma exchange: novel therapies for thrombotic thrombocytopenic purpura. Hematology Am Soc Hematol Educ Program 2018; 2018(1):539–47.
21. Alwan F, Vendramin C, Vanhoorelbeke K, et al. Presenting ADAMTS13 antibody and antigen levels predict prognosis in immune-mediated thrombotic thrombocytopenic purpura. Blood 2017;130(4):466–71.
22. Kremer Hovinga JA, Lammle B. Role of ADAMTS13 in the pathogenesis, diagnosis, and treatment of thrombotic thrombocytopenic purpura. Hematology Am Soc Hematol Educ Program 2012;2012:610–6.
23. Swart L, Schapkaitz E, Mahlangu JN. Thrombotic thrombocytopenic purpura: a 5-year tertiary care centre experience. J Clin Apher 2019;34(1):44–50.
24. Coppo P, Veyradier A. Current management and therapeutical perspectives in thrombotic thrombocytopenic purpura. Presse Med 2012;41(3 Pt 2):e163–76.
25. Masias C, Wu H, McGookey M, et al. No major differences in outcomes between the initial and relapse episodes in patients with thrombotic thrombocytopenic purpura: the experience from the Ohio State University Registry. Am J Hematol 2018;93(3):E73–5.
26. Gurjar M, Saigal S, Azim A, et al. Acute pancreatitis-induced thrombotic thrombocytopenic purpura. JOP 2012;13(1):80–2.
27. George JN, Chen Q, Deford CC, et al. Ten patient stories illustrating the extraordinarily diverse clinical features of patients with thrombotic thrombocytopenic purpura and severe ADAMTS13 deficiency. J Clin Apher 2012;27(6):302–11.
28. Benhamou Y, Boelle PY, Baudin B, et al. Cardiac troponin-I on diagnosis predicts early death and refractoriness in acquired thrombotic thrombocytopenic purpura. Experience of the French Thrombotic Microangiopathies Reference Center. J Thromb Haemost 2015;13(2):293–302.
29. Bendapudi PK, Hurwitz S, Fry A, et al. Derivation and external validation of the PLASMIC score for rapid assessment of adults with thrombotic microangiopathies: a cohort study. Lancet Haematol 2017;4(4):e157–64.
30. Li A, Khalighi PR, Wu Q, et al. External validation of the PLASMIC score: a clinical prediction tool for thrombotic thrombocytopenic purpura diagnosis and treatment. J Thromb Haemost 2018;16(1):164–9.
31. Rock GA, Shumak KH, Buskard NA, et al. Comparison of plasma exchange with plasma infusion in the treatment of thrombotic thrombocytopenic purpura. Canadian Apheresis Study Group. N Engl J Med 1991;325(6):393–7.
32. Scully M, Hunt BJ, Benjamin S, et al. Guidelines on the diagnosis and management of thrombotic thrombocytopenic purpura and other thrombotic microangiopathies. Br J Haematol 2012;158(3):323–35.
33. Schwartz J, Padmanabhan A, Aqui N, et al. Guidelines on the use of therapeutic apheresis in clinical practice-evidence-based approach from the writing committee of the American Society for Apheresis: the seventh special issue. J Clin Apher 2016;31(3):149–62.
34. Bell WR, Braine HG, Ness PM, et al. Improved survival in thrombotic thrombocytopenic purpura-hemolytic uremic syndrome. Clinical experience in 108 patients. N Engl J Med 1991;325(6):398–403.

35. Balduini CL, Gugliotta L, Luppi M, et al. High versus standard dose methylpred-nisolone in the acute phase of idiopathic thrombotic thrombocytopenic purpura: a randomized study. Ann Hematol 2010;89(6):591–6.

36. Benhamou Y, Baudel JL, Wynckel A, et al. Are platelet transfusions harmful in acquired thrombotic thrombocytopenic purpura at the acute phase? Experience of the French thrombotic microangiopathies reference center. Am J Hematol 2015;90(6):E127–9.

37. Scully M, Cataland S, Coppo P, et al. Consensus on the standardization of ter-minology in thrombotic thrombocytopenic purpura and related thrombotic mi-croangiopathies. J Thromb Haemost 2017;15(2):312–22.

38. Page EE, Kremer Hovinga JA, Terrell DR, et al. Rituximab reduces risk for relapse in patients with thrombotic thrombocytopenic purpura. Blood 2016; 127(24):3092–4.

39. Froissart A, Buffet M, Veyradier A, et al. Efficacy and safety of first-line rituximab in severe, acquired thrombotic thrombocytopenic purpura with a suboptimal response to plasma exchange. Experience of the French Thrombotic Microan-giopathies Reference Center. Crit Care Med 2012;40(1):104–11.

40. Scully M, Cohen H, Cavenagh J, et al. Remission in acute refractory and relaps-ing thrombotic thrombocytopenic purpura following rituximab is associated with a reduction in IgG antibodies to ADAMTS-13. Br J Haematol 2007;136(3): 451–61.

41. Lim W, Vesely SK, George JN. The role of rituximab in the management of pa-tients with acquired thrombotic thrombocytopenic purpura. Blood 2015; 125(10):1526–31.

42. Zaja F, Battista ML, Pirrotta MT, et al. Lower dose rituximab is active in adults patients with idiopathic thrombocytopenic purpura. Haematologica 2008; 93(6):930–3.

43. Westwood JP, Thomas M, Alwan F, et al. Rituximab prophylaxis to prevent throm-botic thrombocytopenic purpura relapse: outcome and evaluation of dosing regimens. Blood Adv 2017;1(15):1159–66.

44. Peyvandi F, Scully M, Kremer Hovinga JA, et al. Caplacizumab for acquired thrombotic thrombocytopenic purpura. N Engl J Med 2016;374(6):511–22.

45. Scully M, Cataland SR, Peyvandi F, et al. Caplacizumab treatment for acquired thrombotic thrombocytopenic purpura. N Engl J Med 2019;380(4):335–46.

46. Mazepa MA, Masias C, Chaturvedi S. How targeted therapy disrupts the treat-ment paradigm for acquired TTP: the risks, benefits, and unknowns. Blood 2019;134(5):415–20.

47. Azoulay E, Bauer PR, Mariotte E, et al. Expert statement on the ICU manage-ment of patients with thrombotic thrombocytopenic purpura. Intensive Care Med 2019;45(11):1518–39.

48. Westwood JP, Webster H, McGuckin S, et al. Rituximab for thrombotic thrombo-cytopenic purpura: benefit of early administration during acute episodes and use of prophylaxis to prevent relapse. J Thromb Haemost 2013;11(3):481–90.

49. Kelton JG, Warkentin TE. Heparin-induced thrombocytopenia: a historical perspective. Blood 2008;112(7):2607–16.

50. Kelton JG, Sheridan D, Santos A, et al. Heparin-induced thrombocytopenia: lab-oratory studies. Blood 1988;72(3):925–30.

51. Cuker A. Recent advances in heparin-induced thrombocytopenia. Curr Opin Hematol 2011;18(5):315–22.

52. Warkentin TE, Sheppard JA, Sigouin CS, et al. Gender imbalance and risk factor interactions in heparin-induced thrombocytopenia. Blood 2006;108(9):2937–41.

53. Bloom MB, Zaw AA, Hoang DM, et al. Body mass index strongly impacts the diagnosis and incidence of heparin-induced thrombocytopenia in the surgical intensive care unit. J Trauma Acute Care Surg 2016;80(3):398–403 [discussion: 403–4].

54. Warkentin TE, Sheppard JA, Horsewood P, et al. Impact of the patient population on the risk for heparin-induced thrombocytopenia. Blood 2000;96(5): 1703–8.

55. Lubenow N, Hinz P, Thomaschewski S, et al. The severity of trauma determines the immune response to PF4/heparin and the frequency of heparin-induced thrombocytopenia. Blood 2010;115(9):1797–803.

56. Newall F, Barnes C, Ignjatovic V, et al. Heparin-induced thrombocytopenia in children. J Paediatr Child Health 2003;39(4):289–92.

57. Warkentin TE, Hayward CP, Boshkov LK, et al. Sera from patients with heparin-induced thrombocytopenia generate platelet-derived microparticles with pro-coagulant activity: an explanation for the thrombotic complications of heparin-induced thrombocytopenia. Blood 1994;84(11):3691–9.

58. Cines DB, Tomaski A, Tannenbaum S. Immune endothelial-cell injury in heparin-associated thrombocytopenia. N Engl J Med 1987;316(10):581–9.

59. Rauova L, Hirsch JD, Greene TK, et al. Monocyte-bound PF4 in the pathogenesis of heparin-induced thrombocytopenia. Blood 2010;116(23):5021–31.

60. Kuter DJ, Konkle BA, Hamza TH, et al. Clinical outcomes in a cohort of patients with heparin-induced thrombocytopenia. Am J Hematol 2017;92(8):730–8.

61. Warkentin TE, Kelton JG. A 14-year study of heparin-induced thrombocytopenia. Am J Med 1996;101(5):502–7.

62. Warkentin TE, Levine MN, Hirsh J, et al. Heparin-induced thrombocytopenia in patients treated with low-molecular-weight heparin or unfractionated heparin. N Engl J Med 1995;332(20):1330–5.

63. East JM, Cserti-Gazdewich CM, Granton JT. Heparin-induced thrombocytopenia in the critically ill patient. Chest 2018;154(3):678–90.

64. Warkentin TE, Greinacher A. Heparin-induced anaphylactic and anaphylactoid reactions: two distinct but overlapping syndromes. Expert Opin Drug Saf 2009; 8(2):129–44.

65. Schindewolf M, Kroll H, Ackermann H, et al. Heparin-induced non-necrotizing skin lesions: rarely associated with heparin-induced thrombocytopenia. J Thromb Haemost 2010;8(7):1486–91.

66. Kowalska MA, Krishnaswamy S, Rauova L, et al. Antibodies associated with heparin-induced thrombocytopenia (HIT) inhibit activated protein C generation: new insights into the prothrombotic nature of HIT. Blood 2011;118(10):2882–8.

67. Lo GK, Juhl D, Warkentin TE, et al. Evaluation of pretest clinical score (4 T's) for the diagnosis of heparin-induced thrombocytopenia in two clinical settings. J Thromb Haemost 2006;4(4):759–65.

68. Lee GM, Arepally GM. Heparin-induced thrombocytopenia. Hematology Am Soc Hematol Educ Program 2013;2013:668–74.

69. Pouplard C, Regina S, May MA, et al. Heparin-induced thrombocytopenia: a frequent complication after cardiac surgery. Arch Mal Coeur Vaiss 2007; 100(6–7):563–8.

70. Jones CG, Pechauer SM, Curtis BR, et al. A platelet factor 4-dependent platelet activation assay facilitates early detection of pathogenic heparin-induced thrombocytopenia antibodies. Chest 2017;152(4):e77–80.

71. Lewis BE, Wallis DE, Berkowitz SD, et al. Argatroban anticoagulant therapy in patients with heparin-induced thrombocytopenia. Circulation 2001;103(14): 1838–43.

72. Lubenow N, Warkentin TE, Greinacher A, et al. Results of a systematic evaluation of treatment outcomes for heparin-induced thrombocytopenia in patients receiving danaparoid, ancrod, and/or coumarin explain the rapid shift in clinical practice during the 1990s. Thromb Res 2006;117(5):507–15.

73. Warkentin TE, Pai M, Sheppard JI, et al. Fondaparinux treatment of acute heparin-induced thrombocytopenia confirmed by the serotonin-release assay: a 30-month, 16-patient case series. J Thromb Haemost 2011;9(12):2389–96.

74. Schindewolf M, Steindl J, Beyer-Westendorf J, et al. Use of fondaparinux off-label or approved anticoagulants for management of heparin-induced thrombocytopenia. J Am Coll Cardiol 2017;70(21):2636–48.

75. Schindewolf M, Steindl J, Beyer-Westendorf J, et al. Frequent off-label use of fondaparinux in patients with suspected acute heparin-induced thrombocytopenia (HIT)–findings from the GerHIT multi-centre registry study. Thromb Res 2014;134(1):29–35.

76. Onwuemene OA, Zantek ND, Rollins-Raval MA, et al. Therapeutic plasma exchange for management of heparin-induced thrombocytopenia: results of an international practice survey. J Clin Apher 2019;34(5):545–54.

77. Padmanabhan A, Jones CG, Pechauer SM, et al. IVIg for treatment of severe refractory heparin-induced thrombocytopenia. Chest 2017;152(3):478–85.

78. Park BD, Kumar M, Nagalla S, et al. Intravenous immunoglobulin as an adjunct therapy in persisting heparin-induced thrombocytopenia. Transfus Apher Sci 2018;57(4):561–5.

79. Taylor FB Jr, Toh CH, Hoots WK, et al. Towards definition, clinical and laboratory criteria, and a scoring system for disseminated intravascular coagulation. Thromb Haemost 2001;86(5):1327–30.

80. Matsuda T. Clinical aspects of DIC–disseminated intravascular coagulation. Pol J Pharmacol 1996;48(1):73–5.

81. Sivula M, Tallgren M, Pettila V. Modified score for disseminated intravascular coagulation in the critically ill. Intensive Care Med 2005;31(9):1209–14.

82. Angstwurm MW, Dempfle CE, Spannagl M. New disseminated intravascular coagulation score: a useful tool to predict mortality in comparison with Acute Physiology and Chronic Health Evaluation II and Logistic Organ Dysfunction scores. Crit Care Med 2006;34(2):314–20 [quiz: 328].

83. Toh CH, Downey C. Performance and prognostic importance of a new clinical and laboratory scoring system for identifying non-overt disseminated intravascular coagulation. Blood Coagul Fibrinolysis 2005;16(1):69–74.

84. Cartin-Ceba R, Kojicic M, Li G, et al. Epidemiology of critical care syndromes, organ failures, and life-support interventions in a suburban US community. Chest 2011;140(6):1447–55.

85. Bakhtiari K, Meijers JC, de Jonge E, et al. Prospective validation of the International Society of Thrombosis and Haemostasis scoring system for disseminated intravascular coagulation. Crit Care Med 2004;32(12):2416–21.

86. Gando S, Saitoh D, Ogura H, et al. Natural history of disseminated intravascular coagulation diagnosed based on the newly established diagnostic criteria for critically ill patients: results of a multicenter, prospective survey. Crit Care Med 2008;36(1):145–50.

87. Kushimoto S, Gando S, Saitoh D, et al. Clinical course and outcome of disseminated intravascular coagulation diagnosed by Japanese Association for Acute

Medicine criteria. Comparison between sepsis and trauma. Thromb Haemost 2008;100(6):1099–105.

88. Murata A, Okamoto K, Mayumi T, et al. The recent time trend of outcomes of disseminated intravascular coagulation in Japan: an observational study based on a national administrative database. J Thromb Thrombolysis 2014;38(3): 364–71.

89. Singh B, Hanson AC, Alhurani R, et al. Trends in the incidence and outcomes of disseminated intravascular coagulation in critically ill patients (2004-2010): a population-based study. Chest 2013;143(5):1235–42.

90. Gando S, Levi M, Toh CH. Disseminated intravascular coagulation. Nat Rev Dis Primers 2016;2:16037.

91. Levi M, Ten Cate H. Disseminated intravascular coagulation. N Engl J Med 1999;341(8):586–92.

92. Gando S. Tissue factor in trauma and organ dysfunction. Semin Thromb Hemost 2006;32(1):48–53.

93. Gando S, Sawamura A, Hayakawa M. Trauma, shock, and disseminated intravascular coagulation: lessons from the classical literature. Ann Surg 2011; 254(1):10–9.

94. Wada H, Matsumoto T, Yamashita Y, et al. Disseminated intravascular coagulation: testing and diagnosis. Clin Chim Acta 2014;436:130–4.

95. Wada H, Wakita Y, Nakase T, et al. Outcome of disseminated intravascular coagulation in relation to the score when treatment was begun. Mie DIC Study Group. Thromb Haemost 1995;74(3):848–52.

96. Colling ME, Bendapudi PK. Purpura fulminans: mechanism and management of dysregulated hemostasis. Transfus Med Rev 2018;32(2):69–76.

97. Marlar RA, Neumann A. Neonatal purpura fulminans due to homozygous protein C or protein S deficiencies. Semin Thromb Hemost 1990;16(4):299–309.

98. Dayama A, Dass J, Seth T, et al. Clinico-hematological profile and outcome of acute promyelocytic leukemia patients at a tertiary care center in North India. Indian J Cancer 2015;52(3):309–12.

99. Cordonnier C, Vernant JP, Brun B, et al. Acute promyelocytic leukemia in 57 previously untreated patients. Cancer 1985;55(1):18–25.

100. Wada H, Thachil J, Di Nisio M, et al. Guidance for diagnosis and treatment of DIC from harmonization of the recommendations from three guidelines. J Thromb Haemost 2013. [Epub ahead of print].

101. Charbit B, Mandelbrot L, Samain E, et al. The decrease of fibrinogen is an early predictor of the severity of postpartum hemorrhage. J Thromb Haemost 2007; 5(2):266–73.

102. Rossaint R, Bouillon B, Cerny V, et al. The European guideline on management of major bleeding and coagulopathy following trauma: fourth edition. Crit Care 2016;20:100.

103. Levi M, Toh CH, Thachil J, et al. Guidelines for the diagnosis and management of disseminated intravascular coagulation. British Committee for Standards in Haematology. Br J Haematol 2009;145(1):24–33.

104. Sakuragawa N, Hasegawa H, Maki M, et al. Clinical evaluation of low-molecular-weight heparin (FR-860) on disseminated intravascular coagulation (DIC)–a multicenter co-operative double-blind trial in comparison with heparin. Thromb Res 1993;72(6):475–500.

105. de la Serna J, Montesinos P, Vellenga E, et al. Causes and prognostic factors of remission induction failure in patients with acute promyelocytic leukemia treated with all-trans retinoic acid and idarubicin. Blood 2008;111(7):3395–402.

106. Brown JE, Olujohungbe A, Chang J, et al. All-trans retinoic acid (ATRA) and tranexamic acid: a potentially fatal combination in acute promyelocytic leukaemia. Br J Haematol 2000;110(4):1010–2.
107. Ranieri VM, Thompson BT, Barie PS, et al. Drotrecogin alfa (activated) in adults with septic shock. N Engl J Med 2012;366(22):2055–64.
108. Allingstrup M, Wetterslev J, Ravn FB, et al. Antithrombin III for critically ill patients. Cochrane Database Syst Rev 2016;(2):CD005370.

Thrombocytopenia-Associated Multiple Organ Failure

Trung C. Nguyen, MD[a,b,*]

KEYWORDS

- TAMOF • TTP • HUS • DIC • Platelet • Thrombocytopenia • Shiga toxin
- Plasma exchange

KEY POINTS

- Thrombocytopenia-associated multiple organ failure is a clinical phenotype that encompasses a spectrum of syndromes associated with disseminated microvascular thromboses.
- Patients with thrombocytopenia-associated multiple organ failure with a genetic predisposition leading to dysregulation of the complement pathway and/or von Willebrand factor/platelet-mediated microvascular thrombosis may be more at risk to develop acute kidney injury.
- There are sufficient preliminary data to support design of randomized controlled trials to evaluate the role of therapeutic plasma exchange in patients with thrombocytopenia-associated multiple organ failure.

INTRODUCTION

Thrombocytopenia-associated multiple organ failure (TAMOF) is a clinical phenotype that encompasses a spectrum of syndromes associated with disseminated microvascular thromboses such as the thrombotic microangiopathies, namely, thrombotic thrombocytopenic purpura/hemolytic uremic syndromes (TTP/HUS) and disseminated intravascular coagulation (DIC). TAMOF is characterized by new onset thrombocytopenia with progression to multiple organ failure (MOF) in critically ill patients. The decrease in platelet counts reflects their involvement in causing disseminated microvascular thromboses, which lead to organ ischemia and dysfunction. Autopsy studies from patients who died with TAMOF reveal widespread microvascular thromboses in all organs.[1–4] With current management strategies, mortalities from TAMOF remain high, ranging from 5% to 80%.[5–13]

---

[a] Department of Pediatrics, Critical Care Medicine Section, Texas Children's Hospital/Baylor College of Medicine, 6651 Main Street, MC: E 1420, Houston, TX 77030, USA; [b] The Center for Translational Research on Inflammatory Diseases (CTRID), The Michael E. DeBakey Veteran Administration Medical Center, Houston, TX 77030, USA
* Department of Pediatrics, Critical Care Medicine Section, Texas Children's Hospital/Baylor College of Medicine, 6651 Main Street, MC: E 1420, Houston, TX 77030.
E-mail address: trungn@bcm.edu

Crit Care Clin 36 (2020) 379–390
https://doi.org/10.1016/j.ccc.2019.12.010   **criticalcare.theclinics.com**

The past decade has brought significant advances in our knowledge of the pathophysiologic processes of TTP, HUS, and DIC.[14,15] Von Willebrand factor (VWF) and ADAMTS-13 (or VWF-cleaving protease) play a central role in TTP.[16] Shiga toxins and the complement pathway are vital in the development of HUS.[17,18] Tissue factor is the major protease that drives the pathology of DIC.[19,20]

THROMBOTIC THROMBOCYTOPENIC PURPURA

In 1924, Dr Moschowitz was the first to describe a case of TTP in a girl who suddenly died with petechiae, paralysis, and coma.[21] Autopsy findings revealed that she had disseminated occlusions of her terminal arterioles and capillaries with hyaline thrombi. For decades, the diagnosis of TTP remained a clinical diagnosis with the classic clinical pentad of thrombocytopenia, hemolytic anemia, fever, and neurologic and renal involvement. In 1982, Dr Moake identified ultra-large VWF (ULVWF) as the "powerful poison which had both agglutinative and hemolytic properties" that caused disseminated microvascular thromboses in TTP.[22] Not until 1998 did Drs Tsai and Lammle from 2 different laboratories simultaneously reported that ADAMTS-13 deficiency was the underlying pathophysiologic process in TTP.[23,24] With ADAMTS-13 deficiency, the ULVWF and large plasma VWF remained uncleaved and maintain their prothrombotic properties in the blood.

TTP is divided into 2 categories: congenital and acquired. In both categories, the ADAMTS-13 activity level is less than 10%. In congenital TTP, more than 80 mutations of the *ADAMTS13* gene have been identified.[25,26] In acquired TTP, ADAMTS-13 inhibitors such as IgG autoantibodies to ADAMTS-13 have been reported.[23,24] Autopsies in patients who have died with TTP reveal characteristic VWF/platelet-rich microthrombi in all organs.[1,2,4,27]

Von Willebrand Factor and ADAMTS-13 in Thrombotic Thrombocytopenic Purpura

VWF is the largest multimeric glycoprotein in plasma with molecular weight ranging from 500 to 20,000 kDa.[28] VWF mediates platelet adhesion to sites of vascular damage by binding to the platelet receptor GP Ib-IX-V complex and to exposed subendothelial collagen. VWF is synthesized by endothelial cells and megakaryocytes as monomers with subsequent dimerization and multimerization in the endoplasmic reticulum and Golgi apparatus, respectively. After synthesis, VWF is secreted by either the constitutive pathway of lower molecular mass (approximately 500 kDa) dimers or the inducible pathway of larger and ULVWF.[28,29] The inducible pathway is induced by inflammation.[30–32] VWF adhesiveness is associated with its larger size. Thus, ULVWF is extremely large and hyperadhesive. ULVWF can spontaneously aggregate platelets by forming high strength bonds with platelet receptor GP Ib-IX-V complex.[33] This ULVWF is rapidly and partially cleaved by ADAMTS-13 before being released into the plasma. Consequently, plasma VWF binds and aggregates platelets only in the presence of modulators such as ristocetin or at high shear stress.[34,35] Deficiency of ULVWF proteolysis results in accumulation of ULVWF in plasma and on endothelial surfaces, as observed in patients with TTP.

ADAMTS-13 is a member of the ADAMTS family of proteases (*A* Disintegrin And Metalloproteinase with ThromboSpondin motifs).[25] *ADAMTS13* gene encodes a protein with 1427 amino acids and its messenger RNA is detected in hepatic stellate cells, endothelial cells, platelets, and glomeruli podocytes.[25,36–40] ADAMTS-13 cleaves VWF at a single peptide bond Tyr842-Met843 in the VWF A2 domain. This cleavage reduces the ULVWF, which spontaneously aggregate platelets, to smaller plasma forms that bind to platelets only with modulators or high fluid shear stress. The cleaved VWF is no longer prothrombotic, but maintains hemostatic functions. Increased complement activity interacts with ADAMTS-13 deficiency in patients with TTP to cause renal involvement related to both defective inhibitory complement function and autoimmune disease.[41–44]

Managing Thrombotic Thrombocytopenic Purpura

The clinical pentad of TTP—thrombocytopenia, hemolytic anemia, fever, and neurologic and renal injuries—triggers the clinicians to workup thrombotic microangiopathies (TMA). ADAMTS—13, VWF, and complement assays should be sent. Elevated lactate dehydrogenase and the presence of schistocytes would suggest the pathophysiologic process of TMA. The confirmatory diagnosis of TTP will be made with ADAMTS-13 activity of less than 10%, the presence of ULVWF, and clinical signs and symptoms of TTP. The therapeutic strategies for TTP are to (1) replenish ADAMTS-13 activity, (2) remove ADAMTS-13 inhibitors, and (3) remove ULVWF. Transfusion with fresh frozen plasma, which contains ADAMTS-13, addresses the first strategy. The second strategy is addressed by steroids and/or rituximab (anti-CD20 on B-lymphocytes), which can be given to decrease the synthesis of IgG inhibitory autoantibodies to ADAMTS-13.[45] The third strategy is addressed by therapeutic plasma exchange (TPE), which is now the standard therapy for newly diagnosed TTP. It has decreased TTP mortality from 100% to less than 20%.[7,9]

The recognition that acute kidney injury is prevalent in TTP is important. TTP and HUS need to be differentiated by molecular diagnosis because they have potentially different management strategies. Plasma therapies including TPE are best for TTP, whereas TPE is not recommended for infection-induced HUS. If uncontrolled complement pathway activation is involved, as reported in some patient with TTP-induced acute kidney injury, the anti-C5 monoclonal antibody eculizumab may also have a role. A multidisciplinary approach is warranted, including early involvement from hematology, transfusion medicine, nephrology, and immunology.

HEMOLYTIC UREMIC SYNDROME

The clinical triad of HUS is thrombocytopenia, hemolytic anemia, and acute kidney injury. The majority of the cases requires only supportive care and do not progress into MOF. However, cases with brain injuries such as coma, seizures, and stroke are more likely to develop TAMOF and are associated with higher mortality.[11] HUS is divided into 2 major clinical phenotypes: infection-induced HUS and atypical HUS with complement dysregulation. Autopsies in patients who have died with HUS reveal disseminated fibrin-rich microthrombi in the majority of cases, but a subset of patients do have VWF/platelet-rich microthrombi.[1,27] These HUS autopsies reveal that the kidneys are markedly involved compared with other organs, contrasting with TTP and DIC where all organs are involved.[1]

Infection-induced HUS accounts for 90% of all HUS cases, and the majority (approximately 85%) are caused by Shiga toxin-producing *Escherichia coli* (STEC) and several other bacteria including *Streptococcus pneumonia*.[13,46] HUS develops in 6% to 15% of the infected patients 2 to 10 days after bloody diarrhea.[46] STEC-HUS has commonly been affecting children until the recent 2011 outbreak in Germany that affected mostly adults.[10] Mortality for STEC-HUS ranges from 5% to 9%.[11]

Atypical HUS accounts for approximately 10% of all HUS cases.[13] The complement pathway genetic mutations account for 50% to 60% and thrombomodulin mutations account for 5% of atypical HUS cases. Mortality is approximately 25% for all atypical HUS, but is 50% to 80% for the familial form of atypical HUS.[12,13]

Shiga Toxins and Complement Pathway in Hemolytic Uremic Syndrome

Shiga toxins produced by enterohemorrhagic *E coli* bind to glycosphingolipid surface receptor globotriaosyl ceramide expressed on the renal microvascular endothelium. The toxins are then internalized, leading to protein synthesis inhibition and cell death.[47] In addition, Shiga toxins can cause a prothrombotic state in a host by activating monocytes to release inflammatory cytokines,[48] activating platelets,[49] increasing tissue factor activity on glomerular endothelial cells,[50] inhibiting ADAMTS-13, stimulating ULVWF release from glomerular endothelial cells,[51] and activating the complement alternative pathway.[52] Recently, investigators proposed a link between the ULVWF and the alternative complement pathway in HUS. They show that the endothelial cells can synthesize the alternative complement components that are assembled and activated on the endothelial cell-secreted ULVWF.[53] The activated complement complex on ULVWF could then cause local endothelial damage.

The complement system is essential for immune surveillance and homeostasis.[54] The complement genetic mutations associated with atypical HUS allow for the tightly regulated complement pathway to become unregulated and hyperactive after an inflammatory trigger. This leads to inflammation, and if severe will lead to uncontrolled systemic inflammation, disseminated microvascular thromboses, and MOF. More than 120 complement genetic mutations have been linked to atypical HUS.[16] Autoantibodies to factor H, a regulatory complement protein, can also cause HUS.[55,56]

Managing Hemolytic Uremic Syndrome

Complement pathway interrogation and a genetic workup should be initiated in patients with the clinical triad of HUS. ADAMTS-13 and VWF assays should be sent to rule out TTP. For the majority of patients with STEC-HUS, supportive care is the current recommendation. The American Society for Apheresis gives a category I recommendation "apheresis (ie, TPE) is accepted as a first line therapy" for atypical HUS owing to autoantibody to factor H.[7] The American Society for Apheresis gives TPE a category II recommendation "apheresis is accepted as a second-line therapy" for atypical HUS owing to complement factor gene mutation. Currently, TPE is not recommended for STEC-HUS (category IV recommendation). Direct complement inhibition with the monoclonal antibody eculizumab should be considered for atypical HUS.[57,58]

Diarrhea or infection-associated HUS with brain injuries and/or rapid progression into TAMOF poses a significant therapeutic strategy dilemma for intensivists. These patients may have a mixture of pathologic mechanisms involving Shiga toxins, VWF, ADAMTS-13, platelets, complements, fibrin, and endothelium. Until clinicians have the ability to rapidly tease out the exact pathologic mechanism, there is a biologic plausibility for the benefit of TPE with the aim of restoring the homeostatic milieu of the plasma. More recent case series have highlighted the benefit of TPE in severe diarrhea or infection-associated HUS.[59,60] Eculizumab also have recently been suggested to be beneficial in STEC-HUS.[19,61]

DISSEMINATED INTRAVASCULAR COAGULATION

The consensus definition of DIC by the Scientific Subcommittee on DIC of the International Society of Thrombosis and Haemostasis is "an acquired syndrome characterized by the intravascular activation of coagulation with loss of localization arising from different causes. It can originate from and cause damage to the microvasculature, which if sufficiently severe, can produce organ dysfunction."[62] Conditions that can trigger DIC include sepsis, cancer, trauma, burns, obstetric complications, toxin exposure, and vascular abnormalities. DIC can occur in 39% of patients with severe sepsis with a mortality rate of up to 50%.[5,6] Clinically, the patients present with shock owing to poor perfusion of the organs and petechiae and purpura on the skin. Autopsies in patients who have died with DIC reveal fibrin-rich microthrombi in small and mid-size vessels in all organs.[2,4,27]

Tissue Factor in Disseminated Intravascular Coagulation

Tissue factor plays a key role in the initiation and propagation of DIC. Tissue factor is expressed from 2 major sources—vessel wall and hematopoietic cells. When the vascular wall is injured, extravascular tissue factor is exposed. Monocytes express and release tissue factor after stimulation by inflammatory cytokines or endotoxins during systemic inflammation, such as an infection.[17,63,64] After expression, tissue factor complexes with factor VIIa. This complex then activates factors IX and X, eventually leading to thrombin generation. Because tissue factor propagates thrombin formation, the endogenous anticoagulants in the body such as antithrombin III, protein C, and tissue factor pathway inhibitor are all found to be impaired during DIC. Decreased synthesis, increased consumption and degradation, and the development of inhibitors all contribute to the depletion of anticoagulants activities.[65] Finally, the body's natural fibrinolytic system that is responsible for the breakdown of clots during a prothrombotic state, is also impaired. Plasminogen-activator inhibitor type 1, a potent inhibitor of the fibrinolytic pathway, is pathologically elevated in DIC and MOF.[66–68] Granulocyte elastase can also proteolyze ADAMTS-13 to inactive fragments.[69]

Managing Disseminated Intravascular Coagulation

In 2013, the Scientific Subcommittee on DIC of the International Society of Thrombosis and Haemostasis published a guideline combining the recommendations from the British, Japanese, and Italian DIC treatment guidelines.[70] In summary, this subcommittee recommends that (1) there is no gold standard for the diagnosis of DIC and no single test is capable of diagnosing DIC; (2) the key in DIC treatment is treating the underlying condition; (3) the transfusions of platelets, fresh frozen plasma, fibrinogen, and prothrombin complex concentrate is recommended in actively bleeding patients with low platelet counts, prolonged prothrombin time/activated partial thromboplastin time, hypofibrinogenemia, or contraindicated fresh frozen plasma transfusion, respectively; (4) therapeutic doses of low molecular weight heparin should be considered if thrombosis predominates; (5) prophylaxis for venous thromboembolism with prophylactic doses of unfractionated heparin or low molecular weight heparin is recommended in nonbleeding patients; (6) the administration of antithrombin III, recombinant thrombomodulin, or activated protein C may be considered; (7) generally, antifibrinolytic agents should not be used; and last (8) patients with severe bleeding, characterized by a marked hyperfibrinolytic state such as leukemia and trauma, could be treated with antifibrinolytic agents.

THROMBOCYTOPENIA-ASSOCIATED MULTIPLE ORGAN FAILURE

In the intensive care unit, overt DIC has been observed in 40% of patients with new-onset thrombocytopenia.[71–73] TTP and HUS are rare diagnoses in the intensive care unit. The mechanism of the other 60% of patients with new-onset thrombocytopenia in the intensive care unit is of great interest because new-onset thrombocytopenia has been associated with significantly higher mortality.[73–75] Investigators studying MOF have observed that pediatric patients with TAMOF defined as platelet counts of less than $100,000/mm^3$ and at least 2 failing organs, have clinical, biomarker, and histologic evidences of a thrombotic microangiopathic process.[76] Only 46% of these patients with TAMOF have evidence of an activated fibrin-mediated pathway as in DIC with prolonged prothrombin time. None of these patients with TAMOF have classic TTP, but 89% of the patients have evidence of increased VWF-mediated thrombosis similar to TTP pathophysiology. Mean ADAMTS-13 activity level is 39%, which is abnormally low, but not less than 10% as in classic patients with TTP. ULVWF is observed in 53% of these patients. Histopathologic findings in these patients with TAMOF reveal VWF/platelet-rich and fibrin-rich microthrombi in the brain, lungs, and kidneys. Of note, all these pediatric patients with TAMOF have concurrent sepsis. These investigators suggest that more than one-half of critically ill children with TAMOF have an acquired ADAMTS-13 deficiency, leading to a thrombotic microangiopathic process.

Other investigators have reported that acquired ADAMTS-13 deficiency associated with systemic inflammation have higher morbidity and mortality.[69,77–80] Many molecules associated with systemic inflammation or activated coagulation can inhibit ADAMTS-13. Interleukin-6 can inhibit ADAMTS-13 from cleaving ULVWF.[30] Plasma-free hemoglobin, which is released during hemolysis, can inhibit ADAMTS-13.[81,82] Plasmin and thrombin, products of activated coagulation and inflammation, can proteolyze and inactivate ADAMTS-13.[83] Released by activated neutrophils during systemic inflammation, granulocyte elastase and reactive oxygen species that oxidize VWF can inhibit ADAMTS-13-mediated cleavage.[69,84] VWF proteolytic fragments seem to provide a negative feedback loop by inhibiting ADAMTS-13.[85] Neutralizing IgG autoantibodies to ADAMTS-13 are the first described inhibitors of ADAMTS-13.[23,24]

Managing Thrombocytopenia-Associated Multiple Organ Failure (Not Overt Disseminated Intravascular Coagulation, Thrombotic Thrombocytopenic Purpura, or Hemolytic Uremic Syndrome)

Mounting evidences are suggesting that a nonspecific plasma therapeutic strategy such as TPE may have a role in reversing MOF and improving outcomes in patients with TAMOF. Of note, all of these patients with TAMOF have concurrent sepsis as a diagnosis.[76,86–89] Currently, the American Society for Apheresis gives a category III recommendation—"Optimum role of apheresis therapy is not established. Decision making should be individualized" —for TPE in sepsis with MOF.[7] A randomized, controlled trial for TPE in TAMOF is warranted.

Currently, there is no monotherapy for DIC and TTP. Various agents had been tried without success such as heparin, antithrombin III, recombinant tissue factor pathway inhibitor, recombinant activated protein C, protein C concentrate, and recombinant soluble thrombomodulin.[90–97] Eculizumab, an anti-C5 monoclonal antibody, is a promising drug for atypical HUS and possibly for STEC-HUS with MOF.[19,57,58,61,98]

Investigators continue to search for effective therapeutic strategies for TAMOF clinical phenotype. Phase I recombinant ADAMTS-13 for congenital TTP is ongoing (ClinicalTrials.gov; NCT02216084). Anti-VWF nanobody trial for acquired TTP has been completed and preliminarily reported at the American Society of Hematology meeting in 2014 "Caplacizumab improved standard of care of patients affected with acquired TTP by a more rapid achievement of platelet normalization and lower number of exacerbations with manageable side effects and bleeding episodes" (ClinicalTrials.gov; NCT01151423). N-acetylcysteine has been shown to decrease the size of VWF in human plasma and mice.[99] Recently, N-acetylcysteine was used successfully to treat a case of refractory TTP.[100] We have recently reported using a recombinant VWF A2 polypeptide that inhibit platelet-fibrin(ogen) interaction to reduce disseminated microvascular thromboses and mortality in an endotoxemia-induced DIC murine model.[101]

Armed with a better understanding of the mechanisms of TAMOF clinical pheno-type, innovative therapeutic strategies are being tried to improve the high morbidity and mortality associated with TAMOF.

REFERENCES

1. Hosler GA, Cusumano AM, Hutchins GM. Thrombotic thrombocytopenic pur-pura and hemolytic uremic syndrome are distinct pathologic entities. A review of 56 autopsy cases. Arch Pathol Lab Med 2003;127(7):834–9.
2. Burke AP, Mont E, Kolodgie F, et al. Thrombotic thrombocytopenic purpura causing rapid unexpected death: value of CD61 immunohistochemical staining in diagnosis. Cardiovasc Pathol 2005;14(3):150–5.
3. Kojima M, Shimamura K, Mori N, et al. A histological study on microthrombi in autopsy cases of DIC. Bibl Haematol 1983;(49):95–106.
4. Asada Y, Sumiyoshi A, Hayashi T, et al. Immunohistochemistry of vascular lesion in thrombotic thrombocytopenic purpura, with special reference to factor VIII related antigen. Thromb Res 1985;38(5):469–79.
5. Dhainaut JF, Yan SB, Joyce DE, et al. Treatment effects of drotrecogin alfa (acti-vated) in patients with severe sepsis with or without overt disseminated intravas-cular coagulation. J Thromb Haemost 2004;2(11):1924–33.
6. Khemani RG, Bart RD, Alonzo TA, et al. Disseminated intravascular coagulation score is associated with mortality for children with shock. Intensive Care Med 2009;35(2):327–33.
7. Szczepiorkowski ZM, Winters JL, Bandarenko N, et al. Guidelines on the use of therapeutic apheresis in clinical practice–evidence-based approach from the Apheresis Applications Committee of the American Society for Apheresis. J Clin Apher 2010;25(3):83–177.
8. Bell WR, Braine HG, Ness PM, et al. Improved survival in thrombotic thrombo-cytopenic purpura-hemolytic uremic syndrome. Clinical experience in 108 pa-tients. N Engl J Med 1991;325(6):398–403.
9. Rock GA, Shumak KH, Buskard NA, et al. Comparison of plasma exchange with plasma infusion in the treatment of thrombotic thrombocytopenic purpura. Ca-nadian Apheresis Study Group. N Engl J Med 1991;325(6):393–7.
10. Frank C, Werber D, Cramer JP, et al. Epidemic profile of Shiga-toxin-producing Escherichia coli O104:H4 outbreak in Germany. N Engl J Med 2011;365(19): 1771–80.
11. Garg AX, Suri RS, Barrowman N, et al. Long-term renal prognosis of diarrhea-associated hemolytic uremic syndrome: a systematic review, meta-analysis, and meta-regression. JAMA 2003;290(10):1360–70.
12. Kaplan BS, Meyers KE, Schulman SL. The pathogenesis and treatment of hemo-lytic uremic syndrome. J Am Soc Nephrol 1998;9(6):1126–33.
13. Noris M, Remuzzi G. Atypical hemolytic-uremic syndrome. N Engl J Med 2009; 361(17):1676–87.
14. Moake JL. Thrombotic microangiopathies. N Engl J Med 2002;347(8):589–600.
15. George JN, Nester CM. Syndromes of thrombotic microangiopathy. N Engl J Med 2014;371(7):654–66.
16. Zafrani L, Mariotte E, Darmon M, et al. Acute renal failure is prevalent in patients with thrombotic thrombocytopenic purpura associated with low plasma ADAMTS13 activity. J Thromb Haemost 2015;13(3):380–9.
17. Noris M, Mescia F, Remuzzi G. STEC-HUS, atypical HUS and TTP are all dis-eases of complement activation. Nat Rev Nephrol 2012;8(11):622–33.

18. Trachtman H, Austin C, Lewinski M, et al. Renal and neurological involvement in typical Shiga toxin-associated HUS. Nat Rev Nephrol 2012;8(11):658–69.

19. Levi M, van der Poll T. Disseminated intravascular coagulation: a review for the internist. Intern Emerg Med 2013;8(1):23–32.

20. In JW, Kim JE, Jeong JS, et al. Diagnostic and prognostic significance of neutrophil gelatinase-associated lipocalin in disseminated intravascular coagulation. Clin Chim Acta 2014;430:145–9.

21. Moschcowitz E. A hitherto undescribed disease. Proceedings of New York Pathological Society 1924;(24):21–4.

22. Moake JL, Rudy CK, Troll JH, et al. Unusually large plasma factor VIII: von Willebrand factor multimers in chronic relapsing thrombotic thrombocytopenic purpura. N Engl J Med 1982;307(23):1432–5.

23. Furlan M, Robles R, Galbusera M, et al. von Willebrand factor-cleaving protease in thrombotic thrombocytopenic purpura and the hemolytic-uremic syndrome. N Engl J Med 1998;339(22):1578–84.

24. Tsai HM, Lian EC. Antibodies to von Willebrand factor-cleaving protease in acute thrombotic thrombocytopenic purpura. N Engl J Med 1998;339(22):1585–94.

25. Levy GG, Nichols WC, Lian EC, et al. Mutations in a member of the ADAMTS gene family cause thrombotic thrombocytopenic purpura. Nature 2001;413(6855):488–94.

26. Zhou Z, Nguyen TC, Guchhait P, et al. Von Willebrand factor, ADAMTS-13, and thrombotic thrombocytopenic purpura. Semin Thromb Hemost 2010;36(1):71–81.

27. Tsai HM, Chandler WL, Sarode R, et al. von Willebrand factor and von Willebrand factor-cleaving metalloprotease activity in Escherichia coli O157:H7-associated hemolytic uremic syndrome. Pediatr Res 2001;49(5):653–9.

28. Sadler JE. Biochemistry and genetics of von Willebrand factor. Annu Rev Biochem 1998;67:395–424.

29. Tsai HM, Nagel RL, Hatcher VB, et al. The high molecular weight form of endothelial cell von Willebrand factor is released by the regulated pathway. Br J Haematol 1991;79(2):239–45.

30. Bernardo A, Ball C, Nolasco L, et al. Effects of inflammatory cytokines on the release and cleavage of the endothelial cell-derived ultralarge von Willebrand factor multimers under flow. Blood 2004;104(1):100–6.

31. Sporn LA, Marder VJ, Wagner DD. Inducible secretion of large, biologically potent von Willebrand factor multimers. Cell 1986;46(2):185–90.

32. Wagner DD. Cell biology of von Willebrand factor. Annu Rev Cell Biol 1990;6:217–46.

33. Moake JL, Turner NA, Stathopoulos NA, et al. Involvement of large plasma von Willebrand factor (vWF) multimers and unusually large vWF forms derived from endothelial cells in shear stress-induced platelet aggregation. J Clin Invest 1986;78(6):1456–61.

34. Arya M, Anvari B, Romo GM, et al. Ultralarge multimers of von Willebrand factor form spontaneous high-strength bonds with the platelet glycoprotein Ib-IX complex: studies using optical tweezers. Blood 2002;99(11):3971–7.

35. Chow TW, Turner NA, Chintagumpala M, et al. Increased von Willebrand factor binding to platelets in single episode and recurrent types of thrombotic thrombocytopenic purpura. Am J Hematol 1998;57(4):293–302.

36. Liu L, Choi H, Bernardo A, et al. Platelet-derived VWF-cleaving metalloprotease ADAMTS-13. J Thromb Haemost 2005;3(11):2536–44.

37. Turner N, Nolasco L, Tao Z, et al. Human endothelial cells synthesize and release ADAMTS-13. J Thromb Haemost 2006;4(6):1396–404.
38. Zhou W, Inada M, Lee TP, et al. ADAMTS13 is expressed in hepatic stellate cells. Lab Invest 2005;85(6):780–8.
39. Manea M, Kristoffersson A, Schneppenheim R, et al. Podocytes express ADAMTS13 in normal renal cortex and in patients with thrombotic thrombocytopenic purpura. Br J Haematol 2007;138(5):651–62.
40. Vesely SK, George JN, Lammle B, et al. ADAMTS13 activity in thrombotic thrombocytopenic purpura-hemolytic uremic syndrome: relation to presenting features and clinical outcomes in a prospective cohort of 142 patients. Blood 2003;102(1):60–8.
41. Coppo P, Bengoufa D, Veyradier A, et al. Severe ADAMTS13 deficiency in adult idiopathic thrombotic microangiopathies defines a subset of patients characterized by various autoimmune manifestations, lower platelet count, and mild renal involvement. Medicine 2004;83(4):233–44.
42. Noris M, Bucchioni S, Galbusera M, et al. Complement factor H mutation in familial thrombotic thrombocytopenic purpura with ADAMTS13 deficiency and renal involvement. J Am Soc Nephrol 2005;16(5):1177–83.
43. Yamada R, Nozawa K, Yoshimine T, et al. A case of thrombotic thrombocytopenia purpura associated with systemic lupus erythematosus: diagnostic utility of ADAMTS-13 activity. Autoimmune Dis 2011;2011:483642.
44. Yamashita H, Takahashi Y, Kaneko H, et al. Thrombotic thrombocytopenic purpura with an autoantibody to ADAMTS13 complicating Sjogren's syndrome: two cases and a literature review. Mod Rheumatol 2013;23(2):365–73.
45. Moake J. Thrombotic microangiopathies: multimers, metalloprotease, and beyond. Clin Transl Sci 2009;2(5):366–73.
46. Tarr PI, Gordon CA, Chandler WL. Shiga-toxin-producing Escherichia coli and haemolytic uraemic syndrome. Lancet 2005;365(9464):1073–86.
47. Johannes L, Romer W. Shiga toxins–from cell biology to biomedical applications. Nat Rev Microbiol 2010;8(2):105–16.
48. van Setten PA, Monnens LA, Verstraten RG, et al. Effects of verocytotoxin-1 on nonadherent human monocytes: binding characteristics, protein synthesis, and induction of cytokine release. Blood 1996;88(1):174–83.
49. Karpman D, Papadopoulou D, Nilsson K, et al. Platelet activation by Shiga toxin and circulatory factors as a pathogenetic mechanism in the hemolytic uremic syndrome. Blood 2001;97(10):3100–8.
50. Nestoridi E, Tsukurov O, Kushak RI, et al. Shiga toxin enhances functional tissue factor on human glomerular endothelial cells: implications for the pathophysiology of hemolytic uremic syndrome. J Thromb Haemost 2005;3(4):752–62.
51. Nolasco LH, Turner NA, Bernardo A, et al. Hemolytic uremic syndrome-associated Shiga toxins promote endothelial-cell secretion and impair ADAMTS13 cleavage of unusually large von Willebrand factor multimers. Blood 2005;106(13):4199–209.
52. Morigi M, Galbusera M, Gastoldi S, et al. Alternative pathway activation of complement by Shiga toxin promotes exuberant C3a formation that triggers microvascular thrombosis. J Immunol 2011;187(1):172–80.
53. Turner NA, Moake J. Assembly and activation of alternative complement components on endothelial cell-anchored ultra-large von Willebrand factor links complement and hemostasis-thrombosis. PLoS One 2013;8(3):e59372.
54. Ricklin D, Hajishengallis G, Yang K, et al. Complement: a key system for immune surveillance and homeostasis. Nat Immunol 2010;11(9):785–97.

55. Dragon-Durey MA, Loirat C, Cloarec S, et al. Anti-Factor H autoantibodies associated with atypical hemolytic uremic syndrome. J Am Soc Nephrol 2005;16(2): 555–63.

56. Noris M, Remuzzi G. Hemolytic uremic syndrome. J Am Soc Nephrol 2005; 16(4):1035–50.

57. Legendre CM, Licht C, Muus P, et al. Terminal complement inhibitor eculizumab in atypical hemolytic-uremic syndrome. N Engl J Med 2013;368(23):2169–81.

58. Zuber J, Fakhouri F, Roumenina LT, et al. Use of eculizumab for atypical haemolytic uraemic syndrome and C3 glomerulopathies. Nat Rev Nephrol 2012;8(11): 643–57.

59. Colic E, Dieperink H, Titlestad K, et al. Management of an acute outbreak of diarrhoea-associated haemolytic uraemic syndrome with early plasma exchange in adults from southern Denmark: an observational study. Lancet 2011;378(9796):1089–93.

60. Kielstein JT, Beutel G, Fleig S, et al. Best supportive care and therapeutic plasma exchange with or without eculizumab in Shiga-toxin-producing E. coli O104:H4 induced haemolytic-uraemic syndrome: an analysis of the German STEC-HUS registry. Nephrol Dial Transplant 2012;27(10):3807–15.

61. Lapeyraque AL, Malina M, Fremeaux-Bacchi V, et al. Eculizumab in severe Shiga-toxin-associated HUS. N Engl J Med 2011;364(26):2561–3.

62. Taylor FB Jr, Toh CH, Hoots WK, et al. Towards definition, clinical and laboratory criteria, and a scoring system for disseminated intravascular coagulation. Thromb Haemost 2001;86(5):1327–30.

63. Conkling PR, Greenberg CS, Weinberg JB. Tumor necrosis factor induces tissue factor-like activity in human leukemia cell line U937 and peripheral blood monocytes. Blood 1988;72(1):128–33.

64. van der Poll T, Levi M, Hack CE, et al. Elimination of interleukin 6 attenuates coagulation activation in experimental endotoxemia in chimpanzees. J Exp Med 1994;179(4):1253–9.

65. Levi M, de Jonge E, van der Poll T. Rationale for restoration of physiological anticoagulant pathways in patients with sepsis and disseminated intravascular coagulation. Crit Care Med 2001;29(7 Suppl):S90–4.

66. Madach K, Aladzsity I, Szilagyi A, et al. 4G/5G polymorphism of PAI-1 gene is associated with multiple organ dysfunction and septic shock in pneumonia induced severe sepsis: prospective, observational, genetic study. Crit Care 2010;14(2):R79.

67. Green J, Doughty L, Kaplan SS, et al. The tissue factor and plasminogen activator inhibitor type-1 response in pediatric sepsis-induced multiple organ failure. Thromb Haemost 2002;87(2):218–23.

68. Madoiwa S, Nunomiya S, Ono T, et al. Plasminogen activator inhibitor 1 promotes a poor prognosis in sepsis-induced disseminated intravascular coagulation. Int J Hematol 2006;84(5):398–405.

69. Ono T, Mimuro J, Madoiwa S, et al. Severe secondary deficiency of von Willebrand factor-cleaving protease (ADAMTS13) in patients with sepsis-induced disseminated intravascular coagulation: its correlation with development of renal failure. Blood 2006;107(2):528–34.

70. Wada H, Thachil J, Di Nisio M, et al. Guidance for diagnosis and treatment of DIC from harmonization of the recommendations from three guidelines. J Thromb Haemost 2013;11(11):761–7.

71. Corrigan JJ Jr. Thrombocytopenia: a laboratory sign of septicemia in infants and children. J Pediatr 1974;85(2):219–21.

72. Stephan F, Hollande J, Richard O, et al. Thrombocytopenia in a surgical ICU. Chest 1999;115(5):1363–70.
73. Vanderschueren S, De Weerdt A, Malbrain M, et al. Thrombocytopenia and prognosis in intensive care. Crit Care Med 2000;28(6):1871–6.
74. Akca S, Haji-Michael P, de Mendonca A, et al. Time course of platelet counts in critically ill patients. Crit Care Med 2002;30(4):753–6.
75. Moreau D, Timsit JF, Vesin A, et al. Platelet count decline: an early prognostic marker in critically ill patients with prolonged ICU stays. Chest 2007;131(6): 1735–41.
76. Nguyen TC, Han YY, Kiss JE, et al. Intensive plasma exchange increases a disintegrin and metalloprotease with thrombospondin motifs-13 activity and reverses organ dysfunction in children with thrombocytopenia-associated multiple organ failure. Crit Care Med 2008;36(10):2878–87.
77. Bockmeyer CL, Claus RA, Budde U, et al. Inflammation-associated ADAMTS13 deficiency promotes formation of ultra-large von Willebrand factor. Haematologica 2008;93(1):137–40.
78. Martin K, Borgel D, Lerolle N, et al. Decreased ADAMTS-13 (A disintegrin-like and metalloprotease with thrombospondin type 1 repeats) is associated with a poor prognosis in sepsis-induced organ failure. Crit Care Med 2007;35(10): 2375–82.
79. Ohshiro M, Kuroda J, Kobayashi Y, et al. ADAMTS-13 activity can predict the outcome of disseminated intravascular coagulation in hematologic malignancies treated with recombinant human soluble thrombomodulin. Am J Hematol 2012;87(1):116–9.
80. Nguyen TC, Liu A, Liu L, et al. Acquired ADAMTS-13 deficiency in pediatric patients with severe sepsis. Haematologica 2007;92(1):121–4.
81. Studt JD, Hovinga JA, Antoine G, et al. Fatal congenital thrombotic thrombocytopenic purpura with apparent ADAMTS13 inhibitor: in vitro inhibition of ADAMTS13 activity by hemoglobin. Blood 2005;105(2):542–4.
82. Zhou Z, Han H, Cruz MA, et al. Haemoglobin blocks von Willebrand factor proteolysis by ADAMTS-13: a mechanism associated with sickle cell disease. Thromb Haemost 2009;101(6):1070–7.
83. Crawley JT, Lam JK, Rance JB, et al. Proteolytic inactivation of ADAMTS13 by thrombin and plasmin. Blood 2005;105(3):1085–93.
84. Chen J, Fu X, Wang Y, et al. Oxidative modification of von Willebrand factor by neutrophil oxidants inhibits its cleavage by ADAMTS13. Blood 2010;115(3): 706–12.
85. Nguyen TC, Balll C, Cruz MA, et al. A negative feedback mechanism of regulating VWF proteolysis by ADAMTS-13. J Thromb Haemost 2011;9(Suppl 2):206.
86. Fortenberry JD, Nguyen T, Grunwell JR, et al. Therapeutic plasma exchange in children with thrombocytopenia-associated multiple organ failure: the thrombocytopenia-associated multiple organ failure network prospective experience. Thrombocytopenia-Associated Multiple Organ Failure (TAMOF) network study group. Crit Care Med 2019;47(3):e173–81.
87. Fortenberry JD, Knezevic A, Nguyen TC, et al. Outcome in children on ECMO with TAMOF receiving plasma exchange: results from the prospective pediatric TAMOF Network Study. Crit Care Med 2012;40(12):A520.
88. Sevketoglu E, Yildizdas D, Horoz OO, et al. Use of therapeutic plasma exchange in children with thrombocytopenia-associated multiple organ failure in the Turkish thrombocytopenia-associated multiple organ failure network. Pediatr Crit Care Med 2014;15(8):e354–9.

89. Ruth A, McCracken C, Hall M, et al. Advanced technologies in pediatric severe sepsis: findings from the PHIS database. Crit Care Med 2013;41(12):A1102.

90. Aoki N, Matsuda T, Saito H, et al. A comparative double-blind randomized trial of activated protein C and unfractionated heparin in the treatment of disseminated intravascular coagulation. Int J Hematol 2002;75(5):540–7.

91. Jaimes F, De La Rosa G, Morales C, et al. Unfractioned heparin for treatment of sepsis: a randomized clinical trial (The HETRASE Study). Crit Care Med 2009; 37(4):1185–96.

92. Warren BL, Eid A, Singer P, et al. Caring for the critically ill patient. High-dose antithrombin III in severe sepsis: a randomized controlled trial. JAMA 2001; 286(15):1869–78.

93. Abraham E, Reinhart K, Opal S, et al. Efficacy and safety of tifacogin (recombinant tissue factor pathway inhibitor) in severe sepsis: a randomized controlled trial. JAMA 2003;290(2):238–47.

94. Bernard GR, Vincent JL, Laterre PF, et al. Efficacy and safety of recombinant human activated protein C for severe sepsis. N Engl J Med 2001;344(10):699–709.

95. Ranieri VM, Thompson BT, Barie PS, et al. Drotrecogin alfa (activated) in adults with septic shock. N Engl J Med 2012;366(22):2055–64.

96. de Kleijn ED, de Groot R, Hack CE, et al. Activation of protein C following infusion of protein C concentrate in children with severe meningococcal sepsis and purpura fulminans: a randomized, double-blinded, placebo-controlled, dose-finding study. Crit Care Med 2003;31(6):1839–47.

97. Saito H, Maruyama I, Shimazaki S, et al. Efficacy and safety of recombinant human soluble thrombomodulin (ART-123) in disseminated intravascular coagulation: results of a phase III, randomized, double-blind clinical trial. J Thromb Haemost 2007;5(1):31–41.

98. Nurnberger J, Philipp T, Witzke O, et al. Eculizumab for atypical hemolytic-uremic syndrome. N Engl J Med 2009;360(5):542–4.

99. Chen J, Reheman A, Gushiken FC, et al. N-acetylcysteine reduces the size and activity of von Willebrand factor in human plasma and mice. J Clin Invest 2011; 121(2):593–603.

100. Li GW, Rambally S, Kamboj J, et al. Treatment of refractory thrombotic thrombocytopenic purpura with N-acetylcysteine: a case report. Transfusion 2014;54(5): 1221–4.

101. Nguyen TC, Gushiken F, Correa JI, et al. A recombinant fragment of von Willebrand factor reduces fibrin-rich microthrombi formation in mice with endotoxemia. Thromb Res 2015;135(5):1025–30.

The Inflammatory and Hemostatic Response in Sepsis and Meningococcemia

Navin P. Boeddha, MD, PhD[a], Thomas Bycroft, MD[b],
Simon Nadel, MD[b,c], Jan A. Hazelzet, MD, PhD[d],*

KEYWORDS

- Bacterial infections • Bacteremia • Hemostasis • Host-pathogen interaction
- Inflammation • Meningococcal infections • Physiology • Sepsis

KEY POINTS

- Complex interplays among host, pathogen, and environment determine the severity of infection ranging from harmless nasopharyngeal colonization to bacteremia, meningitis, sepsis, and lethal disease.
- The inflammatory response includes proinflammatory and anti-inflammatory responses in innate and adaptive immunity. The net proinflammatory state causes endothelial dysfunction and activation of the hemostatic response.
- Within the wide range of illness severity, deposition of fibrin throughout the microcirculation could result in multiple organ dysfunction, skin grafts/amputation, and death.
- Meningococci hold unique properties to promote adhesion, colonization, and invasion into the bloodstream.

INTRODUCTION

Despite important reductions in the number of cases as a result of vaccination programs, *Neisseria meningitidis* (meningococcal) disease is still a major cause of invasive bacterial infections globally.[1,2] Complex interplays among host, pathogen, and environment determine the severity of disease.[3–6] The severity of infection ranges from harmless nasopharyngeal colonization to bacteremia, meningitis, sepsis, and lethal disease.

Meningococcemia refers to dissemination of meningococci into the bloodstream and is notorious for its rapid progression to fulminant disease. Meningococcal

[a] Department of Pediatrics, Erasmus MC-Sophia Children's Hospital, University Medical Center Rotterdam, Doctor Molewaterplein 40, 3015 GD Rotterdam, The Netherlands; [b] St Mary's Hospital, Imperial College Healthcare NHS Trust, Praed Street, W21NY London, UK; [c] Department of Paediatrics, Faculty of Medicine, Imperial College London, South Kensington Campus, London SW7 2AZ, UK; [d] Department of Public Health, Erasmus MC, University Medical Center Rotterdam, Doctor Molewaterplein 40, 3015 GD Rotterdam, The Netherlands
* Corresponding author.
E-mail address: j.a.hazelzet@erasmusmc.nl

Crit Care Clin 36 (2020) 391–399
https://doi.org/10.1016/j.ccc.2019.12.005
0749-0704/20/© 2019 The Authors. Published by Elsevier Inc. This is an open access article under the CC BY-NC-ND license (http://creativecommons.org/licenses/by-nc-nd/4.0/).

endotoxins in the bloodstream and the subsequent inflammatory host response induce endothelial damage, excessive coagulation, and downregulation of fibrinolysis. Hence, the delicate balance between coagulation and anticoagulation shifts toward thrombosis and widespread deposition of fibrin throughout the microcirculation with thromboembolism contributing to multiple organ dysfunction and eventually death.[7]

Meningococcal sepsis serves as a unique model to study inflammation and coagulation in sepsis. Because of early recognition of clinical features, such as the characteristic rash and shock syndrome, pathophysiologic processes in the early phase of sepsis can be studied. In addition, meningococcal disease most commonly occurs in previously healthy children and the broad spectrum of illness severity enables the study of risk factors for adverse outcome. Lastly, meningococcal disease is still common, and thus relevant, in many countries across the world.

In this article, we review the pathogenesis of sepsis, in particular the inflammatory and hemostatic response in meningococcal sepsis. Reviews on meningococcal sepsis epidemiology, clinical features, management, and prevention are found elsewhere.[8,9]

INFLAMMATORY RESPONSE IN SEPSIS

The inflammatory response[10–12] to infection is characterized by two stages and includes innate and adaptive immune responses (**Fig. 1**). The first stage, a proinflammatory response, is initiated by pattern-recognition receptors of the innate immune system (eg, monocytes, macrophages, neutrophils, and dendritic cells) sensing pathogens (pathogen-associated molecular patterns) or stress signals (danger-associated molecular patterns). This detection leads to an intracellular signaling with activation of transcription factors, leading to the release of various proinflammatory cytokines (eg, tumor necrosis factor-α, interleukin-1, interleukin-6) and chemokines that attract even more immune cells, enhancing phagocytosis. Additionally, proteins of the complement system (eg, C1q and mannan-binding lectin) bind to the surface of pathogens and augment their destruction.

These proinflammatory factors also mount a more specific adaptive immune response, which depends on antigen presentation via major histocompatibility complex molecules to lymphocytes. Two classes of lymphocytes, T cells and B cells, are responsible for cell-mediated immune responses and antibody responses, respectively. T cells directly recognize and destroy infected cells, whereas the production of antibodies against specific pathogens by B cells provides humoral immunity.

Simultaneous to the proinflammatory response, a systemic inhibition of the immune system occurs to restore homeostasis.[13] The result is that monocytes and macrophages have diminished capacity to release proinflammatory cytokines on stimulation and blood monocytes are reprogrammed with reduced expression of HLA-DR.[14,15] Additionally, there is an increase in T-cell apoptosis and release of anti-inflammatory mediators to counteract continual inflammation. Thus, the innate and adaptive immune system contribute to sepsis-induced immunosuppression.[10]

Usually, the combined proinflammatory and anti-inflammatory response is able to combat the infection, without becoming unbalanced and harmful. However, an excessive proinflammatory response can result in early mortality in sepsis because of cardiovascular collapse and multiple organ dysfunction. In addition, an extended release of anti-inflammatory mediators (termed immunoparalysis) can potentially result in failure to clear primary infections and increases susceptibility to new infections, resulting in late sepsis mortality.

Meningococcemia is the result of meningococci evading the inflammatory host response. Pili are present on meningococci cell membrane and play a key role in

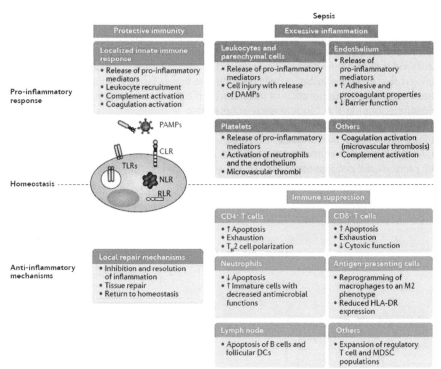

Fig. 1. The inflammatory response to sepsis. The inflammatory response includes a proinflammatory and an anti-inflammatory response. An initial proinflammatory response is initiated by PAMPs sensed by immune cells (eg, leukocytes and parenchymal cells, endothelial cells, and platelets) through an assortment of cell-surface and intracellular pattern recognition receptors (eg, TLRs, NLRs, RLRs, and CLRs). Various proinflammatory cytokines and chemokines are released to neutralize the infection. In addition, an anti-inflammatory compensatory mechanism restrains the initial inflammation, prevents collateral tissue damage, and restores homeostasis. An unbalanced and harmful response may result from prevailing and multiplying of the pathogen despite an activated immune response, leading to a concurrent excessive inflammation (*top right*). Extended release of anti-inflammatory mediators could result in immune suppression (*bottom right*). CLR, C-type lectin receptors; DAMPs, danger-associated molecular patterns; DCs, dendritic cells; MDSC, myeloid-derived suppressor cell; NLR, nucleotide-binding oligomerization domain-like receptors; PAMPs, pathogen-associated molecular patterns; RLR, retinoic acid–inducible gene-like receptors; TLRs, Toll-like receptors. (*From* van der Poll T, van de Veerdonk FL, Scicluna BP, et al. The immunopathology of sepsis and potential therapeutic targets. Nat Rev Immunol. 2017;17(7):407-20; with permission.)

adherence and nasopharyngeal colonization. Epithelial penetration is enhanced by phagocytic vacuoles and outer membrane proteins.[16,17] After invasion into the bloodstream, the outer membrane is further used to evade the host immune response by inhibiting phagocytosis.[16] Meningococci furthermore possess properties to inhibit host complement activation by binding host complement factor H to the meningococcal factor H–binding protein.[18,19] Virulence factors of the meningococcal outer membrane, including outer membrane proteins and surface blebs containing lipopolysaccharide, function as endotoxin, and stimulation of various proinflammatory cytokines results in an excessive proinflammatory response.[20]

HEMOSTATIC RESPONSE IN SEPSIS

The hemostatic response[21–23] is initiated because of endothelial activation and bystander damage after invasion of the bloodstream and inflammation activation by meningococci and endotoxins. Subsequently, tissue factor is released and increasingly expressed by endothelial cells (**Fig. 2**). The tissue factor–factor VII pathway ultimately results in the generation of thrombin, and the conversion of fibrinogen to fibrin.

Meningococci in the bloodstream adhere onto endothelial cells via pili, have the ability to resist high blood velocities, multiply, and form microcolonies on the apical surface of the endothelial cells.[24] Subsequently, the integrity of the endothelium is challenged. Invasion of meningococci through the endothelium involves transcellular and paracellular processes: transcellular, via cell fenestrations or establishment of

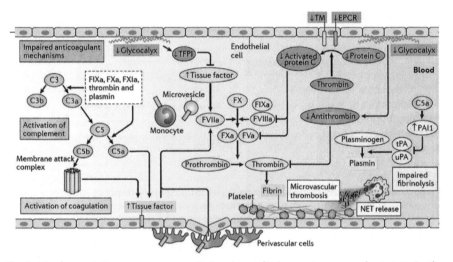

Fig. 2. The hemostatic response to sepsis. Sepsis results in a net procoagulant state in the microvasculature by at least three mechanisms. (1) Inflammatory cytokine-initiated activation of tissue factor generating thrombin (*gray*). Sepsis is accompanied by inflammation-induced vessel injury, which exposes tissue factor to blood coagulation factors, resulting in blood clotting. Tissue factor binds and activates FVII, after which a cascade of proteolytic reactions results in the formation of FXa, thrombin, and fibrin. (2) Insufficient control of anticoagulant pathways (*orange*). The tendency toward thrombosis during sepsis is augmented by the concurrently compromised activity of the three main anticoagulant pathways: antithrombin, TFPI, and the protein C system. Antithrombin is the main inhibitor of thrombin and FXa, whereas TFPI is the main inhibitor of the tissue factor–FVIIa complex. Activated protein C is generated from protein C at the surface of resting endothelial cells, a process that is mediated by the binding of thrombin to TM and is amplified by the EPCR. Activated protein C proteolytically inactivates the coagulation cofactors FVa and FVIIIa, thereby inhibiting coagulation. During sepsis, the protein C system is impaired as a result of multiple factors, most notably the decreased synthesis of protein C by the liver, the increased consumption of protein C, and the impaired activation of protein C as a result of diminished TM expression on endothelial cells. (3) PAI-1-mediated suppression of fibrinolysis (*blue*). The interaction with the complement system (*green*) is outside the scope of this review. EPCR, endothelial cell protein C receptor; NET, neutrophil extracellular traps; PAI, plasminogen activator inhibitor; TFPI, tissue factor pathway inhibitor; TM, thrombomodulin; tPA, tissue-plasminogen activator; uPA, urokinase plasminogen activator. (*From* van der Poll T, van de Veerdonk FL, Scicluna BP, et al. The immunopathology of sepsis and potential therapeutic targets. Nat Rev Immunol. 2017;17(7):407-20; with permission.)

complex systems of vesiculovacuolar organelles, and paracellular based on the coordinated opening and closure of endothelial cell–cell junctions.[25] These processes also account for the ability to cross the blood-brain barrier.[26] Additionally, there is a direct interaction between bacteria and endothelial cells leading to a loss of integrity and increase in endothelial permeability.[26] As a consequence, histology of skin lesions reveal bacteria within the endothelium and thrombi.[27]

In normal circumstances, activation of coagulation is controlled by three important physiologic anticoagulant pathways: (1) the antithrombin system, (2) tissue factor pathway inhibitor, and (3) the activated protein C (PC) pathway. The main function of the PC pathway is to control coagulation by causing inactivation of activated (a) factor V (cofactor of factor Xa) and factor VIIIa (cofactor of factor IX), subsequently preventing thrombin generation.[28] PC also neutralizes plasminogen activator inhibitor (PAI)-1. PAI-1, encoded by *SERPINE1*, is produced by endothelial cells. PAI-1 functions as the principal inhibitor of tissue plasminogen activator and urokinase plasminogen activator, and is the most important fibrinolytic inhibitor in vivo. Thus, PC concomitantly increases fibrinolytic capacity. Thrombomodulin, an endothelial cell surface glycoprotein, binds circulating thrombin and forms a thrombomodulin-thrombin complex (**Fig. 3**). This complex rapidly activates PC bound to the endothelial cell PC receptor. Activated PC then dissociates from the endothelial cell PC receptor, binds to protein S, and forms a complex that inactivates factor Va and factor VIIIa, thus reducing thrombin generation.

In sepsis, decreased activity of all three natural anticoagulant mechanisms results from a combination of impaired synthesis, ongoing consumption, leakage into the interstitial space, and proteolytic degradation. Decreased levels of PC[29] and increased levels of PAI-1[30,31] are associated with a negative outcome in sepsis. In meningococcal disease, it has been shown clearly that 4G/4G homozygotes have higher levels of PAI-1, which is associated with more severe disease.[30]

Altogether, these mechanisms in patients with sepsis result in coagulation abnormalities ranging from subtle derangements only detectable by highly sensitive assays to widespread deposition of fibrin throughout the microcirculation, manifesting as disseminated intravascular coagulation, as typically seen in meningococcal sepsis. Ultimately, disseminated intravascular coagulation contributes to multiple organ dysfunction and to the need for skin grafts, amputation of digits and extremities, and can eventually result in death from multiple organ dysfunction.

Genetic polymorphisms or combination of polymorphisms partly determine interindividual variety in the host response to infection and have been associated with susceptibility and severity of sepsis.[4,32] A genome-wide association study, including approximately 1500 patients with meningococcal disease, reported an association between polymorphisms in the previously mentioned complement factor H region, which play a role in complement activation, and susceptibility.[19] In adults with sepsis caused by pneumonia, a genome-wide association study revealed FER, which encodes a cytosolic nonreceptor tyrosine kinase that influences neutrophil chemotaxis and endothelial permeability, to be associated with a reduced risk of death.[33] Although genetic variations have the potential to affect the host response to an infectious challenge, genetic findings have not been translated to clinical practice.

Neutrophil Extracellular Traps as Cross-link Between Inflammation and Coagulation

Neutrophils are an important part of the innate immune defense. They migrate to the site of infection to release regulatory cytokines, chemokines, and leukotrienes to contribute to microbial killing.[34] One of the tools actively contributing to microbial

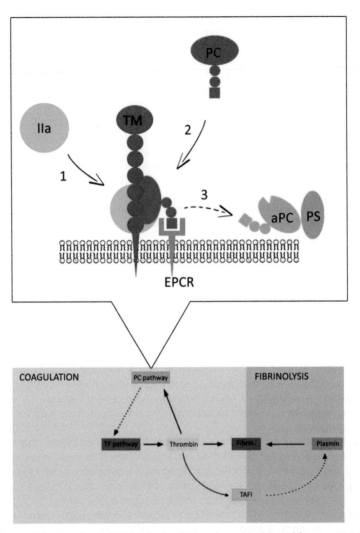

Fig. 3. The protein C pathway. TM binds circulating thrombin (1) and forms a TM-thrombin complex, which activates PC bound to EPCR into aPC (2). APC then dissociates from the EPCR, binds to PS, and forms a complex that inactivates factor Va and factor VIIIa (3). aPC, activated protein C; EPCR, endothelial cell protein C receptor; IIa, thrombin; PS, protein S; TM, thrombomodulin. (*From* Boeddha NP, Emonts M, Cnossen MH, et al. Gene Variations in the Protein C and Fibrinolytic Pathway: Relevance for Severity and Outcome in Pediatric Sepsis. Semin Thromb Hemost. 2017;43(1):36-47; with permission.)

killing is the release of neutrophil extracellular traps (NETs). NETs are extracellular DNA matrix, containing granule proteins and histones to degrade virulence factors and to kill bacteria.[35]

Although NETs are primarily considered as a protective mechanism because of the toxicity of antimicrobial components of the NETs, NETs may contribute to disease severity by causing cell damage via cytotoxic effects of NET-bound histones and by promoting coagulation.[36–38] During systemic inflammation in sepsis, NETs or their components may damage tissue and endothelia, which then initiates the coagulation cascade.

In addition, NETs stimulate platelet adhesion, which may partly account for the thrombocytopenia commonly observed in sepsis.[39] NETs also promote various procoagulant and antifibrinolytic processes,[38] such as fibrin clot formation, factor XII activation, and via histones, interaction with thrombomodulin-dependent PC activation leading to increased thrombin generation. This process named "immunothrombosis" is an important link between inflammation and coagulation.[40] Ideally, a balance in NETs is needed to prevent excess thrombin generation, while preserving adaptive hemostasis.

The currently available literature on NETs or components of NETs in sepsis mostly originates from adult studies or animal studies. Several adult studies demonstrated increased (derivatives of) NETs during infectious conditions: increased neutrophil elastase-DNA in patients with pneumonia and nonpulmonary sepsis compared with critically ill control subjects,[41] increased plasma histone and cell free (cf)-DNA levels in 17 patients with sepsis compared with critically ill patients without sepsis,[42] elevated cf-DNA and myeloperoxidase DNA in patients with influenza A viral infection,[43] and higher serum cf-DNA/NETs levels in 31 patients with sepsis compared with healthy control subjects.[36] In a study including 60 children with meningococcal sepsis, NET levels were higher in the acute phase of disease, that is, at admission to pediatric intensive care unit and at 24 hours after admission, compared with 1 month after admission.[44] Most of these studies reported an association between NET levels and illness severity or mortality.[36,41,43] Thus, in the early phase of infection, NETs are increased and seem to be associated with illness severity.

SUMMARY

This article reviews the inflammatory and hemostatic response in sepsis, illustrating a complex interplay among host, pathogen, and environmental factors. Meningococci hold unique properties to promote adhesion, colonization, and invasion into the bloodstream. The inflammatory host response, including proinflammatory and anti-inflammatory responses in innate and adaptive immunity, skew toward a proinflammatory state. This leads to endothelial dysfunction and activation of hemostatic response. Within the wide range of illness severity, deposition of fibrin throughout the microcirculation could result in multiple organ dysfunction, the need for skin grafts and amputation, and eventually death.

DISCLOSURE

The authors declare no conflicts of interest.

REFERENCES

1. Martinon-Torres F, Salas A, Rivero-Calle I, et al. Life-threatening infections in children in Europe (the EUCLIDS Project): a prospective cohort study. Lancet Child Adolesc Health 2018;2(6):404–14.
2. Boeddha NP, Schlapbach LJ, Driessen GJ, et al. Mortality and morbidity in community-acquired sepsis in European pediatric intensive care units: a prospective cohort study from the European Childhood Life-threatening Infectious Disease Study (EUCLIDS). Crit Care 2018;22(1):143.
3. Wright V, Hibberd M, Levin M. Genetic polymorphisms in host response to meningococcal infection: the role of susceptibility and severity genes. Vaccine 2009; 27(Suppl 2):B90–102.
4. Emonts M, Hazelzet JA, de Groot R, et al. Host genetic determinants of *Neisseria meningitidis* infections. Lancet Infect Dis 2003;3(9):565–77.

5. Loh E, Kugelberg E, Tracy A, et al. Temperature triggers immune evasion by *Neisseria meningitidis*. Nature 2013;502(7470):237–40.

6. Boeddha NP, Driessen GJ, Cnossen MH, et al. Circadian variation of plasminogen-activator-inhibitor-1 levels in children with meningococcal sepsis. PLoS One 2016;11(11):e0167004.

7. Zeerleder S, Hack CE, Wuillemin WA. Disseminated intravascular coagulation in sepsis. Chest 2005;128(4):2864–75.

8. Dwilow R, Fanella S. Invasive meningococcal disease in the 21st century-an update for the clinician. Curr Neurol Neurosci Rep 2015;15(3):2.

9. Nadel S, Ninis N. Invasive meningococcal disease in the vaccine era. Front Pediatr 2018;6:321.

10. Hotchkiss RS, Monneret G, Payen D. Sepsis-induced immunosuppression: from cellular dysfunctions to immunotherapy. Nat Rev Immunol 2013;13(12):862–74.

11. Netea MG, Balkwill F, Chonchol M, et al. A guiding map for inflammation. Nat Immunol 2017;18(8):826–31.

12. van der Poll T, van de Veerdonk FL, Scicluna BP, et al. The immunopathology of sepsis and potential therapeutic targets. Nat Rev Immunol 2017;17(7):407–20.

13. Muszynski JA, Nofziger R, Moore-Clingenpeel M, et al. Early immune function and duration of organ dysfunction in critically Ill children with sepsis. Am J Respir Crit Care Med 2018;198(3):361–9.

14. Boeddha NP, Kerklaan D, Dunbar A, et al. HLA-DR expression on monocyte subsets in critically Ill children. Pediatr Infect Dis J 2018;37(10):1034–40.

15. Venet F, Lukaszewicz AC, Payen D, et al. Monitoring the immune response in sepsis: a rational approach to administration of immunoadjuvant therapies. Curr Opin Immunol 2013;25(4):477–83.

16. Stephens DS, Hoffman LH, McGee ZA. Interaction of *Neisseria meningitidis* with human nasopharyngeal mucosa: attachment and entry into columnar epithelial cells. J Infect Dis 1983;148(3):369–76.

17. Nassif X, So M. Interaction of pathogenic neisseriae with nonphagocytic cells. Clin Microbiol Rev 1995;8(3):376–88.

18. Schneider MC, Prosser BE, Caesar JJ, et al. Neisseria meningitidis recruits factor H using protein mimicry of host carbohydrates. Nature 2009;458(7240):890–3.

19. Davila S, Wright VJ, Khor CC, et al. Genome-wide association study identifies variants in the CFH region associated with host susceptibility to meningococcal disease. Nat Genet 2010;42(9):772–6.

20. van Deuren M, Brandtzaeg P, van der Meer JW. Update on meningococcal disease with emphasis on pathogenesis and clinical management. Clin Microbiol Rev 2000;13(1):144–66, table of contents.

21. Iba T, Levy JH. Inflammation and thrombosis: roles of neutrophils, platelets and endothelial cells and their interactions in thrombus formation during sepsis. J Thromb Haemost 2018;16(2):231–41.

22. Gando S, Levi M, Toh CH. Disseminated intravascular coagulation. Nat Rev Dis Primers 2016;2:16037.

23. Levi M, van der Poll T. Coagulation and sepsis. Thromb Res 2017;149:38–44.

24. Mairey E, Genovesio A, Donnadieu E, et al. Cerebral microcirculation shear stress levels determine *Neisseria meningitidis* attachment sites along the blood-brain barrier. J Exp Med 2006;203(8):1939–50.

25. Nourshargh S, Hordijk PL, Sixt M. Breaching multiple barriers: leukocyte motility through venular walls and the interstitium. Nat Rev Mol Cell Biol 2010;11(5):366–78.

26. Coureuil M, Join-Lambert O, Lecuyer H, et al. Pathogenesis of meningococce-mia. Cold Spring Harb Perspect Med 2013;3(6) [pii:a012393].
27. Pron B, Taha MK, Rambaud C, et al. Interaction of *Neisseria meningitidis* with the components of the blood-brain barrier correlates with an increased expression of PilC. J Infect Dis 1997;176(5):1285–92.
28. Esmon CT. The protein C pathway. Chest 2003;124(3 Suppl):26S–32S.
29. Macias WL, Nelson DR. Severe protein C deficiency predicts early death in se-vere sepsis. Crit Care Med 2004;32(5 Suppl):S223–8.
30. Hermans PW, Hibberd ML, Booy R, et al. 4G/5G promoter polymorphism in the plasminogen-activator-inhibitor-1 gene and outcome of meningococcal disease. Meningococcal Research Group. Lancet 1999;354(9178):556–60.
31. Li L, Nie W, Zhou H, et al. Association between plasminogen activator inhibitor-1 -675 4G/5G polymorphism and sepsis: a meta-analysis. PLoS One 2013;8(1): e54883.
32. Wong HR. Genetics and genomics in pediatric septic shock. Crit Care Med 2012; 40(5):1618–26.
33. Rautanen A, Mills TC, Gordon AC, et al. Genome-wide association study of sur-vival from sepsis due to pneumonia: an observational cohort study. Lancet Respir Med 2015;3(1):53–60.
34. Kovach MA, Standiford TJ. The function of neutrophils in sepsis. Curr Opin Infect Dis 2012;25(3):321–7.
35. Brinkmann V, Reichard U, Goosmann C, et al. Neutrophil extracellular traps kill bacteria. Science 2004;303(5663):1532–5.
36. Czaikoski PG, Mota JM, Nascimento DC, et al. Neutrophil extracellular traps induce organ damage during experimental and clinical sepsis. PLoS One 2016;11(2):e0148142.
37. McDonald B, Davis RP, Kim SJ, et al. Platelets and neutrophil extracellular traps collaborate to promote intravascular coagulation during sepsis in mice. Blood 2017;129(10):1357–67.
38. Papayannopoulos V. Neutrophil extracellular traps in immunity and disease. Nat Rev Immunol 2018;18(2):134–47.
39. Fuchs TA, Brill A, Duerschmied D, et al. Extracellular DNA traps promote throm-bosis. Proc Natl Acad Sci U S A 2010;107(36):15880–5.
40. Kimball AS, Obi AT, Diaz JA, et al. The emerging ROLE of NETs in venous throm-bosis and immunothrombosis. Front Immunol 2016;7:236.
41. Lefrancais E, Mallavia B, Zhuo H, et al. Maladaptive role of neutrophil extracellular traps in pathogen-induced lung injury. JCI Insight 2018;3(3) [pii:98178].
42. Hashiba M, Huq A, Tomino A, et al. Neutrophil extracellular traps in patients with sepsis. J Surg Res 2015;194(1):248–54.
43. Zhu L, Liu L, Zhang Y, et al. High level of neutrophil extracellular traps correlates with poor prognosis of severe influenza A infection. J Infect Dis 2018;217(3): 428–37.
44. Hoppenbrouwers T, Boeddha NP, Ekinci E, et al. Neutrophil extracellular traps in children with meningococcal sepsis. Pediatr Crit Care Med 2018;19(6):e286–91.

Immune Consequences of Endothelial Cells' Activation and Dysfunction During Sepsis

Stéphanie Pons, MD[a], Marine Arnaud, MSc[a], Maud Loiselle, MD[a], Eden Arrii[a], Elie Azoulay, MD, PhD[b], Lara Zafrani, MD, PhD[a,b,*]

KEYWORDS

- Endothelial dysfunction • Hemostasis • Barrier function • Sepsis • Innate immunity
- Adaptive immunity

KEY POINTS

- Endothelial cells have a crucial role in several physiologic processes: blood fluidity, vasomotor tone regulation, osmotic balance, and vascular barrier function.
- Sepsis, a state of systemic inflammation, induces endothelial cell activation but can lead to endothelial dysfunction and multiorgan failure.
- The endothelium has a key role in organizing the innate immune response during sepsis, but it also exhibits properties involved in the activation of adaptive immunity.

INTRODUCTION

The vascular endothelium is a cell monolayer covering the inner layer of the blood vessels providing a direct interface between the circulating blood cells and parenchymal cells. The endothelium is composed of 1 to 6×10^{13} endothelial cells (ECs) covering a surface of 1000 m^2.[1] The vascular endothelium has a fundamental role in multiple physiologic processes such as vasomotor tone regulation, primary hemostasis, osmotic balance, and vascular barrier function.[2,3] ECs also perform important immunologic functions. By sensing pathogens' components present in blood, ECs are capable of initiating the innate immune response.[4] ECs are also conditional antigen-presenting cells (APCs) and allow, in some specific situations, the initiation of adaptive immunity and local recruitment of antigen (Ag)-specific lymphocytes.[5]

Sepsis is defined as a life-threatening organ dysfunction caused by a dysregulated host response to infection.[6] During tissue invasion by a pathogen, the recognition of

[a] INSERM U976, Saint-Louis Teaching Hospital, 1, Avenue Claude Vellefaux, Paris 75010, France;
[b] Medical Intensive Care Unit, Saint-Louis Teaching Hospital, 1, Avenue Claude Vellefaux, Paris 75010, France
* Corresponding author. Medical Intensive Care Unit, Saint-Louis Teaching Hospital, 1, Avenue Claude Vellefaux, Paris 75010, France.
E-mail address: lara.zafrani@aphp.fr

Crit Care Clin 36 (2020) 401–413
https://doi.org/10.1016/j.ccc.2019.12.001
0749-0704/20/© 2019 Elsevier Inc. All rights reserved.

criticalcare.theclinics.com

pathogen-associated molecular patterns (PAMPs) by specific receptors activates a powerful innate inflammatory reaction. The uncontrolled amplification of the host's proinflammatory response can lead to septic shock and the failure of distant, non-infected organs.[7] Thus, sepsis is known to induce severe EC dysfunction leading to dysregulation of homeostasis, tissue edema, and vascular barrier disruption.[8,9] Moreover, sepsis activates the immune properties of ECs, inducing the activation of innate and adaptive immunity.

This review discusses many of the latest insights into the immune functions of ECs and the immune consequences of endothelial cell activation and dysfunction during sepsis.

RESTING ENDOTHELIAL CELLS

In basal conditions, vascular ECs display transport and permeability functions, and maintain and regulate blood flow. All these fundamental homeostatic functions have already been reviewed in depth elsewhere.[10–13]

In brief, the endothelium plays a crucial role in homeostasis. Based on structural aspects, ECs express tight junctions, adherens junctions, and gap junctions.[14–16] Intercellular junctions can dynamically change and allow the passage of cellular elements, fluid, and molecules from the vascular space to the peripheral tissue, via the paracellular pathway.[17,18] However, transport properties are tissue dependent. For example, the permeability of the blood-brain barrier is extremely limited with a high density of inter-EC tight junctions that restrict solute transport and only allow free water to cross paracellularly. Concomitantly, ECs mediate a controlled passage of proteins via vesicular transport (transcellular pathway).[19] Thus, the transcytosis process is regulated by different factors, such as caveolin-1, a component of the vesicles, and different signaling molecules.[20,21] The integrity of the endothelium as a barrier and transporter of solutes is also largely determined by the endothelial cytoskeleton and the glycocalyx. The glycocalyx mediates several other key physiologic processes such as hemostasis, leukocyte and platelet adhesion, and shear-stress transmission to the endothelium.[22]

The endothelium is also involved in blood vessel formation. Vascular endothelial growth factor (VEGF) is the most important molecule involved in vascular formation because it is required to initiate the angiogenesis of immature vessels. Other molecules such as angiopoietins are also important for vessel maturation.[23]

ECs also provide a nonthrombogenic inner layer of the vascular wall that helps to maintain blood fluidity, allowing the blood to flow without systemic bleeding or clotting. Different anticoagulant and antiplatelet mechanisms are essential to prevent thrombosis.[24] The expression of tissue factor pathway inhibitor (TFPI) blocking the initiation of coagulation and the expression of heparan sulfate proteoglycans binding antithrombin III are important anticoagulant mechanisms.[25] Moreover, ECs synthesize thrombomodulin (TM), an anticoagulant protein that binds to thrombin. TM modulates substrate specificity of thrombin and activates protein C, which in association with protein S inactivates factors V and VIII and inhibits coagulation.[26] Activation of coagulation also requires a phospholipid surface, enriched in phosphatidylserine, provided by activated platelets. Resting ECs prevent platelet activation by secreting nitric oxide (NO), prostaglandins and proteases, and a disintegrin and metalloprotease with thrombospondin type I repeats (ADAMTS)-13 or ADAMTS-18, which cleave hyperactive ultralarge von Willebrand factor (vWF) monomers into active vWF fragments.[27] ECs also prevent platelet activation by contact with the basement membrane collagen.[28] Finally, ECs participate in thrombolysis by tissue-plasminogen activator and urokinase synthesis, promoting the conversion of plasminogen to plasmin.[29,30]

ECs play a role in the regulation of vasomotor tone in response to both physiologic and chemical factors circulating in the vascular lumen or secreted by surrounding tissues. The most important vasodilating mediator synthesized by ECs is NO.[31] ECs constitutively express NO synthase 3, which is activated by shear forces sensed by the ECs, inducing a low basal production of NO.[32] Blood flow is also regulated by the inducible synthesis of mediators, such as prostacyclin, endothelin, or platelet-activating factor, which increase or decrease the tone of the surrounding vascular smooth muscle cells[33,34] (**Fig. 1**).

Finally, resting ECs do not interact with leukocytes because leukocyte-interactive proteins (P-selectin and chemokines) are internalized into Weibel-Palade bodies, which are specialized vesicles.[35,36] Resting ECs also suppress the transcription of other adhesion molecules (E-selectin, vascular cell adhesion molecule 1 [VCAM-1], and intercellular adhesion molecule 1 [ICAM-1]). The absence of interaction between circulating leukocytes or platelets and resting ECs is also due to the presence of a healthy glycocalyx layer, which normally is a couple of hundred nanometers taller than typical adhesion molecules and recovers them.[37]

Failure of ECs to adequately perform any of these basal functions constitutes "endothelial cell dysfunction." These dysfunctions activate the innate and adaptive responses and are crucial in the pathophysiology of sepsis-induced organ failure.

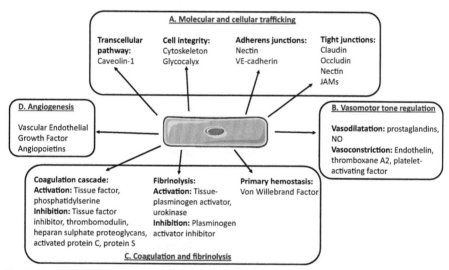

Fig. 1. Physiologic functions of endothelial cells (ECs) depend on secretion and expression of several molecules. ECs exhibit a key role in different physiologic processes, such as molecular and cellular trafficking (A), vasomotor tone regulation (B), coagulation and fibrinolysis (C), and angiogenesis (D). (A) Cell integrity, adherens junctions, and tight junctions are essential to regulate the paracellular and transcellular endothelial trafficking of molecules and cells. (B) ECs display an active role in vasomotor tone regulation. The main vasorelaxant mediator that is synthesized by ECs is NO.[31] Blood flow is also regulated by the inducible synthesis of mediators, such as prostacyclin, endothelin, or platelet-activating factor that increase or decrease the tone of the surrounding vascular smooth muscle cells. (C) Coagulation and fibrinolysis are highly regulated by ECs. Different anticoagulant and antiplatelet mechanisms are necessary to prevent thrombosis or bleeding. (D) The endothelium is also involved in blood vessel formation. Vascular endothelial growth factor is the most important molecule involved in vascular formation, and other molecules such as angiopoietins are important for vessel maturation. JAMs, junctional adhesion molecules; NO, nitric oxide.

ROLE OF ENDOTHELIAL CELLS IN INNATE IMMUNITY

Sepsis, as well as other diseases, induces acute systemic inflammation but overall can lead to homeostasis dysregulation by the loss or inappropriate exaggeration of ECs functions. Acute inflammation induces "endothelial cell activation," defined as the acquisition of new properties by resting ECs.[10] Different stimuli that are released into the blood circulation, such as PAMPs (ie, lipopolysaccharide [LPS]) or proinflammatory cytokines, may activate ECs and provoke proinflammatory responses.[38]

Endothelial Cells in Pathogen Recognition

The first step of innate immunity activation is the recognition of PAMPs or damage associated molecular patterns (DAMPs) through pattern-recognition receptors, such as toll-like receptors (TLRs). TLRs are surface receptors recognizing these biomolecules and initiating signals resulting in proinflammatory gene expression, leukocyte chemotaxis, phagocytosis, and activation of adaptive immune responses.[39] ECs display different TLRs on their surface.[40] In general, TLR-2 and TLR-4 are ubiquitously present within the vasculature, whereas other TLRs are expressed in specific conditions.[41] ECs are heterogeneous, displaying specific phenotypes and functions depending on the organ. Similarly, TLR expression depends on the organic origin of ECs. The activation of ECs through TLRs can occur directly through recognition of DAMPs or PAMPs, or may depend on a prior inflammatory stimulus such as that induced by interferon-γ (IFN-γ), LPS, tumor necrosis factor α (TNF-α), or interleukin (IL)-1b. For instance, TLR-3 is present on human vascular ECs and direct ligation by poly(I:C) upregulates TLR-2, IFN-γ, IL-28, IL-29, and signal transducers and activators of transcription 1 (STAT-1) expression.[42] TLR-4 expression has been found on various ECs and significantly increases under inflammatory conditions. LPS is recognized by TLR-4 and activates nuclear factor κB in microvascular ECs. Moreover, LPS, IFN-γ, and TNF-α upregulate TLR-4 mRNA and protein expression.[43] Other receptors involved in innate immunity have been detected in ECs, such as the NOD-like receptors (NLR)-1 and -2. NLRs are cytosolic proteins that detect microbial peptides and regulate inflammation[44] and, like TLRs, are also upregulated in response to LPS and proinflammatory cytokines.[45]

Inflammation and Endothelial Cells

Vasodilation is one of the first endothelial responses that occur during inflammation. It is regulated by the vasoactive molecules NO and prostacyclin, which are released by stimulated ECs, resulting in the relaxation of surrounding smooth muscle cells.[46] Prostaglandins also induce vasodilatation. They are generated by the action of cyclooxygenase enzymes on arachidonic acid, cross the intercellular space, and elicit the relaxation of muscle cells.[47] Other molecules have been found to cause vasodilation during inflammation, including C-type natriuretic peptide, hydrogen sulfide, or the potassium ion.[48,49]

Mediators of local inflammation, such as kinins, cytokines, histamine, and arachidonic acids, as well as complement components such as C3a and C5a, also increase capillary permeability. Moreover, proinflammatory molecules, such as TNF-α, can lead to the removal of occludin and junctional adhesion molecule A from the tight junctions, increasing permeability.[50] This increase in permeability can result in immune cell infiltration, edema, and severe damage to the endothelium. LPS recognition by ECs can also directly initiate angiogenesis through TNF receptor-associated factor 6-dependent signaling pathways.[51] This angiogenic signaling pathways is also implicated in vascular permeability, via VEGFs/VEGF receptors and angiopoietins/Tie receptors. Thus, VEGF, also known as vascular permeability factor, strongly increases vascular permeability.[52]

On activation by inflammatory factors such as IL-1β and TNF-α, or in response to pathogen detection, ECs increase the expression of adhesion molecules, namely ICAM-1, VCAM-1, and E-selectin, and P-selectin, leading to increased adhesion of leukocytes and platelets and transmigration of leukocytes through the vascular wall. Moreover, in conditions of inflammation and sepsis, cytokines and reactive species induce glycocalyx shedding, exposing the adhesion molecules on EC surface and initiating leukocyte adhesion and their subsequent transmigration to the tissues.[53] The general model for leukocyte recruitment by ECs involves a multistep cascade.[54] First, leukocyte rolling is mediated by L-selectin, P-selectin, and E-selectin, which interact with P-selectin glycoprotein ligand 1 and other glycosylated ligands.[55,56] L-selectin is expressed by most leukocytes, whereas E-selectin and P-selectin are expressed by inflamed ECs. The interactions between selectins and their ligands enable leukocytes to adhere to the endothelium under conditions of blood flow.[57] Leukocyte arrest during rolling is then triggered by chemokines or other chemoattractants and is mediated by the binding of leukocyte integrins to immunoglobulin superfamily members, such as ICAM-1 and VCAM-1, expressed by ECs.[58,59] Transmigration through the endothelium is the final step in the process of leukocyte migration into inflamed tissues and can occur with minimal disruption of vessel walls. Two routes are possible. The first is paracellular migration, which involves the release of EC vascular endothelial cadherin (VE-cadherin) and is facilitated by intracellular membrane compartments containing PECAM-1 (platelet endothelial cell adhesion molecule 1).[60,61] Transcellular leukocyte migration represents the route of migration for only a minority of emigrating cells, occurring in the central nervous system and in *in vitro* models.[62,63] After recruitment to the inflammatory site, neutrophils release antimicrobial peptides and lytic enzymes, and produce reactive oxygen species or initiate phagocytosis to eliminate the pathogen.[64] In addition to classic phagocytosis, neutrophils can release chromatin, nuclear proteins, and serine proteases extracellularly to form neutrophil extracellular traps (NETs). NETs can trap pathogens and limit their dispersion, initiate coagulation, and induce endothelial injury. Increasing experimental and clinical evidence indicates that NET formation during sepsis can lead to the development of multiple organ dysfunction.[65,66]

Finally, during inflammation ECs exhibit antifibrinolytic and procoagulant properties. Inflammatory molecules (TNF-α, LPS) or damaged ECs initiate coagulation by increasing the expression of tissue factor (TF) on monocytes and on ECs *in vitro*.[67,68] Once expressed, TF binds and activates factor VII, which in turn activates factors IX and X. This coagulation cascade leads to thrombin and then clot formation.[69] Moreover, regulatory anticoagulant systems such as protein C or TFPI are defective, which amplifies intravascular thrombus formation. A proinflammatory state may also decrease endothelial expression of TM, leading to a decreased activation of protein C. Moreover, the granulocytes recruited at the inflammatory site release elastases that cleave and inactivate endothelial TM. In addition, the fibrinolytic pathway is suppressed during sepsis by the increased release of plasminogen activator inhibitor by the endothelium.[70] Finally, inflammatory mediators can inactivate ADAMTS-13, increasing the prothrombotic state.[71] Thus, sepsis can lead to disseminated microvascular thrombosis, organ ischemia, and multiple organ failure (**Fig. 2**).

ROLE OF ENDOTHELIAL CELLS IN ADAPTIVE IMMUNITY

ECs may also participate in the activation of adaptive immunity via several pathways. As already mentioned, ECs, like dendritic cells, are reported to express both TLRs and NLRs. Muramyl dipeptide, a bacterial component, is recognized by NLR-2 in ECs,

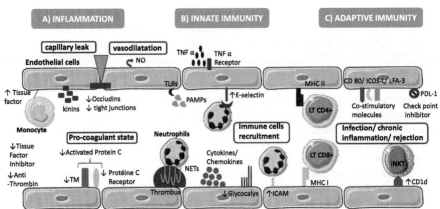

Fig. 2. Role of activated endothelium in inflammation, and innate and adaptive immunity. (A) Endothelial cells (ECs) are activated during inflammation, leading to the dysfunction of physiologic roles of the endothelium. Vasodilation is one of the first endothelial responses that occur during inflammation. It is regulated by the vasoactive molecules NO and prostacyclin, which are released by stimulated ECs. Capillary leak is secondary to the secretion of mediators of local inflammation, such as kinins, cytokines, histamine, and arachidonic acids, but also because occludin is then removed from the tight junctions, leading to increased permeability. Inflammation also induces a procoagulant state by increasing the expression of TF on monocytes and on ECs, inducing the initiation of the coagulation cascade. Moreover, inflammatory conditions decrease the level of antithrombin and of TF inhibitor. Finally, a proinflammatory state may also decrease endothelial expression of thrombomodulin, leading to decreased activation of protein C. (B) ECs may also initiate a powerful innate immune response. On activation by inflammatory factors such as tumor necrosis factor α or in response to the detection of PAMPs by their TLRs, ECs increase the expression of adhesion molecules intercellular adhesion molecule 1, E-selectin, and P-selectin, leading to an increased adhesion of leukocytes and platelets and transmigration of leukocytes through the vascular wall. Moreover, during sepsis, cytokines induce glycocalyx shedding, exposing the adhesion molecules that initiate leukocyte adhesion. During sepsis, in addition to classic phagocytosis, neutrophils can release chromatin, nuclear proteins, and serine proteases extracellularly to form NETs. NETs can trap pathogens and limit their dispersion, initiate coagulation, and induce endothelial injury. (C) In specific conditions, such as prolonged infection, chronic inflammation, and transplant rejection, ECs may initiate an adaptive immune response. ECs express class I MHC and, depending on the vasculature/organ, class II MHC. They are also able to process antigens and can act as antigen-presenting cells. Moreover, some ECs express various molecules, including CD80, lymphocyte function-associated antigen 3, inducible T cell costimulator ligand, which is known to be a lymphocyte T costimulatory molecule, or programmed death ligand 1, a coinhibitory molecule. ECs can also upregulate the expression of CD1d, an MHC-I–like molecule able to present Ag to invariant natural killer T cells. CD, cluster of differentiation; ICAM, intercellular adhesion molecule 1; ICOS-L, inducible T cell costimulator ligand; iNKT, invariant natural killer T cells; LFA-3, lymphocyte function-associated antigen 3; LT, T lymphocyte; MHC, major histocompatibility complex; NETs, neutrophil extracellular traps; NO, nitric oxide; PAMPs, pathogen-associated molecular patterns; PDL-1, programmed death ligand 1; TLR, toll-like receptor; TM, thrombomodulin; TNF-α, tumor necrosis factor α.

leading to the upregulation of IL-6 secretion, which induces CD4$^+$ T helper cell (Th)17 polarization and inhibits CD4$^+$ Th1 and Th2 responses.[72] Moreover, platelet-EC interactions may participate in adaptive immunity activation. Indeed, platelets produce soluble CD40L, which engages the CD40 present on EC surface. This interaction leads to adhesion molecule expression, chemokine and cytokine secretion, and leukocyte recruitment. Thus, activated platelets act like activated T cells, which release CD40L.[73] ECs also express class I major histocompatibility complex (MHC) and depending on the vasculature/organ, class II MHC.[74,75] They are also able to process Ags and can act as APCs.[76] During sepsis, T cell migration into inflamed tissue involves the adhesion of the cells to the microvascular ECs. During cell transmigration, recognition of cognate MHC-peptide complex by specific T lymphocytes may occur. Moreover, some ECs also express various molecules, including CD80, CD86, lymphocyte function-associated antigen 3, inducible T cell costimulator ligand, programmed death ligand (PDL)-1 or -2, CD40, and CD134L, which are known to be lymphocyte T costimulatory or coinhibitory molecules.[77,78] Ag presentation, costimulatory molecules expression and cytokines secretion are necessary to activate T cells. However, CD80 and CD86, costimulators, which are necessary for naïve T cell activation, are absent from most endothelia. Thus, it seems that ECs cannot activate naïve lymphocytes but can mediate Ag-specific stimulation of Ag effector or memory CD4 and CD8 lymphocytes.[79–81] It has also been shown that human ECs could have a role in reinforcing T cell proliferation and increasing T regulator lymphocyte (Treg) suppressor function.[82] Moreover, under inflammatory conditions, human ECs can generate Th17 and Treg.[5] Treg recruitment to the site of inflammation is also induced by their ability to recognize self-Ags presented by the endothelium.[83] ECs can also upregulate the expression of CD1d, an MHC-I–like molecule, able to present Ag to invariant natural killer T cells (iNKT)[84] (see **Fig. 2**). However, the direct evidence of Ag presentation by ECs to iNKT in vivo has not yet been obtained. As explained earlier, ECs also express class I MHC and can present cognate Ag, inducing the activation of memory CD8 cytotoxic T lymphocytes and endothelial cell killing. The expression of both PDL-1 and PDL-2 downregulates CD8 T cell activation and cytolysis.[85–87] Another property of ECs, as conditional APCs, is to either induce inflammation or immune tolerance. Thus, liver sinusoidal ECs can induce Ag-specific CD8$^+$ T cell tolerance, Treg differentiation, and Th17 and Th1 response inhibition.[88,89]

Finally, during endothelial damage, endothelial progenitor cells (EPCs) may be mobilized to repair the vascular lesion.[90] EPCs exhibit the same T cell–activating properties as ECs.[91] EPCs express both endothelial markers (CD31, VEGF receptor 2, and vWF) and monocytic lineage markers (CD14 and several chemokines). EPCs display antigen-presenting capacity similar to that of monocytes and much stronger than in human vascular ECs. EPCs also express costimulatory molecules such as CD80 and CD86 on their surface, being therefore able to significantly activate naïve T cells.[92] It is interesting that circulating EPCs increase during sepsis but their role in T cell activation in this disease has never been studied.[93]

ENDOTHELIAL CELL HETEROGENEITY AND ORGAN DYSFUNCTION DURING SEPSIS

The endothelium plays a central role in the pathogenesis of sepsis leading to multiorgan failure syndrome. The endothelium is highly heterogeneous in morphology and function between different organs, and between different vessels in the same organ. For example, during sepsis, the procoagulant properties of ECs are differentially regulated between vascular beds. Yamamoto and Loskutoff[94] showed that LPS infusion may result in organ-specific deposition of fibrin in the kidney and adrenal gland. In another study, the administration of LPS in mice induced a decrease in TM expression in the lung and brain but not in the kidney. Similarly, Yano and colleagues[95] showed in an experimental model of endotoxemia that ICAM-1 mRNA expression was induced 18-fold in the kidney compared with 6-fold in the heart, 2-fold in the liver, or 2-fold in the lung. The concept of EC heterogeneity is crucial in understanding the pathophysiology of sepsis and multiple organ failure, because different organs will display various responses to sepsis. Such diversity is reflected in the heterogeneity of the response of the various organs during sepsis.

SUMMARY

The endothelium has a fundamental role in many essential physiologic functions. Its heterogeneity in morphology and function explains that its roles can vary from one organ to another or according to the type of vessel. Moreover, owing to their localization, ECs are one of the first cells able to detect circulating pathogens and can initiate a powerful proinflammatory response as well as the recruitment and trafficking of innate immune cells. ECs may also participate in the activation of adaptive immunity by several pathways. Expressing MHC-1 and MHC-2 and a wide range of costimulatory molecules, they may, under specific conditions, initiate Ag-specific lymphocyte recruitment and induce Th17 or Treg generation. In doing so, ECs are active regulators of innate and adaptive immune functions and may become a future target for immunomodulatory therapeutics for sepsis and septic shock.

DISCLOSURE

S. Pons received a research grant from the French Intensive Care Society and one from the European Society of Intensive Care Medicine. L. Zafrani and M. Arnaud received a research grant from Jazz Pharma. E. Arrii has received fees for lectures from MSD, Pfizer, and Alexion. Her institution and research group have received support from Baxter, Jazz Pharma, Fisher & Payckle, Gilead, Alexion, and Ablynx. The remaining authors have disclosed that they do not have any conflicts of interest.

REFERENCES

1. Jaffe EA. Cell biology of endothelial cells. Hum Pathol 1987;18(3):234–9.
2. Roumenina LT, Rayes J, Frimat M, et al. Endothelial cells: source, barrier, and target of defensive mediators. Immunol Rev 2016;274(1):307–29.
3. Daniel AE, van Buul JD. Endothelial junction regulation: a prerequisite for leukocytes crossing the vessel wall. J Innate Immun 2013;5(4):324–35.
4. Salvador B, Arranz A, Francisco S, et al. Modulation of endothelial function by Toll like receptors. Pharmacol Res 2016;108:46–56.
5. Taflin C, Favier B, Baudhuin J, et al. Human endothelial cells generate Th17 and regulatory T cells under inflammatory conditions. Proc Natl Acad Sci U S A 2011; 108(7):2891–6.
6. Singer M, Deutschman CS, Seymour CW, et al. The Third International Consensus definitions for sepsis and septic shock (Sepsis-3). JAMA 2016;315(8):801–10.
7. Delano MJ, Ward PA. The immune system's role in sepsis progression, resolution, and long-term outcome. Immunol Rev 2016;274(1):330–53.
8. Teixeira MM, Williams TJ, Hellewell PG. Role of prostaglandins and nitric oxide in acute inflammatory reactions in Guinea-pig skin. Br J Pharmacol 1993;110(4): 1515–21.
9. Leclerc J, Pu Q, Corseaux D, et al. A single endotoxin injection in the rabbit causes prolonged blood vessel dysfunction and a procoagulant state. Crit Care Med 2000;28(11):3672–8.
10. Pober JS, Sessa WC. Evolving functions of endothelial cells in inflammation. Nat Rev Immunol 2007;7(10):803–15.

11. Busse R, Fleming I. Vascular endothelium and blood flow. Handb Exp Pharmacol 2006;(176 Pt 2):43–78.
12. Muller WA. Transendothelial migration: unifying principles from the endothelial perspective. Immunol Rev 2016;273(1):61–75.
13. Radeva MY, Waschke J. Mind the gap: mechanisms regulating the endothelial barrier. Acta Physiol 2018;222(1).
14. Luscinskas FW, Shaw SK. The biology of endothelial cell-cell lateral junctions. Microcirculation 2001;8(3):141–2.
15. Saez JC, Berthoud VM, Branes MC, et al. Plasma membrane channels formed by connexins: their regulation and functions. Physiol Rev 2003;83(4):1359–400.
16. Aijaz S, Balda MS, Matter K. Tight junctions: molecular architecture and function. Int Rev Cytol 2006;248:261–98.
17. Taveau J-C, Dubois M, Le Bihan O, et al. Structure of artificial and natural VE-cadherin-based adherens junctions. Biochem Soc Trans 2008;36(Pt 2):189–93.
18. Sui XF, Kiser TD, Hyun SW, et al. Receptor protein tyrosine phosphatase micro regulates the paracellular pathway in human lung microvascular endothelia. Am J Pathol 2005;166(4):1247–58.
19. Frank PG, Woodman SE, Park DS, et al. Caveolin, caveolae, and endothelial cell function. Arterioscler Thromb Vasc Biol 2003;23(7):11611168.
20. Machleidt T, Li WP, Liu P, et al. Multiple domains in caveolin-1 control its intracellular traffic. J Cell Biol 2000;148(1):17–28.
21. Shajahan AN, Timblin BK, Sandoval R, et al. Role of Src-induced dynamin-2 phosphorylation in caveolae-mediated endocytosis in endothelial cells. J Biol Chem 2004;279(19):20392–400.
22. Pillinger NL, Kam P. Endothelial glycocalyx: basic science and clinical implications. Anaesth Intensive Care 2017;45(3):295–307.
23. Visconti RP, Richardson CD, Sato TN. Orchestration of angiogenesis and arteriovenous contribution by angiopoietins and vascular endothelial growth factor (VEGF). Proc Natl Acad Sci U S A 2002;99(12):8219–24.
24. Yau JW, Teoh H, Verma S. Endothelial cell control of thrombosis. BMC Cardiovasc Disord 2015;15:130.
25. Wood JP, Ellery PER, Maroney SA, et al. Biology of tissue factor pathway inhibitor. Blood 2014;123(19):2934–43.
26. Anastasiou G, Gialeraki A, Merkouri E, et al. Thrombomodulin as a regulator of the anticoagulant pathway: implication in the development of thrombosis. Blood Coagul Fibrinolysis 2012;23(1):1–10.
27. Giblin JP, Hewlett LJ, Hannah MJ. Basal secretion of von Willebrand factor from human endothelial cells. Blood 2008;112(4):957–64.
28. Watson SP. Platelet activation by extracellular matrix proteins in haemostasis and thrombosis. Curr Pharm Des 2009;15(12):1358–72.
29. Rijken DC, Lijnen HR. New insights into the molecular mechanisms of the fibrinolytic system. J Thromb Haemost 2009;7(1):4–13.
30. Huber D, Cramer EM, Kaufmann JE, et al. Tissue-type plasminogen activator (t-PA) is stored in Weibel-Palade bodies in human endothelial cells both in vitro and in vivo. Blood 2002;99(10):3637–45.
31. Weitzberg E, Hezel M, Lundberg JO. Nitrate-nitrite-nitric oxide pathway: implications for anesthesiology and intensive care. Anesthesiology 2010;113(6):1460–75.
32. Moncada S, Higgs A. The L-arginine-nitric oxide pathway. N Engl J Med 1993;329(27):2002–12.
33. Levin ER. Endothelins. N Engl J Med 1995;333(6):356–63.

34. Lopes-Martins R, Catelli M, Araújo C, et al. Pharmacological evidence of a role for platelet activating factor as a modulator of vasomotor tone and blood pressure. Eur J Pharmacol 1996;308(3):287–94.

35. Shcheglovitova ON, Boldyreva NV, Sklyankina NN, et al. IFN-α, IFN-β, and IFN-γ have different effect on the production of proinflammatory factors deposited in Weibel-palade bodies of endothelial cells infected with Herpes Simplex Virus type 1. Bull Exp Biol Med 2016;161(2):270–5.

36. McCormack JJ, Lopes da Silva M, Ferraro F, et al. Weibel-Palade bodies at a glance. J Cell Sci 2017;130(21):3611–7.

37. Marki A, Esko JD, Pries AR, et al. Role of the endothelial surface layer in neutrophil recruitment. J Leukoc Biol 2015;98(4):503–15.

38. Brevetti G, Giugliano G, Brevetti L, et al. Inflammation in peripheral artery disease. Circulation 2010;122(18):1862–75.

39. Iwasaki A, Medzhitov R. Toll-like receptor control of the adaptive immune responses. Nat Immunol 2004;5(10):987–95.

40. Heidemann J, Domschke W, Kucharzik T, et al. Intestinal microvascular endothelium and innate immunity in inflammatory bowel disease: a second line of defense? Infect Immun 2006;74(10):5425–32.

41. Khakpour S, Wilhelmsen K, Hellman J. Vascular endothelial cell Toll-like receptor pathways in sepsis. Innate Immun 2015;21(8):827–46.

42. Tissari J, Sirén J, Meri S, et al. IFN-alpha enhances TLR3-mediated antiviral cytokine expression in human endothelial and epithelial cells by up-regulating TLR3 expression. J Immunol 2005;174(7):4289–94.

43. Faure E, Thomas L, Xu H, et al. Bacterial lipopolysaccharide and IFN-gamma induce Toll-like receptor 2 and Toll-like receptor 4 expression in human endothelial cells: role of NF-kappa B activation. J Immunol 2001;166(3):2018–24.

44. Opitz B, Püschel A, Beermann W, et al. *Listeria monocytogenes* activated p38 MAPK and induced IL-8 secretion in a nucleotide-binding oligomerization domain 1-dependent manner in endothelial cells. J Immunol 2006;176(1):484–90.

45. Oh H-M, Lee H-J, Seo G-S, et al. Induction and localization of NOD2 protein in human endothelial cells. Cell Immunol 2005;237(1):37–44.

46. Quillon A, Fromy B, Debret R. Endothelium microenvironment sensing leading to nitric oxide mediated vasodilation: a review of nervous and biomechanical signals. Nitric Oxide 2015;45:20–6.

47. Ricciotti E, FitzGerald GA. Prostaglandins and inflammation. Arterioscler Thromb Vasc Biol 2011;31(5):986–1000.

48. Edwards G, Dora KA, Gardener MJ, et al. K^+ is an endothelium-derived hyperpolarizing factor in rat arteries. Nature 1998;396(6708):269–72.

49. Chauhan SD, Nilsson H, Ahluwalia A, et al. Release of C-type natriuretic peptide accounts for the biological activity of endothelium-derived hyperpolarizing factor. Proc Natl Acad Sci U S A 2003;100(3):1426–31.

50. McKenzie JAG, Ridley AJ. Roles of Rho/ROCK and MLCK in TNF-alpha-induced changes in endothelial morphology and permeability. J Cell Physiol 2007;213(1):221–8.

51. Pollet I, Opina CJ, Zimmerman C, et al. Bacterial lipopolysaccharide directly induces angiogenesis through TRAF6-mediated activation of NF-kappaB and c-Jun N-terminal kinase. Blood 2003;102(5):1740–2.

52. Hippenstiel S, Krüll M, Ikemann A, et al. VEGF induces hyperpermeability by a direct action on endothelial cells. Am J Physiol 1998;274(5):L678–84.

53. Uchimido R, Schmidt EP, Shapiro NI. The glycocalyx: a novel diagnostic and therapeutic target in sepsis. Crit Care 2019;23(1):16.

54. Ley K, Laudanna C, Cybulsky MI, et al. Getting to the site of inflammation: the leukocyte adhesion cascade updated. Nat Rev Immunol 2007;7(9):678–89.

55. Kansas GS. Selectins and their ligands: current concepts and controversies. Blood 1996;88(9):3259–87.

56. McEver RP, Cummings RD. Perspectives series: cell adhesion in vascular biology. Role of PSGL-1 binding to selectins in leukocyte recruitment. J Clin Invest 1997;100(3):485–91.

57. Alon R, Hammer DA, Springer TA. Lifetime of the P-selectin-carbohydrate bond and its response to tensile force in hydrodynamic flow. Nature 1995;374(6522): 539–42.

58. Campbell JJ, Qin S, Bacon KB, et al. Biology of chemokine and classical chemo-attractant receptors: differential requirements for adhesion-triggering versus chemotactic responses in lymphoid cells. J Cell Biol 1996;134(1):255–66.

59. Campbell JJ, Hedrick J, Zlotnik A, et al. Chemokines and the arrest of lympho-cytes rolling under flow conditions. Science 1998;279(5349):381–4.

60. Muller WA. Leukocyte-endothelial-cell interactions in leukocyte transmigration and the inflammatory response. Trends Immunol 2003;24(6):327–34.

61. Shaw SK, Bamba PS, Perkins BN, et al. Real-time imaging of vascular endothelial-cadherin during leukocyte transmigration across endothelium. J Immunol 2001;167(4):2323–30.

62. Cinamon G, Shinder V, Shamri R, et al. Chemoattractant signals and beta 2 integ-rin occupancy at apical endothelial contacts combine with shear stress signals to promote transendothelial neutrophil migration. J Immunol 2004;173(12):7282–91.

63. Millán J, Hewlett L, Glyn M, et al. Lymphocyte transcellular migration occurs through recruitment of endothelial ICAM-1 to caveola- and F-actin-rich domains. Nat Cell Biol 2006;8(2):113–23.

64. Nathan C. Neutrophils and immunity: challenges and opportunities. Nat Rev Im-munol 2006;6(3):173–82.

65. Czaikoski PG, Mota JMSC, Nascimento DC, et al. Neutrophil extracellular traps induce organ damage during experimental and clinical sepsis. PLoS One 2016;11(2):e0148142.

66. Dwivedi DJ, Toltl LJ, Swystun LL, et al. Prognostic utility and characterization of cell-free DNA in patients with severe sepsis. Crit Care 2012;16(4):R151.

67. Franco RF, de Jonge E, Dekkers PE, et al. The in vivo kinetics of tissue factor messenger RNA expression during human endotoxemia: relationship with activa-tion of coagulation. Blood 2000;96(2):554–9.

68. Heyderman RS, Klein NJ, Daramola OA, et al. Induction of human endothelial tis-sue factor expression by *Neisseria meningitidis*: the influence of bacterial killing and adherence to the endothelium. Microb Pathog 1997;22(5):265–74.

69. Schouten M, Wiersinga WJ, Levi M, et al. Inflammation, endothelium, and coag-ulation in sepsis. J Leukoc Biol 2008;83(3):536–45.

70. Kinasewitz GT, Yan SB, Basson B, et al. Universal changes in biomarkers of coag-ulation and inflammation occur in patients with severe sepsis, regardless of caus-ative micro-organism [ISRCTN74215569]. Crit Care 2004;8(2):R82–90.

71. Nolasco LH, Turner NA, Bernardo A, et al. Hemolytic uremic syndrome-associated Shiga toxins promote endothelial-cell secretion and impair ADAMTS13 cleavage of unusually large von Willebrand factor multimers. Blood 2005;106(13):4199–209.

72. Manni M, Ding W, Stohl LL, et al. Muramyl dipeptide induces Th17 polarization through activation of endothelial cells. J Immunol 2011;186(6):3356–63.

73. Danese S, Fiocchi C. Platelet activation and the CD40/CD40 ligand pathway: mechanisms and implications for human disease. Crit Rev Immunol 2005;25(2): 103–21.

74. Lozanoska-Ochser B, Peakman M. Level of major histocompatibility complex class I expression on endothelium in non-obese diabetic mice influences CD8 T cell adhesion and migration. Clin Exp Immunol 2009;157(1):119–27.

75. Abrahimi P, Qin L, Chang WG, et al. Blocking MHC class II on human endothelium mitigates acute rejection. JCI Insight 2016;1(1).

76. Savage CO, Brooks CJ, Harcourt GC, et al. Human vascular endothelial cells process and present autoantigen to human T cell lines. Int Immunol 1995;7(3):471–9.

77. Khayyamian S, Hutloff A, Büchner K, et al. ICOS-ligand, expressed on human endothelial cells, costimulates Th1 and Th2 cytokine secretion by memory $CD4^+$ T cells. Proc Natl Acad Sci U S A 2002;99(9):6198–203.

78. Satoh S, Suzuki A, Asari Y, et al. Glomerular endothelium exhibits enhanced expression of costimulatory adhesion molecules, CD80 and CD86, by warm ischemia/reperfusion injury in rats. Lab Invest 2002;82(9):1209–17.

79. Ma W, Pober JS. Human endothelial cells effectively costimulate cytokine production by, but not differentiation of, naive $CD4^+$ T cells. J Immunol 1998;161(5): 2158–67.

80. Perez VL, Henault L, Lichtman AH. Endothelial antigen presentation: stimulation of previously activated but not naïve TCR-transgenic mouse T cells. Cell Immunol 1998;189(1):31–40.

81. Sage PT, Varghese LM, Martinelli R, et al. Antigen recognition is facilitated by invadosome-like protrusions formed by memory/effector T cells. J Immunol 2012;188(8):3686–99.

82. Lim WC, Olding M, Healy E, et al. Human endothelial cells modulate $CD4^+$ T cell populations and enhance regulatory T cell suppressive capacity. Front Immunol 2018;9:565.

83. Fu H, Kishore M, Gittens B, et al. Self-recognition of the endothelium enables regulatory T-cell trafficking and defines the kinetics of immune regulation. Nat Commun 2014;5:3436.

84. Huber SA, Sartini D. Roles of tumor necrosis factor alpha (TNF-alpha) and the p55 TNF receptor in CD1d induction and coxsackievirus B3-induced myocarditis. J Virol 2005;79(5):2659–65.

85. Dengler TJ, Pober JS. Human vascular endothelial cells stimulate memory but not naive $CD8^+$ T cells to differentiate into CTL retaining an early activation phenotype. J Immunol 2000;164(10):5146–55.

86. Grabie N, Gotsman I, DaCosta R, et al. Endothelial programmed death-1 ligand 1 (PD-L1) regulates $CD8^+$ T-cell mediated injury in the heart. Circulation 2007; 116(18):2062–71.

87. Rodig N, Ryan T, Allen JA, et al. Endothelial expression of PD-L1 and PD-L2 down-regulates $CD8^+$ T cell activation and cytolysis. Eur J Immunol 2003; 33(11):3117–26.

88. Kaczmarek J, Homsi Y, van Üüm J, et al. Liver sinusoidal endothelial cell-mediated CD8 T cell priming depends on co-inhibitory signal Integration over time. PLoS One 2014;9(6):e99574. Zimmer J, ed.

89. Klugewitz K, Blumenthal-Barby F, Schrage A, et al. Immunomodulatory effects of the liver: deletion of activated $CD4^+$ effector cells and suppression of IFN-gamma-producing cells after intravenous protein immunization. J Immunol 2002;169(5):2407–13.

90. Siavashi V, Asadian S, Taheri-Asl M, et al. Endothelial progenitor cell mobilization in preterm infants with sepsis is associated with improved survival. J Cell Biochem 2017;118(10):3299–307.
91. Suárez Y, Shepherd BR, Rao DA, et al. Alloimmunity to human endothelial cells derived from cord blood progenitors. J Immunol 2007;179(11):7488–96.
92. Raemer PC, Haemmerling S, Giese T, et al. Endothelial progenitor cells possess monocyte-like antigen-presenting and T-cell-co-stimulatory capacity. Transplantation 2009;87(3):340–9.
93. Tapia P, Gatica S, Cortés-Rivera C, et al. Circulating endothelial cells from septic shock patients convert to fibroblasts are associated with the resuscitation fluid dose and are biomarkers for survival prediction. Crit Care Med 2019;47(7): 942–50.
94. Yamamoto K, Loskutoff DJ. Fibrin deposition in tissues from endotoxin-treated mice correlates with decreases in the expression of urokinase-type but not tissue-type plasminogen activator. J Clin Invest 1996;97(11):2440–51.
95. Yano K, Liaw PC, Mullington JM, et al. Vascular endothelial growth factor is an important determinant of sepsis morbidity and mortality. J Exp Med 2006; 203(6):1447–58.

Coagulation Disorders in Hemophagocytic Lymphohistiocytosis/Macrophage Activation Syndrome

Sandrine Valade, MD*, Eric Mariotte, MD, Elie Azoulay, MD, PhD

KEYWORDS

- Hemophagocytic lymphohistiocytosis • Coagulation • Fibrinolysis • Hemorrhage

KEY POINTS

- Coagulation disorders are common during hemophagocytic lymphohistiocytosis (HLH), the more frequently reported anomaly being an isolated decrease in fibrinogen level.
- Mechanisms leading to hypofibrinogenemia remain incompletely understood but are probably linked to disseminated intravascular coagulation and/or hyperfibrinolysis.
- Hypofibrinogenemia is associated with mortality, and further studies are required to explore this correlation.

WHAT IS HEMOPHAGOCYTIC LYMPHOHISTIOCYTOSIS?
Epidemiology

Hemophagocytic lymphohistiocytosis (HLH, or macrophage activation syndrome, or hemophagocytic syndrome) was first described in 1939.[1] Since the first description of this syndrome, a growing number of cases have been reported, mostly in small series.[2,3] The incidence of HLH is low, estimated around 1 new case per 800,000 people per year in the general population, but the syndrome is probably underdiagnosed. A recent review compiling data from 775 patients with HLH found a sex ratio (M/F) of 1.7 and a median age of 50 years at the time of diagnosis.[4]

Diagnosis

The typical presentation of HLH associates multiple cytopenias with high fever and organ dysfunction.[5–7]

Two main classifications are routinely used to help with the diagnosis of HLH: the HLH 2004 criteria developed by Henter and colleagues[5] and most recently the HScore[8] (**Box 1**, **Table 1**).

Medical ICU, Saint Louis University Hospital, Assistance Publique des Hôpitaux de Paris, 1 Avenue Claude Vellefaux, 75010 Paris, France
* Corresponding author.
E-mail address: sandrine.valade@aphp.fr

Crit Care Clin 36 (2020) 415–426
https://doi.org/10.1016/j.ccc.2019.12.004
0749-0704/20/© 2020 Elsevier Inc. All rights reserved.

criticalcare.theclinics.com

Box 1
HLH 2004 criteria

The diagnosis of HLH can be established if one of either 1 or 2 discussed here is fulfilled

1 .A molecular diagnosis consistent with HLH

2 .Diagnostic criteria for HLH fulfilled (5 out of the 8 following criteria)
    a .Initial diagnostic criteria (to be evaluated in all patients with HLH)
        Fever
        Splenomegaly
        Cytopenias (affecting ≥2 of 3 lineages in the peripheral blood)
            Hemoglobin less than 90 g/L (in infants <4 weeks: hemoglobin <100 g/L)
            Platelets <100 x 10^9/L
            Neutrophils <1.0 x 10^9/L
        Hypertriglyceridemia and/or hypofibrinogenemia:
            Fasting triglycerides ≥3.0 mmol/L (ie, ≥265 mg/dL)
            Fibrinogen ≤1.5 g/L
        Hemophagocytosis in bone marrow or spleen or lymph nodes
        No evidence of malignancy
    b .New diagnostic criteria
        Low or absent NK cell activity (according to local laboratory reference)
        Ferritin ≥500 mg/L
        Soluble CD25 (ie, soluble IL-2 receptor) ≥2400 U/mL

Abbreviations: IL, interleukin; NK, natural killer.

Adapted from Henter J-I, Horne A, Aricó M, et al. HLH-2004: Diagnostic and therapeutic guidelines for hemophagocytic lymphohistiocytosis. Pediatr Blood Cancer. 2007;48(2):124-131. doi:10.1002/pbc.210; with permission.

The HLH 2004 classification was developed for the diagnosis of pediatric forms of HLH. It therefore includes 1 genetic criterion (presence of a genetic anomaly associated with hereditary forms of HLH) and 8 clinical or biological criteria: (1) fever; (2) splenomegaly; (3) Cytopenias (≥2 of the 3 cell lines) with hemoglobin <9 g/dL,

---

Table 1
HScore for diagnosis of hemophagocytic syndrome

Known underlying immunosuppression (HIV or immunosuppressive treatment)	0 (no) or 18 (yes)
Temperature	0 (<38.4°C), 33 (38.4°C–39.4°C) 49 (>39.4°C)

Number of cytopenia
  Leukopenia <5000/mm³
  Platelets <110,000/mm³
  Hb <9.2 g/dL
	0 (1 lineage), 24 (2 lineages), or 34 (3 lineages)

Ferritin (ng/mL)	0 (<2000), 35 (2000–6000), or 50 (>6000)
Triglyceride (mmol/L)	0 (>1.5), 44 (1.5–4), or 64 (>4)
Fibrinogen (g/L)	0 if >2.5 g/L 30 if ≤2.5 g/L
Serum glutamic oxaloacetic transaminase (UI/L)	0 (<30) or 19 (≥30)
Hemophagocytosis features on bone marrow aspiration	0 (no) or 35 (yes)

Adapted from Fardet L, Galicier L, Lambotte O, et al. Development and validation of the HScore, a score for the diagnosis of reactive hemophagocytic syndrome. Arthritis Rheumatol Hoboken NJ. 2014;66(9):2613-2620. doi:10.1002/art.38690; with permission.

platelets <100 x 10^9/L, and PNN less than 1.0 x 10^9/L; (4) hypertriglyceridemia ≥3.0 mmol/L and/or hypofibrinogenemia ≤1.5 g/L; (5) hyperferritinemia ≥500 µg/L; (6) histologic evidence of hemophagocytosis on bone marrow or lymph node examination; (7) low or absent natural killer (NK) cell activity; (8) soluble CD25 ≥2400 U/mL. The last 2 criteria are not available in routine practice, so only 6 out of 8 HLH 2004 criteria are usually used in adult patients. Five out of these 6 criteria are required for the diagnosis of HLH in this population.

The HScore was more recently developed by French investigators for the diagnosis of reactive hemophagocytic syndrome (acquired forms of HLH). Each item of the HScore is attributed a value, and the sum of these values leads to a final score from 90 to 250. Higher scores are correlated with higher probability of HLH. The optimal cut-off value proposed by the investigators was 169, which correctly classifies patients with HLH in 90% of the cases.

These 2 classifications can be used for the diagnosis of HLH. The major caveat, however, is that none of their criteria are specific for HLH, with the exception of soluble CD25 dosage (≥2400 U/mL) when available. A very high level (≥10,000 U/mL) of soluble CD25 seems to be very specific of HLH (specificity >90%).[9] For instance, histologic hemophagocytosis can be observed in the absence of HLH during sepsis, multiorgan failure, or after red blood cell transfusions.[10] Conversely, histologic hemophagocytosis can be absent in the bone marrow biopsies of patients with authentic HLH (in up to 30% of the cases).[7,11,12] However, in very severely ill patients, when the worst or maximal values of each item of the diagnostic scores are considered, the diagnostic performances of the 2 classifications seem to be very good and equivalent: in a retrospective study, 5 HLH 2004 criteria allowed an accurate classification of patients in 91% of the patients (sensitivity 80% and specificity 96%), whereas HScore greater than 185 adequately classified 87% of the patients (sensitivity 85%, specificity 88%).[13] Similarly, in patients who are in intensive care unit (ICU), the HScore and the HLH 2004 criteria seem to be both sensitive and specific (Sandrine Valade, unpublished data, 2020).

Pathophysiology

The pathophysiology of HLH remains incompletely understood. However, based on the pathophysiology of genetic forms of HLH, several points can be raised (**Fig. 1**). First, a defect of NK cells and CD8+ T lymphocytes cytotoxicity is suspected. In the presence of a trigger (eg, an infection), the impaired cytotoxic functions of these immune cells lead to a prolonged and persistent exposure to the pathogen. As a result, NK cells and T lymphocytes proliferate and produce abnormally high levels of cytokines (interferon [IFN] gamma, macrophage colony-stimulating factor, etc.) that in turn activate macrophages. In response, macrophages also release a large number of cytokines including, but not limited to, interleukin (IL) 6, IL10, and tumor necrosis factor (TNF) alpha.[4,6,14–17] These cytokines are responsible for different symptoms such as fever, cytopenia, hepatic cytolysis, high levels of ferritin and triglycerides, coagulation disorders, and histologic hemophagocytosis. Some investigators have suggested that some cytokines are specific of certain organ damage, such as IFN gamma, which seems to be more elevated when coagulation disorders and liver dysfunction are present, or IL10, which seems associated with cytopenias.[18] In addition, macrophages are also able to activate lymphocytes, creating an uncontrolled loop of inflammation and leading to a so-called cytokine storm.

Etiologic Diagnosis

The triggers/underlying conditions responsible of HLH can be classified into 3 main categories: infections, neoplasms, and systemic rheumatic diseases.[4,19,20] The cause

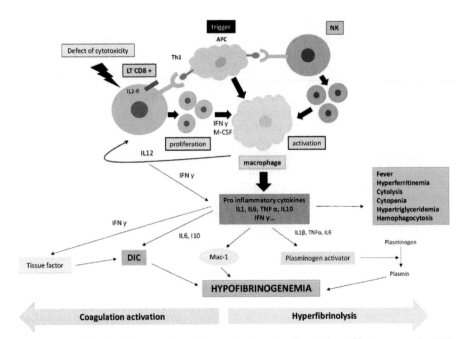

Fig. 1. HLH pathophysiology and possible mechanisms leading to hypofibrinogenemia. APC, antigen-presenting cell; DIC, disseminated intravascular coagulation; IFN, interferon; IL, interleukine; LT, lymphocyte T; M-CSF, macrophage colony-stimulating factor; TNF, tumor necrosis factor.

of HLH remains unknown after an exhaustive workup in a small number of patients. Physicians should keep in mind that several conditions may be found in association in the same patient at the same time.

Infections are probably the most common cause of HLH. They mainly consist of viral infections (by *Herpesviridae* such as Epstein-Barr virus [EBV], cytomegalovirus, herpes simplex virus, varicella zoster virus, human herpes virus 6 [HHV6], HHV8, etc. and human immunodeficiency virus [HIV] in case of an associated opportunistic infection), bacterial (mycobacteria are predominant, *Rickettsia, Salmonella*, etc.), or parasitic/fungal infections (*Leishmania, Histoplasma, Toxoplasma*, etc.).[4,6,21]

The most frequent neoplasms are lymphoproliferative disorders, especially T-cell lymphomas, but also B-cell or Hodgkin lymphomas, and multicentric Castleman disease.[11,21–23] HLH secondary to solid tumors are less frequent but have nevertheless been described.

Systemic rheumatic diseases represent the less frequent underlying condition in adults with HLH. Systemic lupus erythematosus and adult-onset Still disease (AOSD) are the most frequent causes.[24]

No strong data exist regarding the impact of an unknown cause on the outcome in patients with secondary HLH: one retrospective study reported a survival of 16% in this specific group, which was similar to hematological patients.[21] Most of the patients in whom no underlying condition has been found often have hematological malignancies, as some investigators demonstrated it with splenectomy as a diagnostic method.[25] The poor outcome is probably related to a delayed specific treatment. An extensive diagnostic workup must always be performed in order to find and treat the underlying condition: every effort must be made in that sense to improve the outcome in patients with HLH.[26,27]

Treatment

Given the low incidence of HLH, no randomized clinical trials focusing on the optimal management of this condition have been conducted. Therapeutic guidelines are mainly based on observational studies and expert opinions. The first step in the management of patients with HLH consists of the prompt administration of broad spectrum antibiotics in case of organ failures, as these patients are immunocompromised (leukopenia, altered NK/T-cell functions). The specific treatment is targeted to the underlying condition, as soon as it has been identified.[27,28] In patients with severe organ failure, it may sometimes be necessary to initiate targeted treatments based on a probable diagnosis, before confirmation can be attained. In the most severe forms of HLH with life-threatening multiple organ failure, a symptomatic treatment with etoposide should be given. This drug remains the cornerstone of therapy in familial HLH,[5] which aims to promptly limit organ failure, as it effectively reverses the cytokine storm by significantly reducing the level of T lymphocyte activation.[29] Early use of etoposide was associated with better outcome in a study conducted in children with EBV-associated HLH (survival rate 90.2% vs 56.5%).[30] In adult patients, the use of etoposide as a first-line therapy was associated with increased survival in a retrospective study.[31] Systemic corticosteroids and intravenous polyvalent immunoglobulin perfusions can also be considered, especially in cases of infection- or systemic rheumatic disease-related HLH.[32,33]

COAGULATION DISORDERS AND HEMOPHAGOCYTIC LYMPHOHISTIOCYTOSIS
Hemostasis Abnormalities

HLH can be associated with several organ dysfunctions including shock and cardiovascular collapse, respiratory failure, acute kidney injury, liver dysfunction, and coagulation disorders.[20]

Because cytopenias are a cornerstone of the diagnosis of HLH, it is easy to understand that the first element of the coagulation system impaired in HLH is primary hemostasis, defined as the formation of the primary platelet plug. Indeed thrombocytopenia is very frequent because it occurs in close to 80% of patients with HLH.[4,7,11,24,31] The cut-off chosen in the HLH 2004 criteria is 100 x 10^9/L; however, severe thrombocytopenia is rarely observed.[4,22] In a large cohort of patients (n = 117) with a concurrent diagnosis of hematological malignancy for most of them (73%), it is remarkable that all the patients exerted thrombocytopenia.[11] Moreover, Dong and colleagues[34] recently demonstrated in a retrospective study including 11 patients that in most of the cases the decrease in platelets worsens during the course of the disease.

Regarding secondary hemostasis and the coagulation cascade, several biological features have been described during HLH. Coagulation disorders are reported in up to 60% of patients with HLH.[4,11,35,36] A decrease in the plasmatic level of fibrinogen, sometimes isolated, is the most frequently reported anomaly (**Table 2**).[7,11,37] Of note, hypofibrinogenemia also belongs to the diagnostic criteria of HLH, and therefore its prevalence in HLH should be carefully considered because it could be overestimated in comparison to other hemostasis perturbations. Several studies have reported that 50% to 80% of patients with HLH have hypofibrinogenemia (fibrinogen ≤1.5 g/L).[4,7,17,18,21,34,36,38,39] Even if coagulation disorders are most common in patients with hematologic conditions–related HLH, an interesting point is that coagulopathy is also observed in patients with HLH secondary to other causes than lymphoma, such as systemic lupus erythematosus and AOSD[24,37] or infectious diseases.[38]

Table 2
Hypofibrinogenemia in patients with hemophagocytic lymphohistiocytosis

Authors	Patients n =	Country	Fibrinogen ≤1.5 g/L n = (%)	Mortality n = (%)
Park et al,[37] 2012	23	Rep of Korea	8 (38.1)	17 (74)
Arca et al,[31] 2015	162	France	-	33 (20.4)
Han et al,[22] 2007	29	Rep of Korea	14 (54)	20 (69) at day 100
Li et al,[36] 2015	85	China	34 (57)	39/60 (65)
Valade et al,[11] 2015	117	France	61 (52)	44 (38%)
Yang et al,[18] 2016	105	China	65 (61.9)	-
Dong et al,[34] 2019	11	China	9 (81.8)	6 (55)
Buyse et al,[23] 2010	56	France	-	29 (52)
Ramos-Casals et al,[4] 2014	1009	International	39/81 (48)	455 (41)
Li et al,[21] 2014	103	China	56/92 (60.9)	77 (74.8)

Raised D-dimer levels and prolonged prothrombin time (with or without associated decrease in factor V activity) are also reported in 50% of the cases, and nearly half of the patients fulfill disseminated intravascular coagulation (DIC) criteria.[4,11,22,36,38] In a retrospective study, 16 of 29 patients (55%) with lymphoma-related HLH had DIC.[22]

Hypotheses on the Mechanisms of Primary Hemostasis Impairment

Thrombocytopenia may result from several mechanisms, such as severe cytokine-mediated inflammation or excessive consumption.[4,31] Most recently, data suggest that a platelet secretion defect could also play a role in coagulopathy. Several investigators demonstrated that there may be a selective impairment of platelet granule secretion in patients with familial HLH (with mutations in the genes involved in the perforin-containing lytic granules: Munc13-4 or Munc18-2).[40,41] Even if the impact on platelet aggregation was mild, these results highlight that not only the platelet count but also the platelet function can be impaired during HLH, which suggests that both qualitative and quantitative defects in platelets may be involved in HLH-associated coagulopathy.

Endothelial cells may also contribute to the impairment of primary hemostasis, although few data currently support this hypothesis. In one study, Munc13-4 (a protein mutated in familial HLH) was identified to promote exocytosis of Weibel-Palade bodies in which von Willebrand factor is stored.[42] There is no evidence that this feature could be shared between acquired forms and genetic forms of HLH, but this supports the hypothesis of an involvement of endothelial cells in the coagulopathy associated to reactive hemophagocytic syndrome.

Hypotheses on the Mechanisms of Hypofibrinogenemia

Although hypofibrinogenemia is frequent during HLH, the mechanisms leading to a low fibrinogen level are not fully understood. This remains an active field of research, where a link to DIC or hyperfibrinolysis has been suggested, but several hypotheses could be raised (see **Fig. 1**).

DIC can be present in all types of inflammatory states. In sepsis, it has been previously shown that patients with associated overt DIC had an increase in the circulating levels of inflammatory and fibrinolytic markers, especially IL6 and IL10.[43,44] In sepsis cytokines play a major role in the coagulation balance. HLH, like sepsis, is also characterized by a massive release of the same proinflammatory cytokines (IL6 and IL10).[14,15] This suggests that DIC could be one of the mechanisms leading to a decrease in fibrinogen level.[39]

As described previously, stimulated macrophages secrete proinflammatory cytokines. They can also release tissue plasminogen activator in excess.[7,17,45–47] As a consequence, there is an increase in the level of plasmin, the predominant enzyme responsible for fibrinolysis, and this may lead to hypofibrinogenemia. Macrophages in the tissues have also been shown to express receptor for urokinase-type plasminogen activator, and this expression is regulated by several cytokines involved in HLH pathophysiology such as TNF alpha, IL1 beta, and IL6.[48] In addition, the plasmin/plasminogen system seems to have a crucial importance in the proinflammatory immune response, especially by affecting the recruitment of and the phagocytosis by macrophages.[49,50] In a mouse model of fulminant HLH, plasmin was found to be excessively activated, and this supports a key role of plasmin in HLH physiology.[51]

IFN gamma could also contribute to hypofibrinogenemia by inducing tissue factor expression in activated macrophages. Tissue factor initiates blood coagulation and can therefore aberrantly provoke an overconsumption of fibrinogen.[18] In vitro studies have demonstrated that IFN gamma can enhance tissue factor expression, which resulted in a higher procoagulant activity.[52] In mice, some results suggest that tissue factor blockade or depletion in efficient macrophages, which are essential for IFN-gamma signaling, protected animals against the development of hypercoagulation-mediated hepatitis.[53] Given the high rates of IFN gamma in HLH,[14,15] it is likely that this cytokine could be involved in coagulation disorders.

The low level of fibrinogen may also be explained by the activation of an alternative fibrinolytic pathway in activated macrophages, in response to the high level of proinflammatory cytokines. Several preliminary studies have found that monocytes or histiocytes can directly uptake fibrin and/or fibrinogen when activated. Fibrinogen binding to the integrin Mac-1 undergoes internalization and is degraded by lysosomes within monocytes.[54–56]

Another mechanism could be liver dysfunction. However, in one study specifically conducted in patients with hepatic manifestations of HLH, there was no clear correlation between factor V, albumin levels, and histologic assessment of liver cell necrosis. The authors could hypothesize that liver failure was predominantly caused by diffuse liver infiltration with activated T lymphocytes and macrophages (histologic hemophagocytosis was found in all liver biopsies) and cytokine-mediated inflammation.[57]

All these mechanisms, alone or together, may contribute to hypofibrinogenemia, which is a key factor in HLH.

Impact of Hemostasis Disorders

Coagulation impairment is strongly correlated to the prognosis in patients with HLH. Hemostasis disorders confer a higher risk of bleeding, and this complication can be severe. Few studies have specifically focused on hemorrhagic complications occurring during HLH,[11,21,58] but several small case series have been reported. The largest retrospective study, including 117 ICU patients, found an incidence of bleeding of 22%.[11] The median time between the occurrence of hemorrhage and HLH diagnosis was about 3 days. Interestingly, the only coagulation factor significantly associated with a bleeding complication in this study was low fibrinogen level with a cut-off value of 2 g/L. Li and colleagues reported bleeding complications in 17% of patients in a retrospective study of 103 patients with HLH. The gastrointestinal tract was the most frequently involved site of bleeding (n = 15), whereas there were fewer intracranial hemorrhages (n = 3). Sixty-one percent of the patients had hypofibrinogenemia less than or equal to 1.5 g/L, and more than half of the patients who experienced a bleeding complication died.[21] This highlights the severity of this complication.

In the authors' previous study, among 97 ICU patients with an HLH diagnosis who underwent at least one invasive biopsy (including bone marrow, liver, lymph nodes, stomach, or skin samplings) or splenectomy, only 7 patients experienced a bleeding event following the invasive procedure.[11] In the authors' experience coagulopathy should not be a barrier to find the underlying disease, as patients with HLH of unknown origin have a very poor survival rate (17% in the study conducted by Li and colleagues,[21,36] 2015). Indeed, current recommendations support the careful and active investigation for an underlying disease.[26] The benefit/risk ratio of invasive procedures can be acceptable if aggressive transfusion support is provided in order to optimize the coagulation parameters.

Mortality remains high in HLH, reaching 40% in the entire population of patients with HLH, with large variations according to the underlying condition and the severity of the syndrome.[4,21–23,31] In the most severe forms presenting with life-threatening organ failure and requiring ICU management, mortality is even higher, ranging from 40% to more than 80%.[11,23,58,59] Patients with HLH associated to hematological malignancies display the lowest survival rates, especially in case of T-cell lymphoma where mortality rates can reach 80%.[4,19,31,39] In a large cohort of 162 patients, the triggering condition was strongly associated with prognosis, with lymphoma patients displaying the lowest survival rates (odds ratio for death 11.9, $P = .003$).[31]

Impaired coagulation is associated with an increased risk of death in patients with HLH. Severe thrombocytopenia[23,31,36] and DIC[22] have been associated with a worse outcome. A low fibrinogen level has also been shown to be strongly correlated to prognosis, with different thresholds varying between 1.5 and 2 g/L. In several retrospective studies, the level of fibrinogen was associated with a worse outcome and increased mortality rates.[11,36,37] However, the mechanism leading to this higher mortality rate remains unclear, as the occurrence of bleeding complications did not always have an impact on prognosis. One hypothesis could be that the lower fibrinogen level could sometimes only be the reflection of a more severe form of HLH (with a more intense cytokine storm and a more intense hemophagocytic activity). This is supported by one study in which the investigators found that patients with the lowest rates of fibrinogen had the highest levels of ferritin, more frequent histologic hemophagocytosis, and required more invasive life-sustaining therapies.[11]

SUMMARY

HLH is a rare condition that can be responsible of life-threatening organ failure. The pathophysiology relies on a defect of cytotoxicity resulting in an uncontrolled inflammatory state. Coagulation disorders are common during HLH and play a key role, both in the global severity of the disease and in the occurrence of hemorrhagic complications. The most frequently reported anomaly is a decrease in the level of fibrinogen, but platelets and endothelial cells may also be involved. Mechanisms leading to hypofibrinogenemia are still not fully understood, and coagulation impairment in HLH remains a promising field of research. In addition, some coagulation factors such as plasminogen seem to have immunomodulatory functions and deserve additional studies in this context.[49,50] Improvements in the understanding of HLH-associated coagulopathy may translate in better outcomes for patients with HLH.

DISCLOSURE

The authors have nothing to disclose.

REFERENCES

1. Bodley Scott R, Robb-Smith AHT. Histiocytic medullary reticulosis. Lancet 1939; 234(6047):194–8.
2. Hayden A, Park S, Giustini D, et al. Hemophagocytic syndromes (HPSs) including hemophagocytic lymphohistiocytosis (HLH) in adults: a systematic scoping review. Blood Rev 2016;30(6):411–20.
3. Allen CE, McClain KL. Pathophysiology and epidemiology of hemophagocytic lymphohistiocytosis. Hematology Am Soc Hematol Educ Program 2015;2015: 177–82.
4. Ramos-Casals M, Brito-Zerón P, López-Guillermo A, et al. Adult haemophagocytic syndrome. Lancet 2014;26(383):1503–16.
5. Henter J-I, Horne A, Aricó M, et al. HLH-2004: diagnostic and therapeutic guidelines for hemophagocytic lymphohistiocytosis. Pediatr Blood Cancer 2007;48(2): 124–31.
6. Ramachandran S, Zaidi F, Aggarwal A, et al. Recent advances in diagnostic and therapeutic guidelines for primary and secondary hemophagocytic lymphohistiocytosis. Blood Cells Mol Dis 2017;64:53–7.
7. Otrock ZK, Daver N, Kantarjian HM, et al. Diagnostic challenges of hemophagocytic lymphohistiocytosis. Clin Lymphoma Myeloma Leuk 2017;17S:S105–10.
8. Fardet L, Galicier L, Lambotte O, et al. Development and validation of the HScore, a score for the diagnosis of reactive hemophagocytic syndrome. Arthritis Rheumatol 2014;66(9):2613–20.
9. Lin M, Park S, Hayden A, et al. Clinical utility of soluble interleukin-2 receptor in hemophagocytic syndromes: a systematic scoping review. Ann Hematol 2017; 96(8):1241–51.
10. Strauss R, Neureiter D, Westenburger B, et al. Multifactorial risk analysis of bone marrow histiocytic hyperplasia with hemophagocytosis in critically ill medical patients–a postmortem clinicopathologic analysis. Crit Care Med 2004;32(6): 1316–21.
11. Valade S, Azoulay E, Galicier L, et al. Coagulation disorders and bleedings in critically ill patients with hemophagocytic lymphohistiocytosis. Medicine (Baltimore) 2015;94(40):e1692.
12. Rivière S, Galicier L, Coppo P, et al. Reactive hemophagocytic syndrome in adults: a retrospective analysis of 162 patients. Am J Med 2014;127(11):1118–25.
13. Debaugnies F, Mahadeb B, Ferster A, et al. Performances of the H-score for diagnosis of hemophagocytic lymphohistiocytosis in adult and pediatric patients. Am J Clin Pathol 2016;145(6):862–70.
14. Henter JI, Elinder G, Söder O, et al. Hypercytokinemia in familial hemophagocytic lymphohistiocytosis. Blood 1991;78(11):2918–22.
15. Fujiwara F, Hibi S, Imashuku S. Hypercytokinemia in hemophagocytic syndrome. Am J Pediatr Hematol Oncol 1993;15(1):92–8.
16. Filipovich AH, Chandrakasan S. Pathogenesis of hemophagocytic lymphohistiocytosis. Hematol Oncol Clin North Am 2015;29(5):895–902.
17. Janka GE. Hemophagocytic syndromes. Blood Rev 2007;21(5):245–53.
18. Yang S-L, Xu X-J, Tang Y-M, et al. Associations between inflammatory cytokines and organ damage in pediatric patients with hemophagocytic lymphohistiocytosis. Cytokine 2016;85:14–7.

19. Parikh SA, Kapoor P, Letendre L, et al. Prognostic factors and outcomes of adults with hemophagocytic lymphohistiocytosis. Mayo Clin Proc 2014;89(4):484–92.

20. Lemiale V, Valade S, Calvet L, et al. Management of hemophagocytic Lympho-Histiocytosis in critically ill patients. J Intensive Care Med 2018;35(2):118–27.

21. Li J, Wang Q, Zheng W, et al. Hemophagocytic lymphohistiocytosis: clinical analysis of 103 adult patients. Medicine (Baltimore) 2014;93(2):100–5.

22. Han AR, Lee HR, Park B-B, et al. Lymphoma-associated hemophagocytic syndrome: clinical features and treatment outcome. Ann Hematol 2007;86(7):493–8.

23. Buyse S, Teixeira L, Galicier L, et al. Critical care management of patients with hemophagocytic lymphohistiocytosis. Intensive Care Med 2010;36:1695–702.

24. Kumakura S, Murakawa Y. Clinical characteristics and treatment outcomes of autoimmune-associated hemophagocytic syndrome in adults. Arthritis Rheumatol 2014;66(8):2297–307.

25. Ma J, Jiang Z, Ding T, et al. Splenectomy as a diagnostic method in lymphoma-associated hemophagocytic lymphohistiocytosis of unknown origin. Blood Cancer J 2017;7(2):e534.

26. Lehmberg K, Nichols KE, Henter J-I, et al. Consensus recommendations for the diagnosis and management of hemophagocytic lymphohistiocytosis associated with malignancies. Haematologica 2015;100(8):997–1004.

27. La Rosée P. Treatment of hemophagocytic lymphohistiocytosis in adults. Hematology Am Soc Hematol Educ Program 2015;2015:190–6.

28. Janka G, Imashuku S, Elinder G, et al. Infection- and malignancy-associated hemophagocytic syndromes. Secondary hemophagocytic lymphohistiocytosis. Hematol Oncol Clin North Am 1998;12(2):435–44.

29. Johnson TS, Terrell CE, Millen SH, et al. Etoposide selectively ablates activated T cells to control the immunoregulatory disorder hemophagocytic lymphohistiocytosis. J Immunol 2014;192(1):84–91.

30. Imashuku S, Kuriyama K, Teramura T, et al. Requirement for etoposide in the treatment of epstein-barr virus-associated hemophagocytic lymphohistiocytosis. J Clin Oncol 2001;15(19):2665–73.

31. Arca M, Fardet L, Galicier L, et al. Prognostic factors of early death in a cohort of 162 adult haemophagocytic syndrome: impact of triggering disease and early treatment with etoposide. Br J Haematol 2015;168(1):63–8.

32. Lambotte O, Khellaf M, Harmouche H, et al. Characteristics and long-term outcome of 15 episodes of systemic lupus erythematosus-associated hemophagocytic syndrome. Medicine (Baltimore) 2006;85(3):169–82.

33. Brisse E, Matthys P, Wouters CH. Understanding the spectrum of haemophagocytic lymphohistiocytosis: update on diagnostic challenges and therapeutic options. Br J Haematol 2016;174(2):175–87.

34. Dong J, Xie F, Jia L, et al. Clinical characteristics of liver failure with hemophagocytic lymphohistiocytosis. Sci Rep 2019;9(1):8125.

35. Palazzi DL, McClain KL, Kaplan SL. Hemophagocytic syndrome in children: an important diagnostic consideration in fever of unknown origin. Clin Infect Dis 2003;1(36):306–12.

36. Li F, Yang Y, Jin F, et al. Clinical characteristics and prognostic factors of adult hemophagocytic syndrome patients: a retrospective study of increasing awareness of a disease from a single-center in China. Orphanet J Rare Dis 2015;10:20.

37. Park H-S, Kim D-Y, Lee J-H, et al. Clinical features of adult patients with secondary hemophagocytic lymphohistiocytosis from causes other than lymphoma: an analysis of treatment outcome and prognostic factors. Ann Hematol 2012;91(6):897–904.

38. Wang Y-R, Qiu Y-N, Bai Y, et al. A retrospective analysis of 56 children with hemo-phagocytic lymphohistiocytosis. J Blood Med 2016;7:227–31.

39. Créput C, Galicier L, Buyse S, et al. Understanding organ dysfunction in hemo-phagocytic lymphohistiocytosis. Intensive Care Med 2008;34(7):1177–87.

40. Sandrock K, Nakamura L, Vraetz T, et al. Platelet secretion defect in patients with familial hemophagocytic lymphohistiocytosis type 5 (FHL-5). Blood 2010;116(26): 6148–50.

41. Nakamura L, Bertling A, Brodde MF, et al. First characterization of platelet secre-tion defect in patients with familial hemophagocytic lymphohistiocytosis type 3 (FHL-3). Blood 2015;125(2):412–4.

42. Chehab T, Santos NC, Holthenrich A, et al. A novel Munc13-4/S100A10/annexin A2 complex promotes Weibel-Palade body exocytosis in endothelial cells. Mol Biol Cell 2017;28(12):1688–700.

43. Hoppensteadt D, Tsuruta K, Hirman J, et al. Dysregulation of inflammatory and hemostatic markers in sepsis and suspected disseminated intravascular coagu-lation. Clin Appl Thromb Hemost 2015;21(2):120–7.

44. Seo JW, Kim HK, Lee DS, et al. Clinical usefulness of plasma interleukin-6 and interleukin-10 in disseminated intravascular coagulation. Korean J Lab Med 2007;27(2):83–8 [in Korean].

45. Friesecke S, Stecher S-S, Greinacher A. Tranexamic acid for treatment of bleeding in hemophagocytic lymphohistiocytosis. Thromb Res 2015;135(5): 1037–9.

46. Unkeless JC, Gordon S, Reich E. Secretion of plasminogen activator by stimu-lated macrophages. J Exp Med 1974;139(4):834–50.

47. Gordon S, Unkeless JC, Cohn ZA. Induction of macrophage plasminogen acti-vator by endotoxin stimulation and phagocytosis: evidence for a two-stage pro-cess. J Exp Med 1974;140(4):995–1010.

48. Yoshida E, Tsuchiya K, Sugiki M, et al. Modulation of the receptor for urokinase-type plasminogen activator in macrophage-like U937 cells by inflammatory medi-ators. Inflammation 1996;20(3):319–26.

49. Miles LA, Baik N, Lighvani S, et al. Deficiency of plasminogen receptor, Plg-RKT, causes defects in plasminogen binding and inflammatory macrophage recruit-ment in vivo. J Thromb Haemost 2017;15(1):155–62.

50. Das R, Ganapathy S, Settle M, et al. Plasminogen promotes macrophage phago-cytosis in mice. Blood 2014;124(5):679–88.

51. Shimazu H, Munakata S, Tashiro Y, et al. Pharmacological targeting of plasmin prevents lethality in a murine model of macrophage activation syndrome. Blood 2017;130(1):59–72.

52. Scheibenbogen C, Moser H, Krause S, et al. Interferon-gamma-induced expres-sion of tissue factor activity during human monocyte to macrophage maturation. Haemostasis 1992;22(4):173–8.

53. Kato J, Okamoto T, Motoyama H, et al. Interferon-gamma-mediated tissue factor expression contributes to T-cell-mediated hepatitis through induction of hyper-coagulation in mice. Hepatology 2013;57(1):362–72.

54. Ooe K. Pathogenesis of hypofibrinogenemia in familial hemophagocytic lympho-histiocytosis. Pediatr Pathol 1991;11(4):657–61.

55. Simon DI, Ezratty AM, Francis SA, et al. Fibrin(ogen) is internalized and degraded by activated human monocytoid cells via Mac-1 (CD11b/CD18): a nonplasmin fibrinolytic pathway. Blood 1993;82(8):2414–22.

56. Loscalzo J. The macrophage and fibrinolysis. Semin Thromb Hemost 1996;22(6): 503–6.

57. de Kerguenec C, Hillaire S, Molinié V, et al. Hepatic manifestations of hemopha-gocytic syndrome: a study of 30 cases. Am J Gastroenterol 2001;96(3):852–7.

58. Kapoor S, Morgan CK, Siddique MA, et al. Intensive care unit complications and outcomes of adult patients with hemophagocytic lymphohistiocytosis: a retro-spective study of 16 cases. World J Crit Care Med 2018;7(6):73–83.

59. Rajagopala S, Singh N, Agarwal R, et al. Severe hemophagocytic lymphohistio-cytosis in adults-experience from an intensive care unit from North India. Indian J Crit Care Med 2012;16:198–203.

Printed and bound by CPI Group (UK) Ltd, Croydon, CR0 4YY

03/10/2024

01040480-0006